# 1997
## YEAR BOOK OF
# VASCULAR SURGERY®

# Statement of Purpose

## The YEAR BOOK Service

The YEAR BOOK series was devised in 1901 by practicing health professionals who observed that the literature of medicine and related disciplines had become so voluminous that no one individual could read and place in perspective every potential advance in a major specialty. In the final decade of the 20th century, this recognition is more acutely true than it was in 1901.

More than merely a series of books, YEAR BOOK volumes are the tangible results of a unique service designed to accomplish the following:

- to *survey* a wide range of journals of proven value
- to *select* from those journals papers representing significant advances and statements of important clinical principles
- to provide *abstracts* of those articles that are readable, convenient summaries of their key points
- to provide *commentary* about those articles to place them in perspective

These publications grow out of a unique process that calls on the talents of outstanding authorities in clinical and fundamental disciplines, trained literature specialists, and professional writers, all supported by the resources of Mosby, the world's preeminent publisher for the health professions.

## The Literature Base

Mosby and its editors survey more than 1,000 journals published worldwide, covering the full range of the health professions. On an annual basis, the publisher examines usage patterns and polls its expert authorities to add new journals to the literature base and to delete journals that are no longer useful as potential YEAR BOOK sources.

## The Literature Survey

The publisher's team of literature specialists, all of whom are trained and experienced health professionals, examines every original, peer-reviewed article in each journal issue. More than 250,000 articles per year are scanned systematically, including title, text, illustrations, tables, and references. Each scan is compared, article by article, to the search strategies that the publisher has developed in consultation with the 270 outside experts who form the pool of YEAR BOOK editors. A given article may be reviewed by any number of editors, from one to a dozen or more, regardless of the discipline for which the paper was originally published. In turn, each editor who receives the article reviews it to determine whether or not the article should be included in the YEAR BOOK. This decision is based on the article's inherent quality, its probable usefulness to readers of that YEAR BOOK, and the editor's goal to represent a balanced picture of a given field in each volume of the YEAR BOOK. In addition, the editor indicates when to include figures and tables from the article to help the YEAR BOOK reader better understand the information.

Of the quarter million articles scanned each year, only 5% are selected for detailed analysis within the YEAR BOOK series, thereby assuring readers of the high value of every selection.

## The Abstract

The publisher's abstracting staff is headed by a seasoned medical professional and includes individuals with training in the life sciences, medicine, and other areas, plus extensive experience in writing for the health professions and related industries. Each selected article is assigned to a specific writer on this abstracting staff. The abstracter, guided in many cases by notations supplied by the expert editor, writes a structured, condensed summary designed so that the reader can rapidly acquire the essential information contained in the article.

## The Commentary

The YEAR BOOK editorial boards, sometimes assisted by guest commentators, write comments that place each article in perspective for the reader. This provides the reader with the equivalent of a personal consultation with a leading international authority—an opportunity to better understand the value of the article and to benefit from the authority's thought processes in assessing the article.

## Additional Editorial Features

The editorial boards of each YEAR BOOK organize the abstracts and comments to provide a logical and satisfying sequence of information. To enhance the organization, editors also provide introductions to sections or individual chapters, comments linking a number of abstracts, citations to additional literature, and other features.

The published YEAR BOOK contains enhanced bibliographic citations for each selected article, including extended listings of multiple authors and identification of author affiliations. Each YEAR BOOK contains a Table of Contents specific to that year's volume. From year to year, the Table of Contents for a given YEAR BOOK will vary depending on developments within the field.

Every YEAR BOOK contains a list of the journals from which papers have been selected. This list represents a subset of the more than 1,000 journals surveyed by the publisher and occasionally reflects a particularly pertinent article from a journal that is not surveyed on a routine basis.

Finally, each volume contains a comprehensive subject index and an index to authors of each selected paper.

# The 1997 Year Book Series

Year Book of Allergy, Asthma, and Clinical Immunology: Drs. Rosenwasser, Borish, Gelfand, Leung, Nelson, and Szefler

Year Book of Anesthesiology and Pain Management®: Drs. Tinker, Abram, Chestnut, Roizen, Rothenberg, and Wood

Year Book of Cardiology®: Drs. Schlant, Collins, Gersh, Graham, Kaplan, and Waldo

Year Book of Chiropractic®: Dr. Lawrence

Year Book of Critical Care Medicine®: Drs. Parrillo, Balk, Calvin, Franklin, and Shapiro

Year Book of Dentistry®: Drs. Meskin, Berry, Kennedy, Leinfelder, Roser, Summitt, and Zakariasen

Year Book of Dermatologic Surgery®: Drs. Greenway, Papadopoulos, and Whitaker

Year Book of Dermatology®: Drs. Sober and Fitzpatrick

Year Book of Diagnostic Radiology®: Drs. Federle, Gross, Dalinka, Maynard, Rebner, Smirniotopolous, and Young

Year Book of Digestive Diseases®: Drs. Greenberger and Moody

Year Book of Drug Therapy®: Drs. Lasagna and Weintraub

Year Book of Emergency Medicine®: Drs. Wagner, Dronen, Davidson, King, Niemann, and Roberts

Year Book of Endocrinology®: Drs. Bagdade, Braverman, Horton, Kannan, Landsberg, Molitch, Morley, Nathan, Odell, Poehlman, Rogol, and Ryan

Year Book of Family Practice®: Drs. Berg, Bowman, Davidson, Dexter, and Scherger

Year Book of Geriatrics and Gerontology®: Drs. Beck, Burton, Ostwald, Rabins, Reuben, Roth, Shapiro, and Whitehouse

Year Book of Hand Surgery®: Drs. Amadio and Hentz

Year Book of Hematology®: Drs. Spivak, Bell, Ness, Quesenberry, Wiernik, and Blume

Year Book of Infectious Diseases®: Drs. Keusch, Barza, Bennish, Poutsiaka, Skolnik, and Snydman

Year Book of Medicine®: Drs. Klahr, Cline, Petty, Frishman, Greenberger, Malawista, Mandell, and O'Rourke

Year Book of Neonatal and Perinatal Medicine®: Drs. Fanaroff, Maisels, Stevenson

Year Book of Nephrology, Hypertension and Mineral Metabolism: Drs. Schwab, Bennett, Emmett, Hostetter, Kumar, and Toto

Year Book of Neurology and Neurosurgery®: Drs. Bradley and Wilkins

1997

# The Year Book of
# VASCULAR SURGERY®

Editor
**John M. Porter, M.D.**
*Professor of Surgery and Head, Division of Vascular Surgery, Oregon Health
Sciences University, Portland, Oregon*

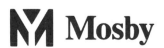 Mosby

St. Louis  Baltimore  Boston  Carlsbad  Chicago  Naples  New York  Philadelphia  Portland
London  Madrid  Mexico City  Singapore  Sydney  Tokyo  Toronto  Wiesbaden

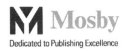

**Mosby**

Dedicated to Publishing Excellence

**A Times Mirror Company**

*Vice President and Publisher, Continuity Publishing:* Kenneth H. Killion
*Director, Editorial Development:* Gretchen C. Murphy
*Developmental Editor:* Kris Horeis, R.N.
*Acquisitions Editor:* Li Wen Huang
*Project Manager, Editing:* Jill C. Waite
*Senior Project Manager, Production:* Max F. Perez
*Freelance Staff Supervisor:* Barbara M. Kelly
*Illustrations and Permissions Coordinator:* Lois M. Ruebensam
*Director, Editorial Services:* Edith M. Podrazik, B.S.N, R.N.
*Information Specialist:* Kathleen Moss, R.N.
*Information Specialist:* Terri Santo, R.N.
*Circulation Manager:* Lynn D. Stevenson

**1997 EDITION**
Copyright © April 1997 by Mosby–Year Book, Inc.

Printed in the United States of America
Composition by Reed Technology and Information Services, Inc.
Printing/binding by Maple-Vail

Mosby–Year Book, Inc.
11830 Westline Industrial Drive
St. Louis, MO 63146
Customer Service: customer.support@mosby.com
　　　　　　　　www.mosby.com/Mosby/CustomerSupport/index.html

Editorial Office:
Mosby–Year Book, Inc.
161 North Clark Street
Chicago, IL 60601
series.editorial@mosby.com

International Standard Serial Number: 0749–4041
International Standard Book Number: 0–8151–6800–4

# Guest Commentators

## William Abbott, M.D.
*Chief, Vascular Surgery, Massachusetts General Hospital, Boston, Massachusetts*

## David Bergqvist, M.D., Ph.D.
*Professor of Vascular Surgery, University Hospital, Department of Surgery, Sweden*

## Jack Cronenwett, M.D.
*Professor of Surgery, Dartmouth-Hitchcock Medical Center, Department of Surgery, Section of Vascular Surgery, Lebanon, New Hampshire*

## Anthony E.B. Giddings
*The Royal Surrey County Hospital, Guildford, United Kingdom*

## Thomas O'Donnell, M.D.
*Professor and Chair, Department of Surgery, New England Medical Center, Boston, Massachusetts*

## William Quiñones-Baldrich, M.D.
*Associate Professor of Surgery, UCLA Center for Health Sciences, Los Angeles, California*

## Rich Yeager, M.D.
*Associate Professor of Surgery, Division of Vascular Surgery, Veterans Administration Medical Center, Portland, Oregon*

# Table of Contents

# Journals Represented

Mosby and its editors survey more than 1,000 journals for its abstract and commentary publications. From these journals, the editors select the articles to be abstracted. Journals represented in this YEAR BOOK are listed below.

American Heart Journal
American Journal of Emergency Medicine
American Journal of Gastroenterology
American Journal of Orthopedics
American Journal of Roentgenology
American Journal of Surgery
American Surgeon
Annals of Internal Medicine
Annals of Surgery
Annals of Vascular Surgery
Archives of Internal Medicine
Archives of Surgery
Arteriosclerosis, Thrombosis, and Vascular Biology
Atherosclerosis
British Journal of Surgery
British Journal of Urology
Cardiovascular Surgery
Chest
Circulation
Circulation Research
European Journal of Vascular and Endovascular Surgery
Journal of Cardiovascular Surgery
Journal of Clinical Investigation
Journal of Computer Assisted Tomography
Journal of Endovascular Surgery
Journal of Internal Medicine
Journal of Nuclear Medicine
Journal of Pediatric Surgery
Journal of Rheumatology
Journal of Surgical Research
Journal of Trauma: Injury, Infection, and Critical Care
Journal of Vascular Surgery
Journal of the American Academy of Dermatology
Journal of the American College of Cardiology
Journal of the American College of Surgeons
Journal of the American Medical Association
Lancet
Neurology
Neuroradiology
New England Journal of Medicine
Quarterly Journal of Medicine
Radiology
Southern Medical Journal
Stroke
Surgery
Thrombosis Research
Thrombosis and Haemostatis

STANDARD ABBREVIATIONS

The following terms are abbreviated in this edition: acquired immunodeficiency syndrome (AIDS), cardiopulmonary resuscitation (CPR), central nervous system (CNS), cerebrospinal fluid (CSF), computed tomography (CT), deoxyribonucleic acid (DNA), electrocardiography (ECG), health maintenance organization (HMO), human immunodeficiency virus (HIV), intensive care unit (ICU), intramuscular (IM), intravenous (IV), magnetic resonance (MR) imaging (MRI), and ribonucleic acid (RNA).

NOTE

The YEAR BOOK OF VASCULAR SURGERY® is a literature survey service providing abstracts of articles published in the professional literature. Every effort is made to assure the accuracy of the information presented in these pages. Neither the editors nor the publisher of the YEAR BOOK OF VASCULAR SURGERY® can be responsible for errors in the original materials. The editors' comments are their own opinions. Mention of specific products within this publication does not constitute endorsement.

To facilitate the use of the YEAR BOOK OF VASCULAR SURGERY® as a reference tool, all illustrations and tables included in this publication are now identified as they appear in the original article. This change is meant to help the reader recognize that any illustration or table appearing in the YEAR BOOK OF VASCULAR SURGERY® may be only one of many in the original article. For this reason, figure and table numbers will often appear to be out of sequence within the YEAR BOOK OF VASCULAR SURGERY®.

# Introduction

As I stated in the introduction to the 1996 YEARBOOK OF VASCULAR SURGERY, I continue to believe that the most important development in the past year has been the ongoing changes in health care delivery, specifically the recruitment of more and more patients into the HMO systems. Many of us have long recognized the primary defect in this system: namely the control of the entire referral pattern by gatekeepers, invariably the least informed group of physicians. These gatekeepers have all too frequently been too uninformed about vascular disease to know when to refer, or have obstinately refused to refer, frequently driven by financial motivation. Interestingly, in the past year important changes have begun to occur, and there are presently a few cracks in the woodwork. Consumer groups have become organized and have loudly protested their perceptions of inadequate health care and refusal to refer. These complaints are being heard by Congress, and important restrictions on HMOs are beginning to be discussed. For the first time in years the profitability of HMOs appears to have declined, and a number of these companies have suffered significant decreases in stock value. May it all continue!

In our field of vascular surgery, some of the most interesting observations have been in the field of epidemiology. The lipid-lowering drug Pravastatin has been convincingly shown to reduce death rate from coronary disease in selected populations, the first clear proof of this ever. This continues to support the position of the National Lipid Consortium, and we will clearly continue to hear a great deal more about cholesterol and lipoproteins in the future. Sadly, the decline in stroke incidence appears to be leveling out, although the significant decline in stroke death continues. Coronary death decline continues, although again, primarily because of increased survival of afflicted patients rather than a decreased incidence of events. Interestingly, the ACAS Study, which I predicted would be so important, has resulted with less impact than I thought. Led by a few prominent nay sayers, increasing numbers of physicians are again questioning the benefit of asymptomatic carotid surgery, pointing out the modest ACAS reduction in stroke with CEA. In the ACAS study benefits were not shown for women, and increasing amounts of stenosis above 60% diameter reduction did not appear associated with an increasing incidence of stroke. Nonetheless, I continue to believe that the ACAS Study was of pivotal importance and clearly must not be ignored.

Sadly, the past year seems to have delivered the death knell to omega-3 fatty acids. Increasing numbers of studies are unable to define clear benefit for this interesting group of fatty acids. Similarly, the beta carotene study has become a cropper with absolutely no benefits detectable. The antioxidants appear destined to a similar fate.

In the field of lipid metabolism there has been increasing interest in the definition of oxidized LDL as a central player in the development of atheromata. Homocysteine continues to occupy center stage in vascular disease epidemiology. It now appears to be a risk factor for deep vein thrombosis, as well as a clear-cut risk factor for atherosclerosis. Lipoprotein(a) has attracted considerable study, but now it appears that its toxic effects primarily occur in association with a significant elevation of low density lipoprotein cholesterol. In other words, patients who have isolate Lp(a) elevation without LDL-C elevation may not be at increased risk.

Atherosclerotic cap erosion continues to be a focus of considerable investigative effort. In the past year, we have learned that mast cell infiltration in the fibrous cap seems to be a near uniform finding, and these cells may elaborate metalloproteases, important in plaque rupture. In a fascinating study of patients dying of sudden cardiac occlusion, investigators found only about half of the fatal thrombi were associated with plaque rupture, while the other half were associated with plaque erosion.

Of great interest in the past year has been the emergence of low molecular weight heparin as a powerful new therapeutic principle in the treatment and prophylaxis of thrombotic disease. Low molecular weight heparin (LMWH) has the benefit of once a day dosing without the need for laboratory monitoring of coagulation status. In fascinating pivotal studies, LMWH has been shown to be at least as effective as unfractionated heparin in both prophylaxis and treatment of venous thrombosis. It has also been shown useful in vascular surgical patients as a substitute for unfractionated heparin during surgery. Of particular importance has been the evidence in the past year that patients with deep vein thrombosis may be treated effectively as outpatients with LMWH without the need for hospitalization at all. I am certain this will have great influence on our future practice patterns concerning the treatment of deep vein thrombosis.

In the endovascular field, the past year has not been particularly noteworthy. We have now had case reports of delayed rupture of aortic aneurysms following endovascular graft stenting. We know that a disappointing percentage, probably about 20%, of endovascular grafts placed in highly selected patients appear to have a leak into the aneurysm sac at 12 months. Many continue to be worried about the potential of the normal infrarenal aortic enlargement with time in aneurysm patients dislodging the proximal fixation of the stent grafts. Dr. Parodi, the putative parent of endovascular grafting, has presented a sobering overview of the field, concluding that much work remains to be done before the technique can be widely applied to patients. I applaud his forthrightness.

Certainly one of the hot topics presently is the use of balloon angioplasty in patients with carotid stenosis. This effort appears to be led primarily by cardiologists with a few fellow travellers. In my opinion, there is insufficient data, including intermediate term follow-up, to justify a prospective randomized trial with carotid endarterectomy at the present time. In other words, I do not believe there is presently a genuine state of equipoise in this important area.

On balance, however, the endovascular juggernaut rolls on, supported in surprising part by invasive cardiologists. Try though I may, to date, I have been unable to generate much enthusiasm for this project. Although endovascular technology remains an extraordinarily appropriate field for investigation, I am very disappointed to note the enthusiasm expressed by many of its proponents to bypass FDA regulations and proceed directly to clinical treatment. I am also extremely disappointed by the many entrepreneurial aspects of this field. I note that many of the primary investigators either own commercial products themselves, or have abundant commercial product funding. The overt conflict of interest in this situation is overwhelming.

A fascinating development in the past year has been the initial articles on the use of power Doppler ultrasonography. I suspect Doppler is going to be an important addition to the vascular laboratory. It indicates the density, as well as the number of red cells per unit volume of tissue, but provides no information concerning velocity or direction of flow. It may be a valuable future adjunct. There continues to be interest in detailed power spectral analysis of venous thrombi in an effort to determine their age. Preliminary results suggest that the technique may actually be useful. If we were able to accurately determine the age of venous thrombi in vascular lab duplex examinations, it would clearly have a significant impact on clinical practice.

Increasing information accumulates that routine detailed coronary investigation and intervention before elective vascular surgery results in little or no objective patient benefit. This is a position now being embraced by conservative vascular internists, indeed a monumental change.

In the field of aortoiliac occlusive disease, axillofemoral grafting appears to provide comparable patency results to aortofemoral grafting, at least in elderly patients. In this patient group there is increasing enthusiasm for selection of the lesser procedure, namely axillobifemoral grafting. In the pharmacologic treatment of claudication, carnitine continues to attract considerable attention. Several major multicenter randomized trials have now shown positive results with the use of propionyl-L-carnitine, and I am certain we shall hear more about this in the future. Postoperative lower extremity graft surveillance received considerable attention in the literature during the past year. The overall consensus appears to be that permanent graft flow velocity surveillance is mandatory in these patients, although the frequency of such studies can be reduced after the first year.

An extremely important topic in the past year has been consideration of thrombolytic therapy in the treatment of acute ischemic stroke. Two important prospective randomized studies using tissue plasminogen activator found modest benefit at three months at the price of increased mortality. Streptokinase, in another study, resulted in no benefit. I conclude that there be minimal benefit from TPA initiated very early in the course of a thrombotic stroke, but I suspect this is going to have minimal clinical impact. The wide lay-press coverage of this topic appears disproportionate to the value of scientific evidence.

Many of you noted the initiation of the Camel Dung Award last year, and it appeared to be well received, with the possible exception of the recipients. I have awarded fewer Camel Dung Awards this year, doubtless reflecting a general uplifting of the vascular surgical literature induced by the CDA itself. I will continue this award in the future, but I warn the candidates that they will have to earn it.

I express appreciation to Dr. Jack Cronenwett, Dr. William Abbott, Dr. Anthony Giddings, and Dr. David Bergqvist, for their excellent efforts as guest editors. Finally, I express profound appreciation to Ms. Heather Morin, who has done all the classification and typing of the contents of this year's YEARBOOK. I point out that she continues to perform this remarkable service despite taking a full course load in college. Her excellence in this role is unparalleled. I also express appreciation to Ms. Kris Horeis of Mosby–Year Book for her usual excellent assistance.

**John M. Porter, M.D.**

# 1 Basic Considerations

## Atherosclerosis

**Tissue Characterisation of Atherosclerotic Carotid Plaques by MRI**
Görtler M, Goldmann A, Mohr W, et al (Univ of Ulm, Germany)
*Neuroradiology* 37:631–635, 1995                                    1–1

*Background.*—Patients with carotid artery plaques associated with intraplaque hemorrhage or atheromatous debris are at elevated risk of embolic stroke. So far, there is no reliable technique to assess plaque morphology in vivo. Magnetic resonance imaging may be capable of distinguishing between various plaque types with different prognostic and treatment implications. The ability of MRI to assess carotid plaque morphology was evaluated in an in vitro study.

*Methods.*—Magnetic resonance imaging scans were obtained of 17 carotid bifurcation plaques that had been removed completely from patients undergoing carotid surgery. Signal intensities were assessed using the contrast-to-noise ratio (CNR). The findings were compared with the histopathologic appearances, which were classified as simple plaques—those made up of fibrous intimal thickening, lipid deposits, and/or atheromatous tissue with cholesterol crystals; largely calcified plaques; and complicated plaques, which included recent intramural hemorrhage or friable atheromatous debris.

*Results.*—These 3 plaque types showed significant differences in mean CNR on T1- and T2-weighted sequences obtained using the FLASH pulse sequence with a 15-degree flip angle. Mean CNR on the T1-weighted sequence was $4.4 \pm 2.3$ for simple plaques, $-4.8 \pm 2.3$ with calcified plaques, and $15.1 \pm 4.3$ for complicated plaques. Every plaque was correctly classified according to the findings on T1-weighted scanning. However, in vivo application of this technique encountered problems with motion artifacts, vessel pulsation triggering, and 6- to 7-minute acquisition times.

*Conclusions.*—Magnetic resonance imaging can correctly classify the morphologic characteristics of carotid plaques in vitro. If scan acquisition times can be shortened and other technical problems dealt with, MRI could become clinically useful for noninvasive assessment of carotid plaque morphology.

▶ Current evidence suggests that as many as one half of acute coronary artery thrombotic occlusions result from plaque rupture without high grade

1

pre-existing stenosis. Certainly plaque rupture in the carotid artery has been implicated as a cause of embolic stroke. Recent editions of the YEAR BOOK OF VASCULAR SURGERY[1] have consistently described increasing interest in the characterization of atherosclerotic plaques in an attempt to determine which appear at greatest risk for rupture. If these could be accurately identified before rupture, early surgery may be indicated. The current study suggests that MRI may be a valuable modality in characterizing such unstable plaques in a prerupture condition. Unfortunately, as the authors accurately observe, the long acquisition time with the accompanying motion artifacts makes the current technique of uncertain clinical significance. Hopefully, future advances in MR technology will overcome these problems. I am certain we shall hear more. See also Abstracts 1–7 and 1–26.

*Reference*

1. 1996 YEAR BOOK OF VASCULAR SURGERY, p 13.

**Serum Total Cholesterol and Long-Term Coronary Heart Disease Mortality in Different Cultures: Twenty-Five-Year Follow-Up of the Seven Countries Study**
Verschuren WMM, Jacobs DR, Bloemberg BPM, et al (Natl Inst of Public Health and Environmental Protection, Bilthoven, The Netherlands; Univ of Minnesota, Minneapolis; Med Ctr of Athens, Greece, et al)
*JAMA* 274:131–136, 1995                                                               1–2

*Objective.*—The relationship between long-term mortality due to coronary heart disease (CHD) and serum total cholesterol in 7 different cultures was compared.

*Design and Main Outcome Measures.*—Baseline and 5- and 10-year follow-up levels of total cholesterol were measured in 12,467 men, aged 40–59, from 7 countries. The relationship between these cholesterol levels and the CHD mortality rates determined 25 years after the start of the study was determined and compared among 6 cohorts that had been formed on the basis of similarities in culture and cholesterol changes during the first 10 years of the study.

*Results.*—The age-standardized CHD mortality rates were linearly related to cholesterol levels in all cultures. The CHD mortality rates ranged from 3% in the Japanese cohort to 20% in the Northern European cohort. A 0.50 mmol/L increase in total cholesterol corresponded to a 12% increase in risk of mortality due to CHD. The absolute levels of CHD mortality were strikingly different among the cohorts studied. For example, there was a threefold range in mortality rates (from 4% to 5% in Japan and the Mediterranean to 10% in Inland Southern Europe, 12% in the United States, and 15% in Northern Europe) for a cholesterol level of 5.45 mmol/L. These differences were not explained by differences in age, smoking, or systolic blood pressure. Differences in diet, biological risk factors other than total cholesterol, and genetic factors may be involved in the differences in absolute risk that were observed.

*Conclusions.*—The relative risk in mortality due to CHD is linearly related to increased serum total cholesterol across cultures. However, the absolute CHD mortality rates at a given cholesterol level vary from culture to culture, indicating that factors such as diet are important with respect to primary prevention.

▶ The anticholesterol consortium strikes again. A 10-year follow-up of a large group of men established an essentially linear relationship between increasing cholesterol and increasing CHD mortality in all cultures except Japanese. The authors' generous concession that other factors in addition to cholesterol must be at work, due to the large cultural differences in absolute mortality, is noted. It appears well established that, within broad limits, increasing serum cholesterol is associated with increasing coronary mortality. It is becoming increasingly apparent, however, that expensive and difficult reductions in serum cholesterol do not necessarily convey protection to the individual.

---

**Patients With Early-Onset Peripheral Vascular Disease Have Increased Levels of Autoantibodies Against Oxidized LDL**
Bergmark C, Wu R, de Faire U, et al (Karolinska Hosp, Stockholm)
*Arterioscler Thromb Vasc Biol* 15:441–445, 1995                    1–3

---

*Background.*—Oxidation of low-density lipoprotein cholesterol (LDL) might be an important early event in the development of atherosclerosis. Healthy subjects and patients with atherosclerosis both show antibodies against oxidatively modified LDL. The level of autoantibodies against oxidized LDL was assessed as a risk factor for peripheral arterial occlusive disease (PAOD) in younger patients.

*Methods.*—The study included 62 patients with PAOD who required surgical reconstruction before the age of 50 years, as well as a group of age- and sex-matched healthy controls. An enzyme-linked immunosorbent assay was used to measure autoantibodies against oxidized LDL. The findings were compared with other risk factors, including smoking, hypertension, family history of premature cardiovascular events, and lipoprotein status.

*Results.*—Levels of autoantibodies against oxidized LDL were significantly higher in the patients than the controls (Fig 1). The patients with PAOD also had significantly higher total cholesterol, LDL, triglycerides, and apolipoprotein A-I and significantly lower levels of high-density-lipoprotein cholesterol. On multivariate analysis, the level of autoantibodies against LDL was more closely associated with PAOD than any of the various lipoprotein findings. In the PAOD patients, elevated levels of autoantibodies against oxidized LDL were significantly associated with the presence of hypertension and a family history of cardiovascular events.

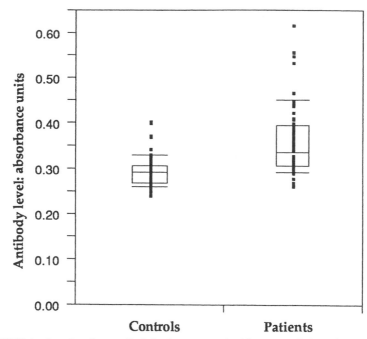

FIGURE 1.—Box plot of autoantibody levels against oxidized lipoprotein cholesterol in patients and control subjects, showing a significant difference ($P < .001$, Wilcoxon) between the 2 groups. The box includes observations from the 25th to the 75th percentile; the horizontal line within the box represents the median value. Lines outside the box represent the 10th and 90th percentiles. The width of the box is proportional to the number of observations. (Courtesy of Bergmark C, Wu R, de Faire U, et al: Patients with early-onset peripheral vascular disease have increased levels of autoantibodies against oxidized LDL. *Arterioscler Thromb Vasc Biol* 15:441–445, 1995. Reproduced with permission, *Arteriosclerosis, Thrombosis, and Vascular Biology*, 1995, American Heart Association.)

*Conclusions.*—Levels of autoantibodies against oxidized LDL are significantly elevated in a group of younger patients with PAOD. The increase in autoantibodies against oxidized LDL is unrelated to the classic risk factors for PAOD, such as age, male sex, and plasma lipoproteins. However, it is significantly associated with hypertension and a family history of premature cardiovascular disease.

▶ When compared to age-matched, nondiseased controls, this group of patients with peripheral vascular disease requiring surgery for occlusive disease before age 50 had the expected increases in cholesterol and triglyceride, and the expected decrease in high-density lipoprotein cholesterol. Interestingly, increased levels of antibodies to oxidized LDL proved to be the best discriminant between the 2 groups. Considerable evidence suggests that LDL must be oxidized before it can be ingested by macrophages, putatively the first step in formation of the atherosclerotic lesion. Thus, as suggested by these authors, LDL oxidation may be both an early and essential step in the development of the atherosclerotic lesion. We are only beginning to understand the complexities of LDL metabolism in human atherosclerosis.

---

**Fish Consumption and Stroke in Men: 30-Year Findings of the Chicago Western Electric Study**
Orencia AJ, Daviglus ML, Dyer AR, et al (Northwestern Univ, Chicago; Univ of Texas, Houston)
*Stroke* 27:204–209, 1996                                                                      1–4

---

*Background.*—Biochemical studies have indicated that n-3 polyunsaturated fish oils reduce platelet aggregation and may protect blood vessel endothelium from ischemic damage. It is not yet clear, however, what practical effect fish consumption has on chronic disease outcomes, such as stroke. Possible effects include increased risk of hemorrhagic strokes, decreased incidence of ischemic events, or no effect. The hypothesis that fish consumption and stroke risk are inversely related was examined.

*Patients and Methods.*—After exclusion, 1,847 men aged 40–55 years, all of whom were free of coronary disease and stroke, were examined. Fish intake was subdivided into 4 levels. These included ≥ 35 g/day or more, 34–18 g/day, 17–1 g/day, and 0 g/day. Combined follow-up was 46,426 patient-years, during which time 76 stroke deaths occurred.

*Results.*—Surprisingly, those who had the largest fish intake also had the highest age-adjusted stroke mortality rate, at 23/10,000 patient-years compared with 15–16/10,000 patient-years among individuals consuming less or no fish. The risk for stroke among those with the greatest fish intake was 34% higher (95% CI, 0.53–3.41) than for those who ate less or no fish. Age-adjusted and multivariate analyses for fatal and nonfatal strokes failed to significantly alter these findings.

*Conclusions.*—The nonsignificantly higher stroke risk for those patients who consumed the greatest amount of fish does not support the hypothesis of an inverse relation between stroke and fish consumption.

▶ The weakness of this study is the retrospective dietary recall data, which may be significantly inaccurate. Nonetheless, the conclusions that men with the highest fish consumption experienced more strokes delivers a major blow to the hypothesis of an inverse relationship between fish consumption and stroke. This study, together with others showing a lack of benefit of omega-3 fatty acids in patients undergoing coronary angioplasty,[1] casts considerable doubt on the relevance of omega-3 fatty acids in atherosclerosis prevention and treatment in Western populations. It is interesting to recall that the putative benefits of omega-3 fatty acids were suggested by studies of isolated, non-Western cultures, which clearly have many differences from Western cultures in addition to diet. Although I am not completely ready to conclude that omega-3 fatty acids have no benefit in Western culture, I am getting close.

*Reference*

1. 1996 YEAR BOOK OF VASCULAR SURGERY, p 11.

## Lipoprotein(a) as a Determinant of the Severity of Angiographically Defined Carotid Atherosclerosis

Watts GF, Mazurkiewicz JC, Tonge K, et al (Univ of Western Australia, Perth; St Thomas' Hosp, London)
*Q J Med* 88:321–326, 1995                                                        1–5

*Background.*—Hyperlipidemia and increased serum concentrations of lipoprotein(a) [Lp(a)] are well-documented risk factors for coronary artery disease. However, it is uncertain whether hyperlipidemia is an important risk factor for stroke and cerebrovascular disease. The relationship between Lp(a) and the severity of underlying carotid artery disease in stroke survivors has not been studied thoroughly. The association of serum Lp(a) concentration with the extent of atherosclerotic lesions, especially in the internal carotid arteries, was investigated.

*Methods.*—Fasting serum lipids, lipoproteins, apolipoproteins, and Lp(a) were measured in 49 white patients with transient ischemic attacks who were undergoing carotid angiography. The severity of extracranial cerebrovascular disease was evaluated by a grading system focusing on the internal carotid artery and carotid bifurcation.

*Findings.*—Compared with a group of healthy persons, patients had significantly greater serum levels of total cholesterol, apolipoprotein B, triglyceride, and Lp(a). Lipoprotein(a) was the only lipoprotein-related variable significantly associated with severity of carotid artery disease, after adjustment for age, sex, blood pressure, and a history of stroke. The concentration of serum Lp(a) was significantly greater in patients with

TABLE 2.—Mean Serum Lipid, Lipoprotein, Apolipoprotein, and Lp(a) Concentrations in the Patient Group vs. the Reference Group of Healthy Subjects

|  | Reference group ($n = 69$) | Patient group ($n = 49$) | 95% CI diff* | | $P$ |
|---|---|---|---|---|---|
| Cholesterol (mmol/l) | 5.57 | 6.19 | 0.09, | 1.14 | 0.02 |
| Triglyceride (mmol/l)† | 1.66 | 2.02 | 0.69, | 0.98 | 0.03 |
| HDL cholesterol (mmol/l) | 1.19 | 1.22 | −0.17, | 0.09 | 0.60 |
| LDL cholesterol (mmol/l) | 3.58 | 3.93 | −0.85, | 0.15 | 0.20 |
| Apolipoprotein Al (g/l) | 1.97 | 2.00 | −0.17, | 0.10 | 0.60 |
| Apolipoprotein B (g/l) | 1.2 | 1.38 | −0.32, | −0.01 | 0.03 |
| Lipoprotein(a) (g/l)† | 0.17 | 0.33 | 0.38, | 0.69 | <0.001 |
| LDL cholesterol/HDL cholesterol | 3.18 | 4.05 | −0.55, | 2.29 | 0.23 |
| Apo B/Apo Al | 0.63 | 0.76 | −0.04, | 0.29 | 0.13 |

* Confidence interval for difference.
† Geometric mean.
(Courtesy of Watts GF, Mazurkiewicz JC, Tonge K, et al: Lipoprotein(a) as a determinant of the severity of angiographically defined carotid atherosclerosis. *Q J Med* 88:321–326, 1995. By permission of Oxford University Press.)

carotid artery disease severity scores above the median value of the sample population compared with those below the median (Table 2).

*Conclusions.*—Increased serum La(a) is a significant determinant of the extent of carotid atherosclerosis. It may be useful for identifying patients at the greatest risk of stroke.

▶ As described in multiple previous editions of the YEAR BOOK OF VASCULAR SURGERY, elevated Lp(a) appears to be a well-defined risk factor for symptomatic atherosclerosis in many areas, including the internal carotid artery. I continue to be mystified by the absence of any clearly defined pathophysiologic relationship between Lp(a) and atherosclerotic disease. Certainly Lp(a) has numerous procoagulant effects, but I wonder if these are sufficient to explain its facilitative role in atherosclerosis. We know that Lp(a) exists as phenotypic isomers of different molecular sizes, and perhaps some of these will prove more important than others in facilitating atherosclerosis. The presence of various pro- and antioxidants may account for some of the observed variations in the effects of Lp(a). In summary, the association of Lp(a) to atherosclerosis appears clear, although not overwhelming, but the pathophysiology remains elusive. See also Abstract 1–29.

---

## Hyperlipidemia: A Novel Etiologic Factor in Deep Vein Thrombosis

Kawasaki T, Kambayashi J-I, Sakon M (Osaka Univ, Japan)
*Thromb Res* 79:147–151, 1995                                    1–6

---

*Objective.*—The association between hyperlipidemia and deep vein thrombosis was investigated.

*Background.*—Deep vein thrombosis resulting in pulmonary embolism is a major health problem in Western countries, but it is not as common in Asian and African countries. This difference may offer information about etiologic factors of this condition in Western countries. A high rate of hyperlipidemia was noted in patients with deep vein thrombosis in the current study.

*Methods.*—In 59 consecutive patients with deep vein thrombosis but no prior history of the problem, and in 59 control subjects, blood tests, lipid analysis, and hemostasis screening tests were performed for hyperlipidemia, thrombocytosis, and erythrocytosis. Tests were done under strict fasting conditions and before any therapeutic drugs were administered.

*Results.*—Values of serum total cholesterol and triglyceride were used. In patients with deep vein thrombosis, the overall incidence of hyperlipidemia was surprisingly high at 59%. The rate of high total cholesterol alone was 25%, and the rate of high triglyceride alone was 8.5% in these patients (Table 1). In control subjects, the overall incidence of hyperlipidemia was 29% (Table 1). Patients with idiopathic deep vein thrombosis had a higher incidence of hypercholesterolemia at 63% than control subjects at 20%. Patients with idiopathic deep vein thrombosis also had higher levels of total cholesterol (255 mg/dL) than control subjects (194

TABLE 1.—Incidence of Hyperlipidemia in Patients With Deep Vein Thrombosis
With or Without Established Risk Factors* and in Normal Subjects

| | No in Group | Hyper-lipidemia | †Hyper-cholesterolemia number of subjects | ‡Hyper-triglyceridemia (percent of group) | Combined |
|---|---|---|---|---|---|
| DVT patients | 59 | 35 (59.3) | 15 (25.4) | 5 (8.5) | 15 (25.4) |
| without risk factors | 24 | 16 (66.7) | 10 (41.7) | 1 (4.2) | 5 (20.8) |
| with risk factors | 35 | 19 (54.3) | 5 (14.3) | 4 (11.4) | 10 (28.6) |
| Normal subjects | 59 | 17 (28.8) | 10 (16.9) | 5 (8.5) | 2 (3.4) |
| DVT patients without risk factors vs normal subjects | | | | | |
| Chi-square | | 10.21 | 5.70 | | |
| P value | | <0.002 | <0.02 | §0.44 | §<0.02 |
| Odds ratios | | 4.9 | 3.5 | 0.47 | 7.5 |
| 95% CI‖ | | 1.7–13.7 | 1.2–10.1 | 0.2–19.3 | 1.3–41.9 |

* Thrombotic disorders, stasis and immobilization, malignancy, and hematologic disorders.
† High cholesterol alone.
‡ High triglyceride alone.
§ Fisher's exact probability.
‖Exact 95% confidence intervals.
(Reprinted from Thrombosis Research, Volume 79, Kawasaki T, Kambayashi J-I, Sakon M: Hyperlipidemia: A novel etiologic factor in deep vein thrombosis, pp 147–151, 1995, with kind permission from Elsevier Science Ltd, The Boulevard, Langford Lane, Kidlington OX5 1GB, UK.)

mg/dL). Of patients with idiopathic deep vein thrombosis, 67% had hyperlipidemia.

*Conclusions.*—Hyperlipidemia may have an important etiologic role in deep vein thrombosis. The possible role of hyperlipidemia has not been previously recognized. The low incidence of deep vein thrombosis in individuals of Asian descent may be associated with their lower levels of cholesterol.

▶ In this small cohort, the prevalence of hyperlipidemia in patients with deep vein thrombosis (DVT) was twice that in normal subjects. These authors conclude that hyperlipidemia should be included as 1 of the major risk factors for DVT, especially idiopathic DVT. I am fascinated to observe the dwindling incidence of truly idiopathic DVT with time. We now know that up to 5% of patients in whom idiopathic DVT is diagnosed have cancer at the time of diagnosis, and another 5% to 10% had cancer develop within 1 year.[1] If hyperlipidemia is firmly established as a risk factor for DVT, truly idiopathic DVT must be a dwindling entity. Contributing to this conclusion is the observation that hyperhomocystinemia is also reported as a risk factor for apparently idiopathic DVT. See also Abstract 1–46.

*Reference*

1. 1994 YEAR BOOK OF VASCULAR SURGERY, pp 405, 409.

## Human Monocyte-Derived Macrophages Induce Collagen Breakdown in Fibrous Caps of Atherosclerotic Plaques: Potential Role of Matrix-Degrading Metalloproteinases and Implications for Plaque Rupture

Shah PK, Falk E, Badimon JJ, et al (Univ of California, Los Angeles; Harvard Med School, Boston)
Circulation 92:1565–1569, 1995                                    1–7

*Objective.*—A key pathologic event that triggers coronary thrombosis is rupture of the fibrous cap of atherosclerotic plaque. The hypothesis that monocyte-derived macrophages induce collagen breakdown in human atherosclerotic fibrous caps by producing matrix-degrading metalloproteinases (MMPs) was tested.

*Methods.*—Ficoll-Plaque density gradient centrifugation was used to isolate mononuclear cells from blood of normal volunteers. The cells were cultured from 4 to 7 days until they transformed into macrophages. Fibrous caps, isolated from atherosclerotic plaques in human abdominal aorta or carotid endarterectomy specimens, were incubated for 48 hours with macrophages in serum-free medium with the MMP inhibitor phosphoramidon (10 samples), with macrophages in serum-free medium without the MMP inhibitor (21 samples), or in medium without macrophages, serum, or inhibitor. Hydroxyproline release, which reflected the amount of collagen degraded in the fibrous caps, was determined spectrophotometrically. Expression of MMP-1 (interstitial collagenase) and MMP-2 (72-kD gelatinase) in the cell culture was identified by immunocytochemistry with specific monoclonal antibodies, and zymography was used to assay MMP activity in the cell culture supernatant.

*Results.*—Hydroxyproline release was significantly greater by the 21 fibrous caps incubated with macrophages than that by the 9 fibrous caps incubated with cell-free medium alone (0.40 vs. 0.02 µg/mL/mg of tissue, respectively). There was no detectable hydroxyproline release by the fibrous caps incubated in the presence of the MMP inhibitor. The production of MMPs was confirmed by immunostaining. Between days 4 and 7 of incubation, cultures without the inhibitor stained positively for MMP-1 and MMP-2. Gelatinolytic (MMP-2) activity, as determined by zymography, was also evident by day 7 of culture in the supernatant of monocyte cultures without inhibitor.

*Conclusions.*—The results support the hypothesis that collagen breakdown is related to MMP expression. Furthermore, monocyte-derived macrophages, by producing MMPs, could induce collagen breakdown in fibrous caps of atherosclerotic plaques and predispose plaques to rupture and subsequent thrombosis.

▶ As noted previously, fibrous cap rupture as an etiologic event in atherosclerotic arterial thromboses is receiving widespread attention.[1, 2] Converging investigations indicate that macrophages are capable of inducing collagen breakdown in the fibrous cap overlying the human atherosclerotic plaque, probably associated with the elaboration of matrix degrading metalloproteinases. This suggests the possibility of future pharmacologic intervention specifically directed at this step in the fibrous cap rupture process. Stay tuned, surely there will be more to follow. See also Abstracts 1–1 and 1–25.

*References*

1. 1995 YEAR BOOK OF VASCULAR SURGERY, p 4.
2. 1996 YEAR BOOK OF VASCULAR SURGERY, p 13.

## Apoptosis in Human Atherosclerosis and Restenosis
Isner JM, Kearney M, Bortman S, et al (Tufts Univ, Boston)
*Circulation* 91:2703–2711, 1995                                    1–8

*Background.*—It has been suggested that apoptosis may play a role in maintaining stable cell populations in tissues with proliferative activity. Apoptosis has been observed in rat vascular smooth muscle cells (SMCs), which have also been shown to maintain high levels of proliferative activity long after injury. The presence of apoptosis in human atherosclerotic or restenotic vascular tissue was investigated, using immunohistochemical methods.

*Methods.*—Fifty-six directional atherectomy specimens, obtained equally from coronary and peripheral arterial sites from patients with primary and restenotic lesions, were studied. Each specimen was sectioned and studied with either histologic analysis to determine the number of intimal cells in specimens with identified apoptosis, or with immunohistochemical analysis, to identify apoptosis. Apoptosis was investigated using DNA nick-end labeling. To further identify apoptotic cells, SMC actin and macrophages were stained with the appropriate antibodies. To investigate associated changes, the *BCL2* and p53 antigens (both often associated with apoptosis in other tissues) were unmasked and proliferative activity was assessed by staining with proliferating cell nuclear antigen (PCNA).

*Results.*—Apoptosis was present in 63% of the 56 specimens, with unequal distributions among the groups of specimens. In the peripheral arterial specimens, apoptosis was identified in 93% of the restenotic specimens and only 43% of the specimens from patients with primary atherosclerosis. In the coronary arterial specimens, apoptosis was identified in 86% of the restenotic specimens and only 29% of the specimens with primary lesions. In these specimens, apoptosis was typically limited to less than 2% of the cells. Apoptosis was seen in both the vascular SMC and the macrophages, which together accounted for less than half of the apoptotic cells. Apoptosis was associated with hypercellular foci and with PCNA staining, indicating ongoing cellular proliferation. There was positive staining for p53 in some of the apoptotic restenotic, but not primary, lesions.

*Conclusions.*—Apoptosis is found in human vascular pathology and is particularly common in restenotic vessels, which generally demonstrate more proliferative activity than primary lesions. The role of apoptosis in modulating the cellularity of lesions causing vascular obstruction is therefore supported.

▶ I have always been fascinated by apoptosis, the apparently genetically encoded cell death program present in many human cell populations. Smooth muscle cells clearly suffer from apoptosis. Interestingly, apoptosis appears more prevalent among restenotic arterial lesions than primary atherosclerotic lesions, and may well modulate the actual cellularity of human vascular obstructions. This suggests the haunting possibility that one may be able to selectively transduce smooth muscle cells in areas of potential restenosis with the *ICE* gene, which has been identified as being associated with apoptosis.

---

**Antibodies Against Endothelial Cells and Cardiolipin in Young Patients With Peripheral Atherosclerotic Disease**
Nityanand S, Bergmark C, de Faire U, et al (Karolinska Hosp, Stockholm; St Görans Hosp, Stockholm; Karolinska Inst, Stockholm)
*J Intern Med* 238:437–443, 1995                                                          1–9

---

*Background.*—Because people who have atherosclerotic disease at an early age have a particularly poor prognosis, identifying any possible additional risk factors for premature vascular occlusion is important. There is increasing evidence of the role of immunologic mechanisms in the pathogenesis of atherosclerosis. In particular, antibodies against endothelial cells (AECA) and antibodies against cardiolipin (ACLA) have been implicated. To investigate the possible role of these autoantibodies, their occurrence was studied in patients younger than 50 years of age undergoing surgical treatment of atherosclerotic peripheral vascular disease.

*Methods.*—Blood samples were obtained from 62 patients undergoing follow-up for the surgical treatment of atherosclerotic peripheral vascular disease before the age of 50 years and from age- and sex-matched, randomly selected controls. The mean age of both groups was 49.3 years, and the mean age at the onset of symptoms in the patient group was 40.3 years. The blood samples were analyzed for routine hematologic and lipoprotein parameters and for the presence of AECA and ACLA.

*Results.*—Antibodies against endothelial cells were detected in 12.9% of the patients and 3% of the controls, and ACLA were detected in 14.5% of the patients and 3% of the controls. Of the 9 patients with ACLA and 8 patients with AECA, 2 had both autoantibodies. Among the patients, those with the antibodies were less likely to have hyperlipidemia or dyslipidemia than those without the antibodies (53% vs. 81%). There were no significant differences in clinical presentation or in the presence of other risk factors between the patients with and without the antibodies.

*Conclusions.*—A subset of patients with premature atherosclerotic peripheral vascular disease has AECA and ACLA. These patients tend to have less hyperlipidemia and dyslipidemia, suggesting that the autoantibodies may play a direct role in the vascular damage. Therefore, patients with premature atherosclerotic disease may have different pathogenetic mechanisms.

▶ Patients with early onset symptomatic peripheral atherosclerosis may have elevated levels of autoantibodies to oxidized low-density lipoprotein as reported in abstract 1–3. They also appear to have a considerably greater prevalence of antibodies against endothelial cells and cardiolipin than controls. The fascinating finding in this study—that patients with symptomatic atherosclerosis and autoantibodies had a distinctly lower prevalence of hyperlipidemia than other patients—suggests that these autoantibodies may be an important atherosclerotic risk factor in this cohort and may be involved in the production of vascular damage. The entire field of antibodies and autoantibodies in human atherosclerosis is deservedly attracting increased attention.

## Coagulation/Thrombolysis

### Low Molecular Mass Heparin Instead of Unfractionated Heparin During Infrainguinal Bypass Surgery

Swedenborg J, Nydahl S, Egberg N (Karolinska Hosp, Stockholm)
*Eur J Vasc Endovasc Surg* 11:59–64, 1996                                           1–10

*Introduction.*—Patients with atherosclerosis receive anticoagulation during vascular reconstructive surgery because they are assumed to have increased coagulability—the result of vessel wall changes, tissue necrosis in the affected limb, and alterations in blood flow and composition. Patients scheduled for infrainguinal bypass surgery took part in a study designed to evaluate low-molecular mass heparin (LMMH) as an anticoagulant and to determine whether such patients show laboratory evidence of hypercoagulation, particularly increased levels of fibrinogen.

*Methods.*—Patients were randomized to receive either unfractionated heparin (UFH), the agent used almost exclusively in this setting, or LMMH. Nine patients were operated for ulcers or gangrene, 6 for rest pain, and 3 for claudication. Femorodistal bypass was the most common procedure, performed in 6 patients with UFH and 7 with LMMH. Blood was drawn from the femoral vein before clamping, during clamping, and after release of the clamps for measurement of coagulation variables.

*Results.*—There were 4 postoperative graft occlusions, 2 in the UFH group and 2 in the LMMH group; 3 could not be salvaged and 1 (from the LMMH group) was successfully thrombectomized. One patient in the UFH group required reoperation for bleeding. All patients had increased levels of fibrinogen, fibrinopeptide A (FPA), fibrin monomers (FM), and thrombin-antithrombin complex (TAT) before surgery. None of these levels increased during surgery. Levels of FM were significantly lower and levels of anti-Xa slightly higher in the LMMH group than in the UFH group. Analysis of the influence of fibrinogen upon levels of FPA and FM demonstrated a strong positive correlation in both instances.

*Discussion.*—Only 2 previous studies have reported the use of LMMH as a perioperative anticoagulant. A derivative of UFH, LMMH mainly inhibits the coagulation cascade as a level above thrombin formation. In these patients undergoing infrainguinal bypass surgery, LMMH was found to be comparable to UFH as an anticoagulant. Potential advantages of LMMH include a lower risk of bleeding and reduction in FM levels. This study also confirmed that patients with arterial occlusive disease have laboratory evidence of a hypercoagulable state.

▶ Few pharmacologic agents in recent years have demonstrated a greater potential impact upon vascular surgery than LMMH. As documented in the next commentary (Abstract 1–11), these agents have the potential to induce considerably less thrombocytopenia than UFH and, as shown in this paper, appear at least as effective as UFH as an anticoagulant during the performance of vascular surgery. I wouldn't be at all surprised to see the use of unfractionated heparin slowly fade away over time.

---

**Heparin-Induced Thrombocytopenia in Patients Treated With Low-Molecular-Weight Heparin or Unfractionated Heparin**
Warkentin TE, Levine MN, Hirsh J, et al (McMaster Univ, Hamilton, Ont, Canada; Hamilton Civic Hosp, Ont, Canada)
*N Engl J Med* 332:1330–1335, 1995                                      1–11

---

*Introduction.*—Thrombocytopenia induced by heparin appears about 5 days after the start of heparin therapy. It is defined by the presence of heparin-dependent IgG antibodies and, paradoxically, can be complicated by thrombolic complications. An analysis of platelet counts and heparin-dependent IgG antibodies was done in a randomized, double-blind, controlled investigation of 665 patients with elective hip surgery receiving prophylaxis against venous thrombosis.

*Methods.*—Patients were randomized to receive twice-daily subcutaneous injections of either low-molecular weight heparin or 7,500 units of unfractionated heparin beginning the day of surgery until 14 days postoperatively, or until discharge. Platelet counts were obtained at baseline and daily. A large subgroup of 387 patients was also tested for heparin-dependent IgG antibodies. Heparin-induced thrombocytopenia was defined as a decrease in the platelet count to below 150,000 per $mm^3$ at 5 or more days after the start of heparin therapy, and a positive test for heparin-dependent IgG antibodies.

*Results.*—Twelve of 665 patients had thrombocytopenia after receiving heparin therapy for 5 or more days. Of these, 9 (2.7%) of the 332 patients receiving unfractionated heparin and none (0%) of the 333 receiving low-molecular weight heparin had heparin-induced thrombocytopenia. Eight of the 9 patients with heparin-induced thrombocytopenia had 1 or more thrombolic events. None of the patients with heparin-induced thrombocytopenia experienced major or minor hemorrhagic events. A higher frequency of heparin-dependent IgG antibodies was detected in patients receiving unfractionated heparin, compared to those receiving low-molecular weight heparin (7.8% vs. 2.2%).

*Conclusion.*—No patients treated with low-molecular weight heparin had heparin-induced thrombocytopenia or thrombotic events. By comparison, 9 patients receiving unfractionated heparin had thrombocytopenia. Eight of 9 had 1 or more thrombotic events. Heparin-induced thrombocytopenia was a strong risk factor for venous thrombosis.

▶ In this prospective, randomized study, no patients receiving low-molecular weight (LMW) heparin had clinical thrombocytopenia develop, and in only 2.2% did IgG heparin-dependent antibodies develop. This was markedly different from the group receiving unfractionated heparin. Whereas it seems clear that the LMW heparins cause heparin-induced thrombocytopenia far less often than does unfractionated heparin, they still do so on occasion. Thus, in a patient with established heparin-induced thrombocytopenia, one cannot simply switch to LMW heparin without first doing detailed coagulation studies because of the low, but real, possibility of cross-reactivity. Perhaps 1 day there will be LMW heparin with zero likelihood of inducing thrombocytopenia.

---

## Mutation in the Gene Coding for Coagulation Factor V and the Risk of Myocardial Infarction, Stroke, and Venous Thrombosis in Apparently Healthy Men

Ridker PM, Hennekens CH, Lindpaintner K, et al (Harvard Med School, Boston; Children's Hosp, Boston; Harvard School of Public Health, Boston; et al)
*N Engl J Med* 332:912–917, 1995                                     1–12

---

*Background.*—A point mutation in the gene coding for coagulation factor V has been associated with a form of activated protein C that resists degradation, and which therefore may increase the risk of venous thrombosis. It is not clear, however, whether healthy individuals are at increased risk. The mutation involves a substitution guanine at nucleotide 1691.

*Objective.*—The G1691A mutation was in 374 initially healthy male physicians enrolled in the Physicians' Health Study who subsequently had myocardial infarction; 209 with stroke; and 121 with deep venous thrombosis and/or pulmonary embolism. The same number of enrollees who remained healthy served as a control group.

*Findings.*—The prevalence of the factor V mutation was 6.1% in men in whom myocardial infarction developed and 4.3% in those with stroke, not significantly different from the 6.0% rate in those who remained free of

TABLE 2.—Relative Risk of Myocardial Infarction, Stroke, and Venous Thrombosis Associated With the Presence of the Factor V Mutation

| VARIABLE | CARDIOVASCULAR DISEASE DURING FOLLOW-UP | | | | |
|---|---|---|---|---|---|
| | NONE ($n = 704$) | MYOCARDIAL INFARCTION ($n = 374$) | STROKE ($n = 209$) | MYOCARDIAL INFARCTION OR STROKE ($n = 583$) | VENOUS THROMBOSIS OR PULMONARY EMBOLISM ($n = 121$) |
| Crude analysis* | | | | | |
| Relative risk | 1.0 | 1.1 | 0.7 | 0.9 | 2.1 |
| 95% CI | — | 0.6–1.8 | 0.3–1.4 | 0.6–1.5 | 1.1–4.0 |
| P value | — | 0.8 | 0.3 | 0.7 | 0.02 |
| Adjusted analysis† | | | | | |
| Relative risk | 1.0 | 1.5 | 1.0 | 1.3 | 2.7 |
| 95% CI | — | 0.8–2.7 | 0.4–2.2 | 0.7–2.2 | 1.3–5.6 |
| P value | — | 0.2 | 0.9 | 0.4 | 0.008 |

\* Adjusted for treatment assignment, age, and smoking status.
† Adjusted for treatment assignment, age, smoking status, history of hypertension, history of elevated cholesterol, family history of myocardial infarction before the age of 60 years, body mass index, presence of diabetes, and frequency of exercise.
*Abbreviation: CI*, confidence interval.
(Reprinted by permission of *The New England Journal of Medicine*. Ridker PM, Hennekens CH, Lindpaintner K, et al: Mutation in the gene coding for coagulation factor V and the risk of myocardial infarction, stroke, and venous thrombosis in apparently healthy men. *N Engl J Med* 332:912–917, 1995, Massachusetts Medical Society.)

cardiovascular disease (Table 2). The mutation was, however, found in 11.6% of men in whom venous thrombosis or pulmonary embolism developed during follow-up. The adjusted relative risk of thrombosis/embolism in heterozygous subjects was 2.7, and the risk of primary venous thrombosis was 3.5. The increased relative risk was apparently chiefly in older men. One fourth of men older than 60 years who had primary venous thrombosis exhibited the mutation.

*Conclusion.*—The G1691A mutation of the factor V gene is the most common inherited factor known to predispose to venous thrombosis.

▶ In men with heterozygosity for mutation in the gene coding for factor V, making it resistant to degradation by activated protein C, the relative risk for idiopathic deep vein thrombosis was 3.5 times the risk in men without the defect. Interestingly there was no increased risk of myocardial infarction or stroke. Thus, the conclusion of this study is that the clinical effect of this point mutation is the increased relative risk of venous thrombosis and pulmonary embolism, not arterial thrombosis. These authors observe, accurately I suppose, that this mutation is the most frequently inherited factor recognized to date that predisposes patients to venous thrombosis. Isn't it again fascinating to note how, with our increasing ability to detect risk factors for venous thrombosis, the incidence of truly idiopathic deep vein thrombosis continues a remarkable decline. See also Abstract 1–13.

### Factor V Leiden and Risks of Recurrent Idiopathic Venous Thromboembolism

Ridker PM, Miletich JP, Stampfer MJ, et al (Harvard Med School, Boston; Washington Univ, St Louis, Mo)
*Circulation* 92:2800–2802, 1995                                    1–13

*Background.*—The factor V Leiden mutation is found in 4% to 6% of the population, and people who are heterozygous for this mutation appear to be at elevated risk for venous thrombosis. It is uncertain whether factor V Leiden plays a role in recurrent idiopathic venous thromboembolism (VTE), however. This information will have a major impact on the consideration of genetic screening programs for secondary prevention of thromboembolic disease. The link between factor V Leiden and risk of recurrent idiopathic VTE was assessed.

*Methods.*—The study included 77 men from the Physicians' Health Study who had an initial idiopathic VTE. Each subject's DNA sample was analyzed for the presence of factor V Leiden. During an average follow-up of 68 months, 11 (14%) of the men had a recurrent idiopathic VTE, all of which occurred after anticoagulation therapy was stopped. Recurrence rates were compared in men with and without factor V Leiden.

*Results.*—Fourteen subjects were heterozygous for factor V Leiden and 63 were genetically unaffected. The incidence rate of recurrent VTE among the subjects with factor V Leiden was 29%, or 7.46/100 person-years. By comparison, the incidence rate for subjects without the mutation was 11%, or 1.8/100 person-years. Factor V Leiden was associated with a crude relative risk of 4.1 for recurrent VTE and an age- and smoking-adjusted relative risk of 4.7. Genotype did not affect the timing of the recurrence. Three fourths of the recurrent VTEs in men with factor V Leiden were attributable to the mutation.

*Conclusions.*—Heterozygosity for factor V Leiden may increase the risk of recurrent idiopathic VTE by four- to fivefold among men who have had an initial episode of thrombosis. The finding of factor V Leiden in a patient with 1 idiopathic VTE may signal the need for more prolonged anticoagulant therapy to prevent recurrent thrombosis.

▶ A very small salami slice of the study described in this abstract concludes that patients with factor V Leiden have a four- to fivefold increased risk of recurrent venous thrombosis after the primary deep vein thrombosis episode and after cessation of anticoagulants. The authors appropriately suggest that such patients may benefit by more prolonged anticoagulation. For polluting the literature with a thin salami slice that could have been easily covered in the preceding article by the same authors, I hereby award them the prestigious Camel Dung Award, which was so well received after its introduction last year.

### The Management of Thrombosis in the Antiphospholipid-Antibody Syndrome

Khamashta MA, Cuadrado MJ, Mujic F, et al (Rayne Inst, London; St Thomas's Hosp, London)
*N Engl J Med* 332:993–997, 1995        1–14

*Background.*—The antiphospholipid-antibody syndrome is a thrombophilic disorder in which venous or arterial thrombosis or both may occur in patients with antiphospholipid antibodies. Although the prevention of thrombosis in this syndrome is important, there is no consensus on the duration and extent of prophylactic treatments. The efficacy of several different methods of antithrombotic treatment in the antiphospholipid-antibody syndrome—warfarin, low-dose aspirin, or a combination of both—was assessed.

*Method.*—A total of 147 patients were classified into 3 groups: 62 patients in whom the syndrome was primary; 66 in whom the syndrome was associated with systemic lupus erythematosus; and 19 in whom it was associated with lupus-like disease. The antithrombotic treatment history of these patients with either warfarin, low-dose aspirin, or both was retrospectively reviewed, and the rates of recurrent thrombosis were analyzed.

*Results.*—One hundred one patients (69%) had a total of 186 episodes of recurrent thrombosis. The median time between the initial thrombosis and the first recurrence was 12 months. Treatment with high-intensity warfarin (international normalized ratio of 3 or above), with or without low-dose aspirin (75 mg per day) was significantly more effective in preventing thrombosis than treatment with low-intensity warfarin (producing an international normalized ratio of less than 3) with or without low-dose aspirin, or aspirin alone (recurrence rates per patient-year were 0.013, 0.23, and 0.18, respectively). The first 6 months after the cessation of warfarin therapy were associated with the highest rate of recurrence of thrombosis. Nonfatal complications of treatment included bleeding in 29 patients during warfarin treatment, with severe symptoms in 7 patients.

*Conclusion.*—This study demonstrates the high risk of recurrent thrombosis in patients with the antiphospholipid-antibody syndrome. Long-term anticoagulation therapy with or without low-dose aspirin, in which an international normalized ratio of 3 or above is maintained, is recommended for these patients.

▶ Just what is the risk of thrombosis in patients with antiphospholipid antibodies? Interestingly, in this study the first thrombotic event was venous in 54% of patients and arterial in 46%. Recurrences were significantly less if the patients were vigorously anticoagulated with warfarin. All the patients in this study met the diagnostic criteria for the antiphospholipid-antibody syndrome. This requires considerably more than the presence of antiphospholipid (anticardiolipin) antibody alone. We have previously shown from our clinic that the presence of anticardiolipin antibody alone conveys little or no risk of arterial thrombosis.[1] Clearly, patients with the antiphospholipid syndrome are much more at risk than those who simply have the anticardiolipin antibody. One must be very careful in interpreting the nuances of clinical presentation in this complex patient population. Semantics are important. Words mean everything. Although vascular surgeons are unlikely to encounter many patients with antiphospholipid syndrome, they are going to encounter a large number of patients with anticardiolipin antibody. These 2 conditions, although similar, are most assuredly not the same thing.

*Reference*

1. Lee R, Taylor LM: *J Vasc Surg,* in press.

---

**Randomized Double-Blind Comparison of Two Doses of Hirulog With Heparin as Adjunctive Therapy to Streptokinase to Promote Early Patency of the Infarct-Related Artery in Acute Myocardial Infarction**
Théroux P, Pérez-Villa F, Waters D, et al (Montreal Heart Inst, Canada)
*Circulation* 91:2132–2139, 1995                                              1–15

---

*Background.*—In patients with acute myocardial infarction (AMI), rapid and complete restoration of coronary artery blood flow improves myocardial salvage and reduces mortality. Recent studies have shown that Hirulog (a direct thrombin inhibitor), when used with tissue-type plasminogen activator or streptokinase, can facilitate thrombolysis and prevent reocclusion better than heparin. In patients with AMI, who first received aspirin and streptokinase, the effects of 2 different doses of Hirulog on angiographic patency were compared with those of heparin.

*Methods.*—During the 11-month study period, 70 of 180 patients with AMI were enrolled in this double-blind, randomized, prospective trial. Inclusion criteria included the onset of chest pain within the previous 6 hours, ST-segment elevation on 2 adjacent ECG leads (or left bundle branch block), and no contraindication to anticoagulation. Coronary artery patency was assessed angiographically 90 and 120 minutes after initiation of aspirin and streptokinase therapy, and again after 2–6 days. Patients were randomized to low-dose Hirulog (0.5 mg/kg per hour for 12 hours, followed by 0.1 mg/kg per hour), to high-dose Hirulog (1 mg/kg per hour for 12 hours, followed by placebo), or to heparin (5,000 U bolus followed by 1,000 U per hour).

*Results.*—At 90 minutes, thrombin inhibition in myocardial infarction (TIMI) flow grade 2 or 3 was present in 96% of patients receiving low-dose Hirulog, in 79% receiving high-dose Hirulog, and in 46% receiving heparin. At 120 minutes, the corresponding figures were 100%, 82%, and 62%. At 90 minutes, the relative risk for restoring TIMI grade 3 was 2.77 for low-dose Hirulog compared with heparin and 1.4 for low-dose compared with high-dose Hirulog. During the next 4 days, patients who received high-dose Hirulog (followed by a placebo infusion after 12 hours) had more clinical events and reocclusion than patients in the 2 other groups. Overall, recurrent ischemia or MI occurred in 7% of the patients who received low-dose Hirulog, in 18% of those given high-dose Hirulog, and in 23% of those given heparin. Serious bleeding complications occurred in 18% to 31% of patients, but none had intracranial bleeding or stroke.

*Conclusions.*—When used as adjunct therapy to aspirin and streptokinase in the early phase of AMI, Hirulog improves early coronary artery patency rates better than heparin. Low doses of Hirulog are at least as effective as high doses. The patency rates (with the combination of low-dose Hirulog and streptokinase) in this study were better than those reported for the combination of front-loaded tissue-type plasminogen activator and heparin.

▶ I have repeatedly stated that the direct thrombin inhibitors, of which Hirulog is representative, will be very important in the future treatment of coagulation abnormalities. Currently, these drugs appear to have a very narrow therapeutic window and, when used in the higher dose ranges, have a disturbing propensity to produce hemorrhagic stroke. The observation reported herein that Hirulog appears superior to heparin when used as adjunctive therapy to streptokinase and aspirin in the early treatment of AMI is noteworthy. Interestingly, high doses were not required and may actually be less effective than lower doses.

## Hirulog in the Treatment of Unstable Angina: Results of the Thrombin Inhibition in Myocardial Ischemia (TIMI) 7 Trial

Fuchs J, and the TIMI 7 Investigators (Harvard Med School, Boston)
*Circulation* 92:727–733, 1995                                                    1–16

*Background.*—Direct antithrombins are a new class of drugs that have shown promise in the treatment of unstable angina. Hirulog is a synthetic, highly specific, direct inhibitor of free and clot-bound thrombin designed with the natural leech-derived compound hirudin as a model. The Thrombin Inhibition in Myocardial Ischemia (TIMI) 7 trial was a randomized, double-blind, dose-finding pilot study of Hirulog used together with aspirin in patients with unstable angina.

*Patients.*—A total of 410 patients with unstable angina were randomized to receive 1 of 4 doses of Hirulog administered in a constant infusion during a 72-hour period. All patients were also given aspirin at a dose of 325 mg/day. The Hirulog doses were 0.02, 0.25, 0.50, and 1.0 $mg \cdot kg^{-1} \cdot h^{-1}$. The primary efficacy end point was "unsatisfactory outcome," defined as the occurrence of death, nonfatal myocardial infarction (MI), rapid clinical deterioration, or recurrent ischemic pain at rest with ECG changes at 72 hours. The secondary efficacy end point was defined as death or nonfatal MI at hospital discharge and after 6 weeks.

*Outcome.*—There was no significant difference in the incidence of unsatisfactory outcome at 72 hours among the 4 dose groups: 8.1%, 6.2%, 11.4%, and 6.2%. However, the secondary end point of death or nonfatal MI at hospital discharge occurred in 10.0% of patients treated with the lowest dose, compared with 3.2% of those treated with any of the 3 higher doses of Hirulog. Similarly, at 6 weeks, the secondary end point had occurred in 12.5% of patients in the low-dose group, compared with 5.2% of patients in any of the 3 higher-dose groups. Only 2 patients (0.5%) had a major spontaneous hemorrhage attributed to the study drug.

*Conclusions.*—Hirulog appears to be a promising new anticoagulant for use in the treatment of unstable angina. However, its efficacy and safety still need to be compared with those of heparin in a much larger, definitive trial.

▶ This dose-ranging study concludes that low-dose Hirulog is superior to higher doses, but clearly the low dose must be above a certain minimum. Thus 0.02 mg/kg/hr was not as effective as 0.25 mg/kg/hr. However, the 0.25 was at least as effective as the 1.0. If there is a lesson here, it is that Hirulog and its associated antithrombins should be used in the lowest possible doses. Not only are higher doses associated with an increased risk of hemorrhagic stroke, they paradoxically appear also to be associated with an increased risk of peripheral arterial occlusions, an observation for which I have absolutely no explanation. See also Abstract 1–15.

## Bleeding Complications With the Chimeric Antibody to Platelet Glycoprotein IIb/IIIa Integrin in Patients Undergoing Percutaneous Coronary Intervention

Aguirre FV, Topol EJ, Ferguson JJ, et al (St Louis Univ, Mo; Cleveland Clinic, Ohio; Texas Heart Inst, Houston; et al)
*Circulation* 91:2882–2890, 1995                                                      1–17

*Background.*—The addition of new antithrombin and antiplatelet drugs to the standard regimen of heparin and aspirin may have an incremental effect on bleeding complications of percutaneous transluminal coronary revascularization (PTCR). In the Evaluation of c7E3 Fab in Preventing Ischemic Complications of High-Risk Angioplasty (EPIC) trial, the periprocedural use of aspirin, heparin, and the chimeric antibody to the platelet glycoprotein IIb/IIIa integrin c7E3 Fab was associated with a significant reduction in postprocedural ischemic complications and 6-month clinical restenosis, but also was related to increased bleeding complications. These complications are reviewed, as are various clinical and procedural variables that were related to increased bleeding complications in the EPIC trial.

*Patients and Methods.*—A total of 2,099 patients younger than age 80 with high-risk clinical or lesion morphologic traits were enrolled. Patients were randomly assigned to placebo bolus plus placebo infusion, c7E3 Fab

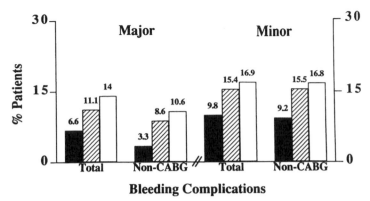

**Bleeding Complications**

FIGURE 1.—Bar graph showing frequency of major and minor bleeding complications among the 3 treatment groups. Values are given for all bleeding complications (Total) and for bleeding complications not related to coronary artery bypass graft surgery (Non-CABG). *Solid bars* indicate placebo (*n* = 696); *hatched bars,* bolus (*n* = 695); and *open bars,* bolus plus infusion (*n* = 708). (Aquirre FV, Topol EJ, Ferguson JJ, et al: Bleeding complications with the chimeric antibody to platelet glycoprotein in IIb/IIIa integrin in patients undergoing percutaneous coronary intervention. *Circulation* 1995; 91:2882–2890. Reproduced with permission *Circulation.* Copyright 1995 American Heart Association.)

bolus plus placebo infusion, or c7E3 Fab bolus plus c7E3 Fab infusion. Periprocedural aspirin and IV heparin also were administered for at least 12 hours after the procedure. Transfusions, decreased hemoglobin, and an index including both parameters were measured.

*Results.*—Major bleeding complications not associated with bypass surgery were noted in 3.3% of the patients treated with placebo, 8.6% of those receiving bolus c7E3 Fab, and 10.6% of those given bolus plus infusion of c7E3 Fab. Blood product transfusions were used in 7.5%, 14.0%, and 16.8% of the patients, respectively. The majority of major bleeding complications occurred at the femoral access site across all 3 treatment groups. Major bleeding complications resulted in intracranial hemorrhage in only 0.3% and in death in only 0.09% of the population. Variables that were significantly and independently associated with major complications on multivariate analysis included increased age, female sex, lower weight, c7E3 Fab therapy, and duration and complexity of the index procedure. No significant increases in major bleeding complications or blood loss were observed among patients receiving bolus plus infusion, compared with those given bolus c7E3 only. Minor bleeding complications not related to bypass surgery occurred in 291 patients and were more commonly observed among those receiving c7E3 (Fig 1).

*Conclusions.*—Bleeding complications not associated with bypass surgery were 2 to 3 times more common among c7E3-treated patients, compared with placebo-treated patients. Most complications were, however, transient and well tolerated. Additional studies should focus on strategies aimed at reducing bleeding complications and improving clinical benefit among patients treated with c7E3 Fab during PTCR.

▶ A whole host of powerful new coagulation-modifying drugs is becoming available. This study describes complications associated with use of the c7E3 Fab antibody to the platelet glycoprotein IIb/IIIa integrin in the EPIC study previously reported. Although the bleeding complications unrelated to bypass surgery were 2 to 3 times higher in patients receiving c7E3 Fab than in patients receiving placebo, these authors describe most complications as transient and well tolerated. Careful attention to risk factor analysis and modification of concomitant anticoagulant therapy will probably reduce associated bleeding complications. At present, neither the long-term utility of this powerful antiplatelet drug nor its role in clinical medicine has been defined.

---

**Attenuation of the Synthesis of Plasminogen Activator Inhibitor Type 1 by Niacin: A Potential Link Between Lipid Lowering and Fibrinolysis**
Brown SL, Sobel BE, Fujii S (Washington Univ, St Louis, Mo; Univ of Vermont, Burlington)
*Circulation* 92:767–772, 1995                                                  1–18

---

*Objective.*—Increased concentrations of plasminogen activator inhibitor type I (PAI-1) have been implicated in the development of atherosclerosis and coronary thrombosis. Gemfibrozil, a lipid lowering agent, has been shown to attenuate PAI-1 expression both in vivo and in vitro. Results of a study to determine if another lipid lowering agent, niacin, could attenuate PAI-1 synthesis in highly differentiated human hepatoma (Hep G2) cells are presented.

*Methods.*—Plasminogen activator inhibitor type 1 activity in plasma and PAI-1 mRNA expression in parenchymal liver cells of niacin-fed Sprague-Dawley rats was determined. Plasminogen activator inhibitor type 1 antigen from Hep G2 cells with and without exposure to niacin and to transforming growth factor-β (TGF-β) was quantified by ELISA. Then, PAI-1 mRNA was isolated from cells with and without preincubation with niacin, transferred by Northern blotting, incubated with α-$^{32}$P-dCTP, subjected to autoradiography, and quantitated by laser densitometry. Washed cells were incubated with $^{35}$S-methionine, and newly synthesized PAI-1 was immunoprecipitated with a mouse monoclonal anti-human PAI-1 antibody.

*Results.*—In Hep G2 cells exposed to niacin, PAI-1 expression was significantly decreased (Fig 1). In Hep G2 cells exposed to TGF-β, PAI-1 increased by a factor of 3.4. When niacin was added, the increase was diminished by 65%. Niacin also reduced the synthesis of PAI-1 in Hep G2 cells by 39% and reduced the augmentation of PAI-1 synthesis in TGF-β fed Hep G2 cells by 44%. Decreased PAI-1 synthesis was the result of a significant reduction in the steady-state mRNA concentration. Whereas mRNA expression increased by a factor of 4.4 at 6 hours in the presence of TGF-β, expression was attenuated by 22% with the addition of niacin. Increased PAI-1 synthesis and PAI-1 mRNA concentrations in the livers of rats treated with dexamethasone were also diminished by pretreatment with niacin.

**A**

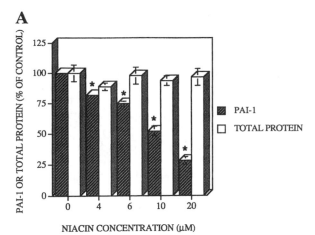

FIGURE 1.—Graphs showing relation between amount of PAI-1 (*hatched bars*) or total protein (*open bars*) in the conditioned medium of Hep G2 cells and concentration of niacin. After serum starvation, confluent monolayers were exposed to 0, 4, 6, 10, or 20 μmol/L niacin for 48 hours. Conditioned medium was harvested and assayed for PAI-1 (*n* = 3 for each condition) and, in separate experiments, for total protein (*n* = 3 for each condition). *Abbreviation: PAI*, plasminogen activator inhibitor. (Brown SL, Sobel BE, Fujii S; Attenuation of the synthesis of plasminogen activator inhibitor type 1 by niacin: A potential link between lipid lowering and fibrinolysis. *Circulation* 1995; 92:767–772. Reproduced with permission *Circulation.* Copyright 1995 American Heart Association.)

*Conclusion.*—Niacin decreases the amount of PAI-1 produced by Hep G2 cells in vitro by attenuating its synthesis. Niacin may help to prevent atherosclerosis by altering intracellular lipid metabolism and may potentiate fibrinolysis, thereby shifting the balance between thrombosis and thrombolysis.

▶ Our old friend niacin has been around for years. It has had a small but well-defined role in secondary prevention, and it does inhibit both triglyceride and cholesterol synthesis. The observation that it may also potentiate fibrinolysis suggests that this drug may be even more important in the future.

## Aspirin Improves the Outcome of Intraarterial Thrombolysis With Tissue Plasminogen Activator

Braithwaite BD, Jones L, Yusuf SW, et al (Gloucestershire Royal Hosp, England; Queens Med Centre, Nottingham, England; Royal Free Hosp, London; et al)
*Br J Surg* 82:1357–1358, 1995                                    1–19

*Objective.*—Although aspirin is an effective antithrombotic agent after myocardial infarction, the result of combining it with tissue plasminogen activator (t-PA) for peripheral intra-arterial thrombolysis is not known.

Results of a retrospective study of aspirin and t-PA treatment in peripheral thrombosis for acute limb ischemia are reported.

*Methods.*—The records from 8 hospitals of 329 patients, aged 44 to 92 years, treated with intra-arterial t-PA for acute limb ischemia, 82 of whom took aspirin before thrombolysis, were retrospectively reviewed for outcome after 30 days, after 12 months and incidence of stroke, rethrombosis, and major hemorrhage.

*Results.*—There were significantly higher limb salvage rates in patients taking aspirin before the event (80% vs. 69%). There were nonsignificant differences between patients taking aspirin and those not taking aspirin in amputation rates (10% vs. 17%) and mortality (10% vs. 14%). Stroke rates, major hemorrhage, and rates of rethrombosis were unaffected. There were 89 infusions during the 12-month follow-up period because of occlusion, 26% of those in patients taking aspirin. Incidences of claudication in aspirin-taking vs. t-PA-only patients were 22% and 36%, and 78% and 63% for limb-threatening ischemia. Ischemia was caused by thrombosis in 73% of patients and by embolism in the remainder. Thirteen percent of aspirin-treated patients required amputation within 30 days. None died. Thirteen percent of t-PA patients required amputation, and another 10% died. In patients taking aspirin, 9% had a major hemorrhage, none had a stroke, and 17% had a rethrombosis. In patients taking t-PA only, 13% had a major hemorrhage, 5 had a stroke, and 16% had a rethrombosis.

*Conclusion.*—In this small study, aspirin did not prevent rethrombosis but did improve limb salvage rates after rethrombosis (86% vs. 72%). Although improved thrombolysis may be the result of impaired platelet activity within the thrombus, this does not explain the reduced mortality in patients taking aspirin.

▶ This rather small study concludes that patients receiving aspirin with intra-arterial thrombolytics in the treatment of acute limb ischemia have significantly higher rates of limb salvage than those receiving thrombolytics without aspirin. I am not particularly surprised by this, as numerous coronary studies have shown that the use of anticoagulant drugs produces results superior to placebo when used with thrombolytics. As always, it is good to have our prejudices confirmed. It is important, however, to note that this was not a randomized trial, and many undefined variables may have had an important role.

---

### Activated Protein C Resistance and Graft Occlusion After Coronary Artery Bypass Surgery

Eritsland J, Gjønnes G, Sandset PM, et al (Ulleval Univ Hosp, Oslo, Norway)
*Thromb Res* 79:223–226, 1995                                                    1–20

---

*Objective.*—Risk factors for arterial thrombosis, as a result of activated protein C (APC) resistance, an inherited genetic defect, are unknown.

TABLE 1.—One Year Incidence of Vein Graft (1 or More Occluded Vein Grafts) Occlusion and IMA Graft Occlusion in Patients With and Without APC Resistance

|  | APC resistance | No APC resistance | *P* value |
|---|---|---|---|
| Vein graft occlusion | 4/10 (40%) | 237/493 (48.1%) | 0.75 |
| IMA graft occlusion | 2/9 (22.2%) | 59/423 (13.9%) | 0.37 |

*Abbreviations: IMA*, internal mammary artery; *APC*, activated protein C.

(Reprinted from *Thrombosis Research* 79, Eritsland J, Gjønnes G, Sandset PM, et al: Activated protein C resistance and graft occlusion after coronary artery bypass surgery, pp 223–226, Copyright 1995, with kind permission from Elsevier Science Ltd, The Boulevard, Langford Lane, Kidlington OX5 1GB, UK.)

Results of a study relating the incidence of 1-year graft occlusion in patients undergoing coronary artery bypass grafting (CABG) to the presence of APC resistance are presented.

*Methods.*—Activated Protein C resistance in 610 patients (87% men), assessed using an automated test method, was defined as an activated partial thromboplastin time (APTT) ratio (in the presence or absence of APC) of less than 2.1 using blood samples from 100 healthy volunteers as controls.

*Results.*—Of 587 samples analyzed, anticoagulant use or the presence of lupus disqualified 41. Activated protein C was diagnosed in 12 of the remaining 546 patients. The prevalence of APC resistance in patients with myocardial infarction (5/281) was similar to that of patients with no myocardial infarction (7/265), or 0.57. Of the 530 patients receiving CABG, 1-year patency was 94.9%. Of the 452 patients receiving internal mammary artery (IMA) grafts, 1-year patency was 95.6%. Graft occlusion in patients with and without APC resistance was compared (Tab 1). Whether patients received aspirin or warfarin as antithrombic treatment had no effect on graft occlusion. Two patients with APC resistance, 1 receiving aspirin and the other warfarin, had IMA occlusion. Seven other patients, 3 receiving aspirin and 4 warfarin, had open IMA grafts. The 2.2% prevalence of APC resistance in this study was lower than anticipated in a normal population but compares with another recent large study that found no association between factor V gene and an increased risk of myocardial infarction.

*Conclusion.*—In this study of patients with atherosclerotic disease, the prevalence of APC resistance was similar to that in the normal population. Incidences of thrombotic complications in patients with and without APC resistance were also similar.

► This study concludes that factor V resistance to APC is not associated with an increase in either myocardial infarction or coronary bypass graft occlusion. Results such as this indicate we are still in the early stages of accurately defining the clinical import of factor V resistance to APC. See also Abstracts 1–12 and 1–13, which reached generally similar conclusions.

## Protein Z Deficiency: A New Cause of Bleeding Tendency

Kemkes-Matthes B, Matthes KJ, (Universität Gießen, Giessen, Germany)
Thromb Res 79:49–55, 1995                                    1–21

*Background.*—The clinical relevance of protein Z, a vitamin K-dependent protein synthesized by the liver, is unknown. Because protein Z promotes the association of thrombin with phospholipid surfaces, it may help keep thrombin from diffusing away from the site of injury. Thus, low plasma concentrations of protein Z might cause a bleeding tendency. Thirty-six patients with an idiopathic bleeding tendency and normal liver functions were prospectively investigated for protein Z deficiency.

*Methods.*—Most of the 36 patients (mean age 43 years, range 10–86 years; 32 women) had a mild-to-moderate bleeding tendency, but 3 of 28 had required blood transfusions during surgery. The patients were com-

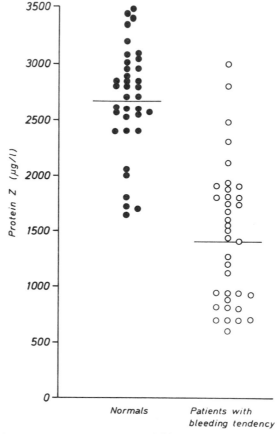

**FIGURE 1.**—Protein Z (µg/L) in 36 patients with bleeding complications of unknown origin in comparison to 36 age- and sex-matched healthy controls. (Reprinted from *Thrombosis Research* 79, Kemkes-Matthes B, Matthes KJ, Protein Z deficiency: A new cause of bleeding tendency, pp 49–55, Copyright 1995, with kind permission from Elsevier Science Ltd, The Boulevard, Langford Lane, Kidlington OX5 1GB, UK.)

pared with 36 healthy, age- and sex-matched control subjects. Appropriate tests were used to exclude defects in the plasma coagulation system, platelet disorders, and von Willebrand's disease.

*Results.*—The mean plasma protein Z levels were significantly lower in the patients than the controls (1,400 ± 610 vs. 2,680 ± 490 µg/L). Twenty-one of the 36 patients had protein Z levels below the lowest value in the control subjects (Fig 1). Thirty-one patients had protein Z levels less than 2,000 µg/L, vs. only 4 of the healthy control subjects. No significant differences were found between the patients and the control subjects in routine coagulation tests (prothrombin time, activated partial thromboplastin time platelet counts) or tests for other vitamin K-dependent factors (II, X, and protein C). However, the patients had longer bleeding times than the controls (10.26 ± 5.05 vs. 6.08 ± 1.74 minutes). Most of the patients with low protein Z levels also had a positive Rumpel-Leede test.

*Conclusions.*—Protein Z deficiency is a newly described bleeding disorder that may cause a mild-to-moderate bleeding tendency and the "capillary fragility syndrome." It is not detected by routine coagulation tests. The higher incidence in women than men is unexplained, but may be due to either a special mode of inheritance or to a patient selection bias.

▶ This novel contribution suggests the existence of another vitamin K-dependent coagulation factor known as protein Z. This hepatic-produced substance appears to promote the association of thrombin with phospholipid surfaces. The authors produce rather weak evidence that protein Z deficiency may be of clinical significance in certain patients with bleeding tendencies. Unfortunately, no tests were done to confirm that coagulation studies returned to normal when protein Z was given. I shall not accept this as a proven condition, but I incude it in the YEAR BOOK because of its potential importance. Stay tuned. I suspect we shall hear more about this.

---

## Reduced Thrombogenicity of Type VI Collagen as Compared to Type I Collagen

Zangari M, Kaplan KL, Glanville RW, et al (Mount Sinai School of Medicine, New York; Shriners Hosp for Crippled Children, Portland, Ore)
*Thromb Res* 79:429–436, 1995                                                    1–22

*Objective.*—The secretory and platelet aggregating activities of recently identified type VI collagen, a subendothelial collagen that interacts with von Willebrand factor (vWF) and would be exposed after vessel injury and de-endothelialization, are evaluated and compared with those of type I collagen in samples of normal human blood.

*Methods.*—Type I collagen from calf skin was purchased and type VI collagen was isolated from human umbilical cord according to an established procedure. Platelet aggregation in blood samples from healthy volunteers was studied by changes in light transmission and by platelet counts. Platelet secretion was determined by measuring the release of radiolabeled serotonin from dense granules by liquid scintillation counting and the release of beta-thromboglobulin (BTG) from alpha-granules by radioimmunoassay.

*Results.*—Significant differences between types VI and I collagen were noted in all measured parameters. The lag time to platelet aggregation was significantly greater and the extent of platelet aggregation was significantly less with type VI than type I collagen. In addition, the mean secretion of both radiolabeled serotonin and BTG was significantly greater with type I than with type VI collagen.

*Conclusions.*—Type VI collagen is a much weaker platelet agonist than type I collagen under in vitro conditions. Type VI may play a modulating role in the platelet thrombotic response of blood vessels following injury.

▶ An enormously complex relationship prevails in the arterial wall surrounding the interaction of vWF and platelets and their associated membrane glycoprotein receptors. von Willebrand factor is necessary for platelet adherence to the subendothelium, at least at high wall shear rates, and platelet membrane glycoprotein receptors clearly have a role in this process. The subendothelial binding protein for vWF is apparently type VI collagen. The current study suggests that type VI collagen induces a significantly diminished platelet activation and aggregation response, compared with type I collagen, indicating that type VI collagen may have a role in normally limiting the platelet thrombotic response after injury at the level of the vascular subendothelium. This appears to be another demonstration of the yin and yang we have come to expect in coagulation factor interactions.

## Coronary Disease

**Prevention of Coronary Heart Disease With Pravastatin in Men With Hypercholesterolemia**
Shepherd J, Cobbe SM, Ford I, et al (Univ of Glasgow, Scotland; Robertson Centre for Biostatistics, Glasgow, Scotland; Galloway District Gen Hosp, Dumfries, Scotland)
*N Engl J Med* 333:1301–1307, 1995                    1–23

*Introduction.*—Previous trials of lipid-lowering drugs suggest that middle-aged men with high cholesterol levels are at a lower risk of myocardial infarction, but there was no definite effect on the risk of death from coronary heart disease. A new type of lipid-lowering drug now is available, the 3-hydroxy-3-methylglutaryl-coenzyme A reductase inhibitors. They block cholesterol synthesis and lower levels of low-density-lipoprotein (LDL) cholesterol.

*Objective.*—A double-blind study of 1 of these agents, pravastatin, was carried out in 6,595 men, 45 to 64 years of age, whose initial plasma cholesterol averaged 272 mg/dL and was at least 252 mg/dL.

*Trial Design.*—Participants were randomly assigned to receive either 40 mg of pravastatin or a placebo each evening, and were followed up for nearly 5 years on average. The 2 groups were well balanced with respect

A

## Definite Nonfatal Myocardial Infarction

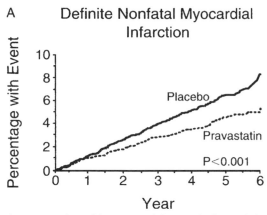

FIGURE 3.—Kaplan-Meier analysis of the time to a definite nonfatal mycardial infarction. (Reprinted by permission of *The New England Journal of Medicine*, Shepherd J, Cobbe SM, Ford I, et al: Prevention of coronary heart disease with pravastatin in men with hypercholesterolemia. *New Engl J Med* 333:1301–1307, 1995, Massachussetts Medical Society.)

to age and initial plasma total cholesterol, LDL cholesterol, and high-density-lipoprotein (HDL) cholesterol levels.

*Results.*—Pravastatin treatment lowered plasma cholesterol levels by 20% and LDL cholesterol levels by 26%. Triglycerides declined 12%, whereas levels of HDL cholesterol increased 5%. No comparable changes took place in placebo recipients. The combined risk of nonfatal myocardial infarction and coronary death declined 31% in the pravastatin-treated patients (Fig 3). The risk of death from all cardiovascular causes decreased 32%, and the overall risk of death decreased 22% in the treated patients. There were 116 incident cancers in the pravastatin group and 106 in the placebo group.

*Implication.*—It is estimated that, if 1,000 middle-aged men with hypercholesterolemia and no history of myocardial infarction were to receive pravastatin for 5 years, there would be 20 fewer nonfatal infarctions and 7 fewer cardiovascular deaths.

▶ This pristine, prospective, randomized trial sought to determine if reducing cholesterol in a large number of men 45–64 years of age, with moderate cholesterol elevation, followed up for almost 5 years, would reduce the combined incidence of nonfatal myocardial infarction and death from coronary disease. None of the study patients had any history of myocardial infarction. They were randomized to pravastatin or placebo. A relatively dramatic risk reduction of 31% occurred in the pravastatin treated patients, with a significant *P* value. Without question, the treatment of hypertension and hypercholesterolemia in selected patients results in a reduction in clinically significant morbid events. It is interesting, however, that the results are really rather modest despite their statistical significance. In fact, these authors estimate that treating 1,000 middle-aged men with hypercholesterolemia with this regimen for 5 years will result in 7 fewer deaths from cardiovascular causes. I wonder how the bean counters will assess such modest benefit at so great a cost?

## Effects of Lipid Lowering by Pravastatin on Progression and Regression of Coronary Artery Disease in Symptomatic Men With Normal to Moderately Elevated Serum Cholesterol Levels: The Regression Growth Evaluation Statin Study (REGRESS)

Jukema JW, on behalf of the REGRESS Study Group (Univ Hosp, Leiden, The Netherlands; Univ Hosp, Groningen, The Netherlands; St Antonius Hosp, Nieuwegein, The Netherlands; et al)
*Circulation* 91:2528–2540, 1995                                                          1–24

*Backgound.*—Previous studies have demonstrated the clinical value of lowering cholesterol, specifically low-density lipoprotein (LDL) in the treatment of coronary atherosclerosis, both in regard to prevention of disease progression and regression of disease already present. However, most of these studies were restricted to select groups of patients who had marked hypercholesterolemia, familial atherosclerosis, a previous history of coronary bypass surgery or angioplasty, or a history of previous myocardial infarction.

*Objective.*—The objective of this study, The Regression Growth Evaluation Statin Study (REGRESS) conducted by a group of 11 hospitals in The Netherlands, was to treat and assess the effects of a hypocholesterolemic agent in a broad range of coronary atherosclerotic patients with normal to moderately elevated serum cholesterol levels.

*Methods.*—The REGRESS was a multicenter, double-blind, palcebo-controlled study. The active agent used was pravastatin, a 3-hydroxy-3 methylglutaryl coenzyme A reductase inhibitor. The duration of the study was 2 years. All patients were men and selected on the basis of a review of their hospital records, indicating that they were candidates for coronary arteriography. Quantitative standards for arteriography findings were established as criteria for inclusion into the study. A serum cholesterol level between 155 and 310 mg/dL was an additional inclusion criterion. Primary end points were: (1) change in the average mean segment diameter (MSD) per patient as determined by coronary arteriography; and (2) change in average minimum obstructive diameter (MOD) per patient as determined by coronary arteriography. Clinical events were also analyzed. Patients were randomized to receive either pravastatin, 40 mg daily, or a placebo, and were seen regularly during the study period. Dietary, alcohol intake, and smoking status were monitored. Laboratory studies were done at baseline and repeated at 2, 4, 6, 12, and 24 months. Coronary arteriography was repeated at 24 months.

*Results.*—Of the 885 males entering the study, 778 (88%) had an evaluable final arteriogram. Table 4 and Figure 5 display data on the incidence of clinical events occurring in the 2 treatment groups over the 24-month treatment period. There were significantly fewer unscheduled

TABLE 4.—Clinical Events

| Clinical Event | Pravastatin | Placebo |
|---|---|---|
| Nonfatal myocardial infarction | 7 | 12 |
| Fatal myocardial infarction | 1 | 1 |
| Coronary heart disease death | 2 | 4 |
| Death due to known nonatherosclerotic cause | 2 | 2 |
| Nonscheduled PTCA | 20 | 47 |
| Nonscheduled CABG | 24 | 22 |
| Stroke and transient ischemic attack | 3 | 5 |
| Total | 59 | 93 |

PTCA indicates percutaneous transluminal coronary angioplasty; CABG, coronary artery bypass graft surgery. (Jukema JW, on behalf of the REGRESS Study Group: Effects of lipid lowering by pravastatin on progression and regression of coronary artery disease in symptomatic men with normal to moderately elevated serum cholesterol levels: The Regression Growth Evaluation Statin Study [REGRESS]. *Circulation* 1995; 91:2528–2540. Reproduced with permission *Circulation.* Copyright 1995 American Heart Association.)

percutaneous transluminal coronary angioplasties (PCTA) in the pravastatin group than in the placebo group and fewer overall clinical events in the pravastatin group compared to the placebo group (89% and 81%, respectively). Otherwise, there were no significant differences in clinical events between the 2 treatment groups. There were significantly greater decreases, both in MSD and MOD in the placebo group compared to the pravastatin group. The effect of pravastatin on MSD and MOD was directly proportional to baseline cholesterol levels, i.e., the higher the baseline cholesterol level, the greater the beneficial effect of pravastatin. No serious adverse effects to pravastatin were noted.

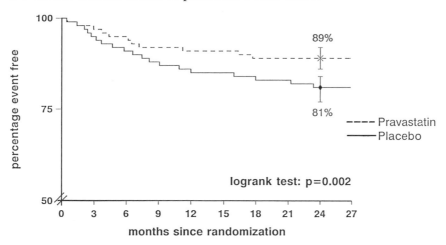

all events: myocardial infarction, death, CABG/PTCA, cerebral vascular accident

FIGURE 5.—Kaplan-Meier curves for time to first clinical event for the 2 treatment groups. All events: myocardial infarction, death, coronary artery bypass graft surgery/percutaneous transluminal coronary angioplasty, cerebral vascular accident. (Jukema JW, on behalf of the REGRESS Study Group: Effects of lipid lowering by pravastatin on progression and regression of coronary artery disease in symptomatic men with normal to moderately elevated serum cholesterol levels: The Regression Growth Evaluation Statin Study [REGRESS]. *Circulation* 1995; 91:2528–2540. Reproduced with permission *Circulation.* Copyright 1995 American Heart Association.)

*Conclusions.*—In symptomatic male patients with coronary atherosclerosis and normal to moderately elevated serum cholesterol levels, pravastatin therapy resulted in less progression and greater regression of coronary atherosclerotic lesions, as well as fewer clinical events than did placebo.

▶ Whereas Abstract 1–23 examined the effects of pravastatin on clinical events, this study focused on its effects in men using quantitative coronary arteriography. During 2 years, generally favorable results were noted in the pravastatin group in reference to quantitative changes in the coronary arteriogram. Although interesting in its own right, the real message is contained in the previous abstract, namely that pravastatin appears to prolong life, at least a little bit, in selected populations.

---

**Infiltrates of Activated Mast Cells at the Site of Coronary Atheromatous Erosion or Rupture in Myocardial Infarction**
Kovanen PT, Kaartinen M, Paavonen T (Univ of Helsinki)
*Circulation* 92:1084–1088, 1995                                  1–25

---

*Objective.*—To determine the role of mast cells in acute coronary syndromes by calculating the number of mast cells at eroded or ruptured sites of coronary atheromas.

*Background.*—Most acute coronary syndromes are preceded by erosion and rupture of coronary atheromas. Mast cells accumulate in the shoulder regions of atheromas, which is where erosion or rupture is most likely to occur. Mast cells are filled with neutral proteases that can trigger extracellular matrix degradation by activating matrix metalloproteinases.

*Methods.*—In 20 patients who died of acute myocardial infarction, specimens of coronary arteries were obtained. The site of atheromatous erosion or rupture was identified. Specimens were stained with monoclonal antibodies against tryptase and chymase, and against macrophages, T lymphocytes, and smooth muscle cells.

*Results.*—Mast cells made up 6% of all nucleated cells at the immediate site of erosion or rupture, 1% of all nucleated cells in the adjacent atheromatous area, and 0.1% of all nucleated cells in the unaffected intimal area. The amount of mast cells that had been stimulated to degranulate and release some of their tryptase and chymase was 86% at the site of erosion or rupture, 63% in the adjacent atheromatous area, and 27% in the unaffected intimal area. There was an increased number of macrophages and T lymphocytes at the site of erosion or rupture, but fewer smooth muscle cells.

*Conclusions.*—There were 200-fold more activated mast cells at the site of atheromatous erosion or rupture than in the unaffected coronary intima. This indicates that the role of mast cells in thrombotic coronary occlusion is significant.

▶ See also Abstracts 1–1 and 1–7. Herein, these authors expand upon their previously published observations that mast cells may have a significant role in the rupture of fibrous caps overlying coronary atheromata.[1] In the previous study they showed mast cells were there, whereas in this study they purport to show that the mast cells are activated and releasing their contained proteases. The authors suggest, and I suspect correctly, that mast cells are an integral component of the inflammatory infiltrate of ruptured coronary plaques. This suggests the obvious therapeutic strategy of inhibiting mast cell activity. Perhaps some day.

*Reference*

1. 1996 YEAR BOOK OF VASCULAR SURGERY, p 13.

## Coronary Plaque Erosion Without Rupture Into a Lipid Core: A Frequent Cause of Coronary Thrombosis in Sudden Coronary Death

Farb A, Burke AP, Tang AL, et al (Armed Forces Inst of Pathology, Washington, DC)
*Circulation* 93:1354–1363, 1996                                         1–26

*Introduction.*—Important mechanisms of thrombosis and in the clinical presentation of unstable angina, acute myocardial infarction, and sudden death are changes in coronary plaque luminal surface morphology consisting of plaque fissure or rupture. "Vulnerable" plaques have been the focus of much attention in determining the cause of coronary thrombosis, which occurs most frequently in lipid-rich plaques with rupture of a thin fibrous cap and contact of the thrombus with a pool of extracellular lipid. However, in sudden coronary death, the frequency of coronary artery thrombosis with or without fibrous cap rupture is not known. The incidence and morphologic characteristics of coronary thrombosis associated with plaque rupture were compared with those of thrombosis in eroded plaques without rupture.

*Methods.*—Histology and immunology were used to study 50 consecutive cases of sudden death due to coronary artery thrombosis.

*Results.*—In 28 patients, plaque rupture of a fibrous cap with communication of the thrombus with a lipid pool was identified. In 22 patients, thrombi without rupture were identified, all of which had superficial erosion of a proteoglycan-rich plaque. In plaque rupture patients, the mean age of death was $53 \pm 10$ years, whereas in patients with eroded plaques without rupture, the mean age was $44 \pm 7$ years. In the eroded plaque group, the number of women was 11 of 22 (50%) compared to 5 of 28 (18%) in the plaque rupture group. In the superficial erosion group, the mean percent luminal area stenosis was $70 \pm 11\%$ compared to $78 \pm 12\%$ in the plaque rupture group. In 23% of the erosions, plaque calcification was present, whereas it was found in 69% of the ruptures. Superficial erosions showed that the fibrous cap was infiltrated by macrophages in 50% of cases and by T cells in 32% of cases, whereas the plaque ruptures were infiltrated by macrophages in 100% of the cases and by T cells in 75% of the cases. In 33% of the ruptures, clusters of smooth muscle cells adjacent to the thrombi were present, compared to 95% of the erosions.

*Conclusion.*—A frequent finding in sudden death due to coronary thrombosis is erosion of proteoglycan-rich and smooth muscle cell-rich plaques lacking a superficial lipid core or plaque rupture, which was found in 44% of the patients studied. More often seen in younger individuals and women, these lesions have less luminal narrowing, calcification, foci of macrophages, and T cells than plaque ruptures. In the formation of coronary thrombi, rupture of a thin fibrous cap overlying a lipid core is not necessarily the only final common pathway.

▶ Although we have been inundated in recent years with the suggestion that rupture of the fibrous cap overlying atheromata is the most frequent cause of coronary thrombosis, we have to date no quantitative estimate of event frequency. In 50 cases of sudden cardiac death, these investigators found that 44% of the fatal thrombi occurred without detectable rupture of a fibrous cap. The patients without rupture were more likely to be younger and female and to have less luminal narrowing and less calcification than their counterparts. Nonetheless, these authors conclude that certain non-ruptured plaques are prone to thrombus, and these they characterize as "eroded." The authors conclude that overt rupture is not essential for thrombosis, but superficial erosion without rupture may be adequate to cause thrombosis and death. This is an interesting permutation and suggests, perhaps, that cap thinning without overt rupture may be all that is required. Cap rupture is becoming the hottest topic in vascular pathology.

---

**Effect of Intravenous Glucagon on Intestinal Viability After Segmental Mesenteric Ischemia**
Gangadharan SP, Wagner RJ, Cronenwett JL (Dartmouth-Hitchcock Med Ctr, Lebanon, NH)
*J Vasc Surg* 21:900–908, 1995                                                    1–27

---

*Objective.*—Vasoactive agents, such as intravenous glucagon, improve survival in rats with acute occlusive mesenteric ischemia. Whether the rat model is relevant to humans and whether the effect of glucagon is the result of direct cardiac inotropic support or selective mesenteric vasodilation are not known. The results of a rat study investigating the effect of intravenous glucagon on intestinal viability per se, after acute occlusive ischemia are presented.

*Methods.*—An 8-cm segment of the midileum in 18 anesthetized Sprague-Dawley rats was made ischemic by clamping both vascular arcades and both ends of the midileum for 105 to 120 minutes. Eight control animals received saline only for 2 hours after declamping, and 10 animals received intravenous glucagon for 2 hours after declamping. After 24

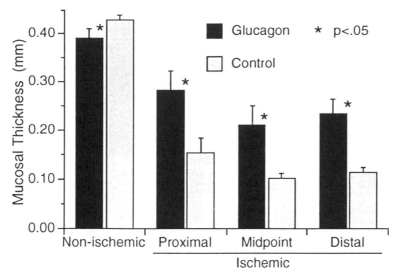

FIGURE 3.—Comparison of ileal mucosal thickness in control and glucagon-treated rats after segmental mesenteric ischemia (mean ± standard error of the mean). (Courtesy of Gangadharan SP, Wagner RJ, Cronenwett JL: Effect of intravenous glucagon on intestinal viability after segmental mesenteric ischemia. *J Vasc Surg* 21:900–908, 1995.)

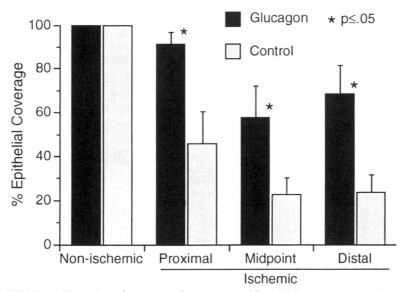

FIGURE 4.—Comparison of percentage of mucosa covered by epithelium in control and glucagon-treated rats after segmental mesenteric ischemia (mean ± standard error of the mean). (Courtesy of Gangadharan SP, Wagner RJ, Cronenwett JL: Effect of intravenous glucagon on intestinal viability after segmental mesenteric ischemia. *J Vasc Surg* 21:900–908, 1995.)

hours, ischemic and nonischemic ileum segments were examined by blinded investigators and compared.

*Results.*—Compared with nonischemic ileum, ischemic segments sustained severe mucosal injury with significant reduction of mucosal thickness as a result of sloughing of almost all the villi (Fig 3). At midpoint, mucosal thickness was significantly reduced by half, epithelial coverage from 100% to 23%, and villar surface from 3.0 to 1.1, compared with treated animals. In glucagon-treated animals, mucosal thickness and epithelial coverage was more than double that found in control animals (Fig 4). The villar surface ratio was also significantly increased in treated animals.

*Conclusion.*—Intravenous glucagon administered early after release of superior mesenteric artery occlusion significantly improves intestinal viability in the rat after segmental mesenteric ischemia.

▶ Clearly, when treating a rat for colonic segmental ischemia, one should consider glucagon.

---

**Extracoronary Atherosclerotic Plaque at Multiple Sites and Total Coronary Calcification Deposit in Asymptomatic Men: Association With Coronary Risk Profile**
Simon A, Giral P, Levenson J (Hôpital Broussais, Paris)
*Circulation* 92:1414–1421, 1995                                        1–28

---

*Objective.*—One hypothetical measure of cardiovascular risk in individuals with subclinical atherosclerosis is the extent of arterial plaque formation observed using high-resolution imaging techniques. The results of the clinical usefulness of extracoronary plaque evaluated with ultrasound imaging and of total coronary calcification deposit detected by ultrafast CT and their relation to risk of coronary events are reported.

*Methods.*—Risk factors, including age, serum cholesterol levels, existence of hypertension, smoking history, presence of left ventricular hypertrophy, and blood glucose levels were evaluated in 618 symptom-free, at-risk men, aged 30 to 70 years. Multifactorial risk factors at 10 years were calculated for each man. Vascular lesions were measured echographically at both coronary arteries, abdominal aorta, and both femoral arteries and numbered as none, 1, 2, or 3 sites. Coronary calcifications were detected tomographically in the left trunk main, left circumflex, left anterior descending coronary, and right coronary artery and graded as 0, 1, or 2 in severity.

*Results.*—In the study population, 246 men had 1 risk factor, 277 had 2, and 95 had 3. There were 170 men with no extracoronary disease sites, 205 with 1 disease site, 168 with 2, and 75 with 3. There were 228 men with no calcification, 144 with grade 1, 131 with grade 2, and 115 with grade 3 calcifications. The number of extracoronary disease sites was significantly associated with age, systolic blood pressure, smoking, and the number of risk factors. The number of calcifications was significantly

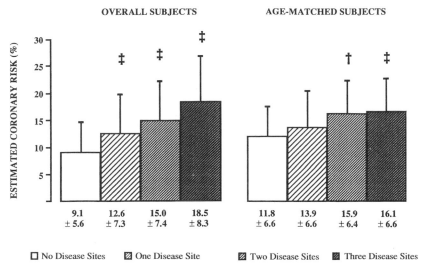

FIGURE 1.—Bar graphs of comparison of the estimated multifactorial risk of coronary events at 10 years according to the number of extraordinary disease sites in all subjects of the study (**left**) and in 4 age-matched (mean age, 50 ± 7 years) subgroups of 52 subjects with no, 1, 2, or 3 disease sites (**right**). Group comparisons are vs. the No Disease Site group: †$P$ < .01, ‡$P$ < .001. (Courtesy of Simon A, Giral P, Levenson J: Extracoronary atherosclerotic plaque at multiple sites and total coronary calcification deposit in asymptomatic men. *Circulation* 92:1414–1421, 1995.)

associated with age, systolic blood pressure, and the number of risk factors. Coronary risk was significantly related to the number of extracorporeal disease sites and the grade of coronary calcification (Fig 1). The odds ratio of coronary risk between 3 disease sites and no disease sites was 2.37; between men with grade 3 coronary calcification deposit and men with no calcification, it was 1.79.

*Conclusion.*—In asymptomatic, at-risk men, the risk of cardiovascular disease is more accurately assessed by B-mode ultrasound at multiple sites than by CT detection of coronary calcification deposits.

▶ This is an ambitiously designed study analyzing various risk factors in relation to B-mode detected plaques in asymptomatic men. The statistical analysis repeats well-known facts: age, systolic blood pressure, and smoking are risk factors for extracoronary arteriosclerotic disease, and with increased extracoronary arteriosclerosis, the risk for coronary disease increases. Not very surprising!

**D. Bergqvist, M.D., Ph.D.**

▶ I agree with Dr. Bergqvist. I find it interesting that the ultrasound detection of extracoronary atherosclerosis was more accurate than total coronary calcium determined by ultrafast CT in reflecting the multifactorial coronary risk profile. However, ultrafast coronary artery calcium CT detection still appears useful as a population screening device.[1]

**J.M. Porter, M.D.**

*Reference*

1. 1995 YEAR BOOK OF VASCULAR SURGERY, p 124.

### Effects of Lowering Elevated LDL Cholesterol on the Cardiovascular Risk of Lipoprotein(a)

Maher VMG, Brown BG, Marcovina SM, et al (Univ of Washington, Seattle)
*JAMA* 274:1771–1774, 1995                                                1–29

*Background.*—There is disagreement as to the contribution of elevated lipoprotein(a) (Lp[a]) levels to coronary artery disease (CAD). Research suggests that reducing low-density-lipoprotein cholesterol (LDL-C) levels could weaken the pathogenicity of elevated LDL-C and Lp(a) levels. This question was addressed as part of a randomized, double-blind, placebo-controlled trial of lipid-reducing therapy for CAD.

*Methods.*—The post hoc analysis included 146 men from the Familial Atherosclerosis Treatment Study. All had CAD, were 62 years old or younger, and had Lp(a) levels of 125 mg/dL or greater. The patients were randomized to receive 1 of 3 treatments: a Step II Diet plus lovastatin, 40 mg/day, and colestipol, 30 g/day; niacin, 4 g/day, plus colestipol; or placebo, plus colestipol for men whose LDL-C level was at the 90th percentile or higher. Treatment continued for 2.5 years. The LDL-C response was characterized as minimal for 36 men with a decrease of 10% or less from baseline and substantial for 84 men with a decrease of more than 10%. The effects of LDL-C reduction on cardiac event rate and on the CAD change associated with elevated Lp(a) were assessed.

*Results.*—Multivariate analyses suggested that Lp(a) was the factor most closely related to baseline CAD severity, r = 0.30. The only factor related to CAD progression for the men with minimal LDL-C reduction was in-treatment Lp(a) levels (r = 0.45). For the patients with substantial LDL-C reduction, disease regression was related to in-treatment LDL-C but not to Lp(a), (r = 0.24 and r = −0.05, respectively). Patients with and without a significant reduction in LDL-C had no significant change in Lp(a) levels. Among the patients with Lp(a) at the 90th percentile or higher, the cardiac event rate was 39% for those who had a minimal reduction in LDL-C vs. 9% in those with a substantial reduction (relative risk 0.23).

*Conclusions.*—The Lp(a) level is a major indicator of baseline disease severity, disease progression, and cardiac event rate in men with CAD and elevated LDL-C levels. If a significant reduction in LDL-C can be achieved, a persistently elevated Lp(a) level is not associated with cardiac events or CAD progression. Men with CAD who have elevated Lp(a) and LDL-C may need particularly close clinical attention.

▶ The message of this article is potentially important. Lipoprotein(a) may only be an important risk factor in patients who also have significant elevation of LDL-C. In patients with low or substantial reductions of LDL-C, persistent elevations of Lp(a) no longer appear atherogenic or clinically threatening. This suggests that Lp(a) treatment should not be considered in a vacuum but in association with other lipid components, especially LDL-C. See also Abstract 1–5.

---

**Endothelial Release of Nitric Oxide Contributes to the Vasodilator Effect of Adenosine in Humans**
Smits P, Williams SB, Lipson DE, et al (Harvard Med School, Boston; Univ Hosp Nijmegen, The Netherlands)
*Circulation* 92:2135–2141, 1995                                                    1–30

---

*Background.*—Adenosine, an endogenous nucleoside, is important in the regulation of vascular tone, particularly during ischemia. Animal research suggests that nitric oxide (NO) contributes to adenosine's vasodilator effect. The current study determined whether the endothelial release of NO contributes to adenosine-induced vasodilation in humans.

*Methods and Findings.*—Thirty-nine healthy volunteers were included. Forearm blood flow (FBF) responses to graded intra-arterial adenosine infusions were assessed by venous occlusion plethysmography. Dose-response curves were created before and during intra-arterial infusion of vehicle or $N^G$-monomethyl-L-arginine (L-NMMA), an NO synthase inhibitor. Before L-NMMA infusion, adenosine induced a dose-dependent FBF increase, from 2.3 to 15.9 mL·min$^{-1}$·dL$^{-1}$. When L-NMMA was infused concurrently, adenosine raised FBF from 1.7 to 10 mL·min$^{-1}$·dL$^{-1}$. This change was significantly decreased compared with that before L-NMMA. The FBF response to adenosine was attenuated by L-NMMA when the NO donor sodium nitroprusside was coinfused to prevent the basal constrictor effect of L-NMMA. By contrast, the FBF response to intra-arterial infusion of the endothelium-independent vasodilator, verapamil, was unaffected by L-NMMA. To determine whether the adenosine-induced release of NO is mediated by the activation of endothelial potassium channels, putatively coupled to adenosine receptors, the FBF response to adenosine was determined before and during infusion of tolbutamide, an adenosine triphosphate (ATP)-dependent potassium channel blocker, or quinidine, a potassium channel blocker. Neither potassium channel blocker attenuated the adenosine-mediated increments in FBF.

*Conclusions.*—Endothelial release of NO at least partly mediates adenosine-induced vasodilation in humans. Although the transducing mechanism is unknown, it does not seem to involve activation of ATP-dependent or quinidine-sensitive potassium channels.

► The endogenous nucleoside, adenosine, appears an important cardiovascular regulatory substance, adapting blood flow to match alterations in tissue oxygen supply or demand. Whereas it was previously thought that adenosine directly influenced second messenger cyclic adenosine monophosphate by an endothelium-independent mechanism, the current study suggests that a significant part of, or perhaps all, adenosine-induced vasodilation in humans is mediated by endothelial release of NO, a mechanism of potentially profound importance in vascular homeostasis in humans.

---

**Effect of Thromboxane A₂ Blockade on Clinical Outcome and Restenosis After Successful Coronary Angioplasty: Multi-Hospital Eastern Atlantic Restenosis Trial (M-HEART II)**
Savage MP, Goldberg S, Bove AA, et al (Thomas Jefferson Univ, Philadelphia)
*Circulation* 92:3194–3200, 1995                                                    1–31

---

*Objective.*—Restenosis, as a result of mechanical injury, is not an uncommon complication after percutaneous transluminal coronary angioplasty (PTCA). Platelet-thromboxane $A_2$ is thought to play a role in this process. Because aspirin reduces the incidence of some coronary events, its long-term effect on restenosis prevention was investigated and compared with that of sulotroban, a selective antagonist of the thromboxane $A_2$ receptor.

*Methods.*—The 752 patients in the double-blind, placebo-controlled Multi-Hospital Eastern Atlantic Restenosis Trial ((M-HEART II) study were randomly assigned to receive either 325 mg/d aspirin ($n = 248$), 800 mg QID sulotroban, or placebo at least 6 hours before PTCA and continuing for 6 months. Angiography was performed before and 6 months after PTCA. Percutaneous transluminal coronary angioplasty was considered successful if stenosis was improved by at least 10%. Patients were examined at 2, 6, 12, 18, and 26 weeks. Clinical failure at 6 months was defined as death, myocardial infarction, or restenosis.

*Results.*—After the procedure, 57 patients were discontinued from the study as a result of side effects and 74 because of protocol violations. There were 112 patients excluded from the study as a result of unsuccessful PTCA. Success rates were similar among treatment groups. Clinical failure was recorded for 30% of the aspirin group, 44% of the sulotroban group, and 41% of the placebo group. The differences were significant among treatment groups. Aspirin, but not sulotroban, was significantly associated with a reduced failure rate compared with placebo. There was no difference among treatment groups with respect to restenosis. Antithromboxane therapy significantly reduced the incidence of myocardial infarction, which was 1.2% in the aspirin group, 1.8% in the sulotroban group, and 5.7% in the placebo group.

*Conclusion.*—At least 6 months of thromboxane $A_2$ blockage significantly reduces late coronary events, although it does not appear to affect the restenosis rate significantly. The overall clinical outcome was superior for aspirin as compared with sulotroban.

▶ Aspirin selectively inhibits thromboxane A₂ synthesis, whereas sulotroban selectively blocks the thromboxane A₂ receptor. Does that make
these substances substantially interchangeable, or even suggest that sulotroban is superior? These investigators conclude that after coronary angioplasty, aspirin is superior to sulotroban, and significantly so. The mysteries
of aspirin continue.

---

**Dietary Intake of Marine n-3 Fatty Acids, Fish Intake, and the Risk of
Coronary Disease Among Men**
Ascherio A, Rimm EB, Stampfer MJ, et al (Harvard Med School, Boston)
*N Engl J Med* 332:977–982, 1995                                    1–32

---

*Background.*—The low rates of coronary heart disease in areas where
fish is a fundamental part of the diet suggest that consumption of fish may
have a protective effect against such disease. The ability of n-3 polyunsaturated fatty acids to decrease plasma levels of very-low-density lipoprotein
cholesterol, increase vasodilation, and reduce platelet aggregation may be
a possible explanation for this protective effect, given that n-3 fatty acids
are abundant in fish. Few epidemiologic studies, however, have examined
this hypothesis. Associations between dietary intake of marine n-3 fatty
acids, fish intake, and the risk of coronary disease among men were
therefore prospectively investigated.

*Participants and Methods.*—In 1986, 44,895 male health professionals
completed detailed and validated dietary questionnaires as part of the
Health Professional Follow-up Study. All participants were free of known
cardiovascular disease. During a 6-year follow-up period, 1,543 coronary
events were recorded in this group. Of these, 264 deaths were associated
with coronary disease, 547 with nonfatal myocardial infarctions, and 732
with coronary artery bypass or angioplasty procedures.

*Results.*—No significant associations between dietary intake of n-3 fatty
acids or fish intake and risk of coronary disease were noted after adjusting
for age and several coronary risk factors. When examining the group in
terms of intake of n-3 fatty acids, the multivariate relative risk of coronary
heart disease was 1.12 for men in the top fifth of the group (median daily
intake, 0.58 g), compared with those in the bottom fifth (median daily
intake, 0.07 g). The multivariate relative risk of coronary disease was 1.14
for men who consumed 6 or more servings of fish per week, compared
with those who consumed 1 serving or less per month. The risk of death
caused by coronary heart disease among men who ate any amount of fish
vs. those who consumed no fish was 0.74. The risk did not decrease as fish
consumption increased.

*Conclusions.*—Among men without pre-existing cardiovascular disease,
an increase in fish intake from 1 to 2 servings per week to 5 or 6 servings
per week does not substantially decrease the risk of coronary heart disease.
The effects of fish or fish oil at lower or higher levels of intake or among

individuals with dietary habits or other risk factors that are considerably different from those in this cohort cannot, however, be entirely excluded.

▶ Another study fails to demonstrate any clinical benefit from eating fish. In this case, increased fish consumption did not significantly reduce the risk of coronary heart disease in the patient cohort under study. This is similar to the material presented in Abstract 1–4. This information, combined with the previously reported lack of benefit of the omega-3 fatty acids in reducing restenosis after coronary angioplasty leads to but 1 conclusion—omega-3 fatty acids have yet to be associated with any proven clinical benefit. [1,2] I suspect the omega-3 craze will slowly fade away.

*References*

1. 1995 YEAR BOOK OF VASCULAR SURGERY, p 4.
2. 1996 YEAR BOOK OF VASCULAR SURGERY, p 11.

**Development and Characterization of a Rapid Assay for Bedside Determinations of Cardiac Troponin T**
Müller-Bardorff M, Freitag H, Scheffold T, et al (Medizinische Universitätsklinik, Heidelberg, Germany)
*Circulation* 92:2869–2875, 1995                                          1–33

*Objective.*—In 20% to 40% of patients, a diagnosis of acute myocardial cell necrosis depends on the appearance of cardiac enzymes. Because measurement of these cardiac markers is a time-consuming process, a whole-blood rapid assay for cardiac troponin T (cTnT) that yields reliable and accurate test results within 20 minutes was developed.

*Methods.*—Cardiac troponin T and skeletal muscle TnT were isolated from human myocardium or skeletal muscle less than 10 hours after death. Cardiospecific antihuman cTnT antibody M7 was labeled with gold, and high-affinity monoclonal antibody 1B10 was conjugated with biotin. The complexed antibodies and buffers were adsorbed onto a paper fleece. Heparinized blood is placed in a well below the fleece, dissolving buffers and antibodies that reacted with TnT in the blood. Blood cells were separated from plasma using a glass-fiber fleece. The resulting immunocomplexes were trapped by binding of biotin-labeled antibodies to immobilized streptavidine. Sensitivity was determined using blood from 5 patients with acute myocardial infarction (AMI), and specificity was tested using purified TnT. The assay was valid within the range of 0.1 to 0.18 µg/L. Precision was determined by quintuplicate measurements at different cTnT concentrations and times.

*Results.*—None of the 25 healthy volunteers had positive results. There were no false positive results in 62 patients without clinical evidence of AMI except for 2 patients with elevated creatine kinase levels of 6,500 and 10,000. The assay was positive for 32 of 35 patients with myocardial cell damage, including 24 patients with radiofrequency-induced myocardial cell damage, and in 7 of 35 patients with unstable angina.

*Conclusion.*—The new rapid assay for cTnT is a sensitive and specific method for detecting minor myocardial cell damage after acute myocardial infarction.

▶ As noted previously, the diagnosis of AMI is not always easy.[1] In recent years it has become clear that the determination of serum troponin has a considerable advantage in the diagnosis of AMI. Until now, laboratory analyis of this substance has taken a long time. This important article reports the results of a rapid assay that yielded reliable and accurate results of serum troponin within 20 minutes. I suspect this will become the diagnostic method of choice for MI.

*Reference*

1. 1995 YEAR BOOK OF VASCULAR SURGERY, p 56.

## Limb Ischemia

**Thromboxane and Neutrophil Changes Following Intermittent Claudication Suggest Ischaemia-Reperfusion Injury**
Khaira HS, Nash GB, Bahra PS, et al (Queen Elizabeth Hosp, Birmingham, England; Univ of Birmingham, England; Selly Oak Hosp, Birmingham, England)
*Eur J Vasc Endovasc Surg* 10:31–35, 1995                                    1–34

*Background.*—Intermittent claudication (IC) is associated with a high cardiovascular mortality rate. Patients with IC may have a series of ischemia-reperfusion injuries that activate neutrophils and release mediators (e.g., thromboxane), which in turn cause systemic increases in vascular permeability and enhanced atherogenesis. The effects of exercise on patients with IC were investigated by assessing neutrophil activation, thromboxane levels, and microalbuminuria (a marker of generalized endothelial permeability).

*Methods.*—Thirty men (median age, 63 years) with IC were recruited from vascular outpatient clinics. Ten control subjects (median age, 64 years) were recruited from a male choir. Studies were done at baseline and repeated for up to 1 hour after maximum tolerated exercise on a treadmill.

*Results.*—After exercise, the patients with IC had a significant increase in their transit time for neutrophils (reflects decreased deformability) in systemic blood, especially in the population of slower flowing cells (90th percentile). Neutrophil transit times did not change after exercise in the control subjects. After exercise, the patients with IC also had a significant increase in their urine albumin/creatinine ratio; the control patients had no change. After exercise in both groups, the plasma concentrations of thromboxane were elevated at 10, 20, and 60 minutes. However, the concentrations were much higher in the patients with IC (Fig 1). Sixty minutes after

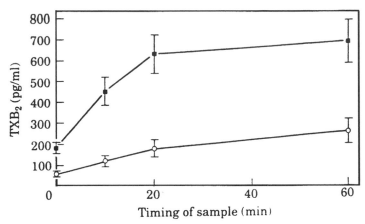

**FIGURE 1.**—Systemic plasma thromboxane levels (mean ± standard error of the mean) at pre-exercise (time point 0) and at 10, 20, and 60 minutes postexercise in patients with intermittent claudication (*solid square n* = 30) and controls (*open circle n* = 10). (Reprinted from the *European Journal of Vascular and Endovascular Surgery* 10, Khaira HS, Nash GB, Bahra PS, et al: Thromboxane and neutrophil changes following intermittent claudication suggest ischaemia-reperfusion injury, pp 31–35, 1995 by permission of the publisher, Academic Press Limited London.)

the patients with IC exercised, their plasma thromboxane concentrations and the percentage change in their median neutrophil transit times were positively correlated.

*Conclusions.*—Patients with intermittent claudication appear to have repeated bouts of ischemia and reperfusion, which is associated with neutrophil activation, thromboxane production, and systemic vascular permeability (due to endothelial injury or dysfunction). These changes may contribute to the increased cardiovascular mortality seen in such patients.

▶ I am impressed by the authors' suggestion that intermittent claudication may be regarded as a series of small ischemia-reperfusion events. They find evidence that episodes of claudication result in a predictable series of reperfusion biochemical changes, including vascular hyperpermeability, plasma thromboxane elevation, and increase in neutrophil transit time. They suggest, without convincing evidence, that such biochemical changes induced by claudication may have a role in patient mortality. I wonder.

---

**L-Arginine Induces Nitric Oxide-Dependent Vasodilation in Patients With Critical Limb Ischemia: A Randomized, Controlled Study**
Bode-Böger SM, Böger RH, Alfke H, et al (Inst of Clinical Pharmacology, Hannover, Germany)
*Circulation* 93:85–90, 1996                                                    1–35

---

*Background.*—Nitric oxide (NO), a potent vasodilator derived from L-arginine, acts intracellularly via a second messenger, cyclic quanosine monophosphate (cGMP). Prostaglandin (PG) $E_1$ also induces peripheral vasodilation, stimulating prostacyclin receptors. The ability of the 2 agents to cause vasodilation in critically ischemic limbs was compared.

*Methods.*—L-Arginine or $PGE_1$ was given intravenously to 10 men with critical ischemia of a limb. Production of NO was established by measurement of urinary $NO_3$ −, its excreted metabolite, and of urinary cGMP. Image-directed duplex ultrasonography was used to measure femoral blood flow velocity. Six men with ischemic limbs received intravenous saline, 0.9%, to serve as a control group.

*Results.*—There was a significant increase in femoral arterial flow during infusion of L-arginine and $PGE_1$. This was due to increased blood flow velocity, inasmuch as the femoral artery diameter did not increase. Placebo caused no increase. Urinary markers of NO activity, $NO_3^-$ and cGMP, both increased significantly during infusion of L-arginine but not $PGE_1$. Placebo caused no change.

*Conclusion.*—Intravenous administration of L-arginine causes peripheral vasodilation in ischemic limbs, apparently through the action of NO and cGMP.

▶ The primary message I take from this article is that even in critically ischemic limbs, further vasodilatation is possible. The old adage that many of us grew up with, namely that severe ischemia induces maximal regional vasodilation, clearly requires re-examination. This and many other studies prove that even maximally ischemic tissue still has the capacity for additional vasodilatation. The question is whether this can be turned to any therapeutic advantage. I am unconvinced.

## Effect of Pentoxifylline on Tissue Injury and Platelet-Activating Factor Production During Ischemia-Reperfusion Injury

Adams JG Jr, Dhar A, Skukla SD, et al (Univ of Missouri, Columbia)
*J Vasc Surg* 21:742–749, 1995                                                    1–36

*Objective.*—The mechanism of ischemia-reperfusion injury (IRI) is unknown, although interaction of the leukocyte with the microvascular endothelium or the lumen of the capillaries may play a role. Because platelet activating factor (PAF) is a mediator of leukocyte-endothelial cell interaction in IRI, the effect on tissue injury and PAF production of pentoxifylline, a platelet aggregation inhibitor, was tested in a skeletal muscle model of IRI.

*Methods.*—Isolated gracilis muscles in 22 female mongrel dogs were subjected to 5 hours of ischemia and 20 hours of reperfusion. Six dogs (group 2) received a 15 mg/kg- and 6 dogs (group 3) received a 25 mg/kg-systemic bolus infusion 10 minutes before reperfusion. Heart rate and arterial blood pressure were monitored. Muscle necrosis was calculated, and levels of PAF were determined by scintillation proximity assay.

# PAF LEVELS

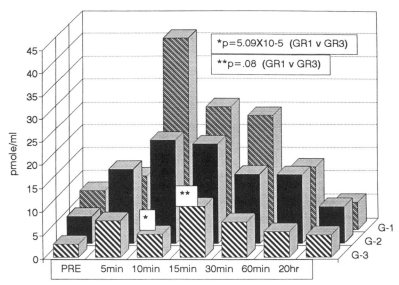

*p=5.09X10-5 (GR1 v GR3)

**p=.08 (GR1 v GR3)

FIGURE 3.—Platelet activating factor levels in group 2 muscles were decreased at 10, 15, and 30 minutes of reperfusion; platelet activating factor levels in group 3 muscles were decreased at all time intervals during the first hour of reperfusion. (Courtesy of Adams JG, Dhar A, Shukla SD, et al: Effect of pentoxifylline on tissue injury and platelet-activating factor production during ischemia-reperfusion injury. *J Vasc Surg* 21:742–749, 1995.)

*Results.*—There was a significant increase in heart rate in groups 2 and 3. The PAF levels decreased nonsignificantly at 10, 15, and 30 minutes in group 2 and significantly at 10 minutes only in group 3, compared with group 1 (Fig 3). There were no significant differences in muscle weights among groups. No significant differences in amount of necrosis were observed between groups 1 and 2. There was significantly less muscle necrosis in group 3, than in group 2.

*Conclusion.*—Pentoxifylline (25 mg/kg) administered before reperfusion of ischemic skeletal muscle significantly decreased the amount of muscle necrosis and 10-minute PAF levels, possibly decreasing tissue injury.

▶ Pentoxifylline, a methylxanthine derivative, has abundant pharmacologic actions in humans. It is well known to have a small effect on claudication, but its actions in other areas may ultimately prove more interesting. Herein is presented evidence that pentoxifylline administered after muscle ischemia, but before reperfusion, has favorable effects as measured by alterations in coagulation factors and a decrease in the amount of muscle necrosis. This interesting drug is also finding uses in shock treatment and transplantation. We have not yet heard the last of this.

## Antioxidant Consumption During Exercise in Intermittent Claudication

Khaira HS, Maxwell SRJ, Shearman CP (Queen Elizabeth Hosp, Birmingham, England)
*Br J Surg* 82:1660–1662, 1995                                               1–37

*Background.*—It has been proposed that patients with intermittent claudication have bouts of ischemia and reperfusion every time they walk. The first step in this ischemia-reperfusion cascade is the formation of oxygen-derived free radicals (ODFR). These are difficult to detect directly, but consumption of antioxidants can be used to monitor their presence. An enhanced chemiluminescent assay for total antioxidant activity in body fluids was used to test the hypothesis of recurrent ischemia-reperfusion with walking in claudicant patients.

*Methods.*—Twenty normotensive non-diabetic claudicants and 9 age- and sex-matched controls were included in this study. After a 90-minute rest period, the subjects gave a urine sample and a blood sample, and blood pressure was recorded. The subjects then exercised to maximum capacity on a treadmill. Blood pressure was then monitored and blood samples taken at 1, 10, and 60 minutes after exercise. Urine was also collected after 60 minutes.

*Results.*— After exercise, microalbuminuria increased in the patient group but not in the control group. Although antioxidant levels were similar in controls and patients at rest, after exercise there was a significant decrease in antioxidants in the patients, which returned to normal within 10 minutes. Controls had a slight increase in antioxidants after exercise. The patients with the largest decreases in antioxidant concentrations also had the highest increases in microalbuminuria.

*Conclusions.*—Patients with intermittent claudication had an increase in microalbuminuria and a decrease in antioxidants after exercise when compared with controls. These results suggest that recurrent ischemia-reperfusion occurs with walking in patients with intermittent claudication, causing systemic damage to endothelium, as detected by microalbuminuria. The potentially injurious effect of exercise is counteracted by an increase in antioxidants in normal individuals, but claudicants have a decrease in antioxidant levels after exercise. This implies that conservative management may be insufficient for some of these patients. The benefits of antioxidant therapy need to be investigated in this patient group.

▶ Continuing the observations reported in Abstract 1–34, Dr. Khaira and associates restate their theory that episodes of claudication are similar to ischemia-reperfusion. They again document microalbuminuria as reported before but now show that there is a decrease in total antioxidant concentration in claudicants immediately after a claudication episode. So what?

## Assessment of Skeletal Muscle Viability by PET

Smith GT, Wilson TS, Hunter K, et al (Univ of Tennessee, Knoxville)
*J Nucl Med* 36:1408–1414, 1995                                    1–38

*Background.*—Positron-emission tomography has been shown to have clinical utility in evaluating tissue viability when used with radiolabeled glucose, which demonstrates the metabolic status of the tissue of interest. Therefore, the utility of PET scans using [18F]fluoro-2-deoxyglucose (FDG) in the assessment of skeletal muscle viability in patients with complications of peripheral vascular disease and in patients with skeletal muscle transfer grafts was examined.

*Methods.*—Thirty patients hospitalized with complications of peripheral vascular disease or after skeletal muscle transfer flap surgery underwent FDG-PET evaluation of skeletal muscle viability. The FDG uptake was compared between the affected muscle region and the same muscle in the contralateral limb. The PET findings were correlated with long-term muscle viability in the patients who had skeletal muscle transfer and with wound healing and limb survival in patients who had skeletal muscle transfer.

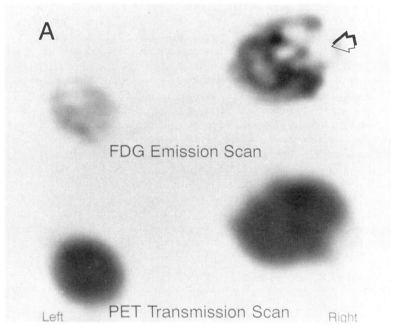

FIGURE 4.—**A,** positron-emission tomography emission and transmission scans from patient 1 show decreased tracer uptake in the lateral compartment of the right lower leg (*arrow*). The uptake ratio of 0.46 was consistent with nonviable tissue. (Reprinted by permission of the Society of Nuclear Medicine from: Smith GT, Wilson TS, Hunter K, et al: Assessment of skeletal muscle viability by PET. *J Nucl Med* 1995, 36:1408–1414.)

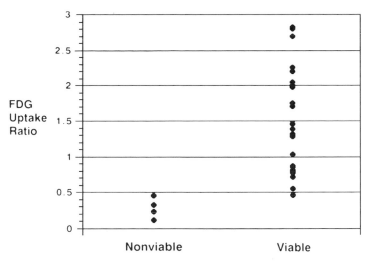

**N** = 31

**FIGURE 5.**—The FDG uptake ratios for peripheral vascular disease and skeletal muscle transfer nonviable (*n* = 6) and viable muscle (*n* = 26) groups as defined by the clinical outcome. All muscles with uptake ratios above 3.0 were viable and are not shown in the graph. The nonviability threshold is 0.46. Patients with ratios below this value ultimately required debridement or amputation; patients with ratios above this value had viable muscles with tissue. One patient with peripheral vascular disease and an FDG uptake ratio of 1.72, who is included in the viable group, had ulcers that healed during the initial hospitalization but underwent distal extremity amputation for recurrent ulcers 3 months later. One patient with viable muscle and an FDG uptake ratio of 0.47 required extensive medical therapy for salvage. *Abbreviation*: FDG, [18][F]fluoro-2-deoxyglucose. (Reprinted by permission, Smith GT, Wilson TS, Hunter K, et al: Assessment of skeletal muscle viability by PET. *J Nucl Med* 36:1408–1414, 1995.)

*Results.*—The patients with peripheral vascular disease had FDG uptake ratios between 0.12 and 1.72. The 6 patients with tissue subsequently found to be nonviable had FDG uptake ratios of 0.46 or lower (Fig 4, A), whereas the 10 patients with viable tissue had FDG uptake ratios of 0.47 or higher (Fig 5). Among the 14 patients with skeletal muscle transfer, the FDG uptake ratios were between 0.12 and 7.88 and demonstrated higher values in the early postoperative period. The viable muscle flaps had FDG uptake ratios of 0.73 or higher.

*Conclusions.*—Positron-emission tomography scanning using FDG is a highly accurate technique for evaluating the viability of the muscle and may be useful in determining long-term prognosis of the muscle tissue in patients undergoing free-flap muscle transfer or with complications of peripheral vascular disease.

▶ The authors have identified the need for a more accurate method of assessing the viability of skeletal muscle after electrical or burn injury, or other trauma in which the skin may be more viable than the deeper tissues. This may also apply to free-muscle transfer in which early swelling precludes accurate assessment of viability, and occasionally after vascular bypass, although in these cases, skin necrosis usually precedes muscle death. The application of PET scanning is logical for the detection of skeletal muscle viability, because glucose uptake can be used as a marker of functioning tissue. Not surprisingly, the authors found that glucose uptake in dead muscle was lower than in viable muscle. Is this helpful? To be worth the 2-hour, $1,500 investment that is required for this study (assuming you have already purchased the PET scanner!), this test would need to detect ischemic muscle prior to death so that timely corrective intervention could be carried out. In the final analysis, application of this technique to humans, even in the experimental setting, seems premature. An animal study in which different degrees of ischemic muscle injury could be carefully quantitated with established techniques (including histology), and compared with glucose uptake by PET scanning, would be far more informative than this eclectic analysis of dead vs. living muscle in a small group of patients. It seems unlikely that this cumbersome and expensive technique will ever be more than a research tool to investigate skeletal muscle metabolism and ischemia.

**J. Cronenwett, M.D.**

## Intimal Hyperplasia

**University of Wisconsin Solution Effects on Intimal Proliferation in Canine Autogenous Vein Grafts**
Cavallari N, Abebe W, Hunter WJ III, et al (Creighton Univ, Omaha, Neb; La Sapienza Univ, Rome)
*J Surg Res* 59:433–440, 1995                                           1–39

*Background.*—Although recent years have seen many improvements in autologous vein harvesting and implantation designed to reduce endothelial injury, no new preservation media have been introduced. The University of Wisconsin solution (UWs) is widely used to preserve organs for transplantation. The UWs solution was evaluated for use in long-term preservation of autogenous vein grafts (AVG).

*Methods.*—A "no-touch" technique was used to obtain autogenous jugular and femoral vein specimens from dogs. One segment was immediately reimplanted, and 3 others were stored for 24 hours at 4°C in 1 of 3 solutions: UWs, normal saline (NS), or autologous whole blood (AWB). The preserved grafts were then placed as reversed interposition grafts in the common carotid or femoral artery positions, as the control grafts were earlier. Light and scanning electron microscopic studies were performed at 6 weeks' follow-up, along with other tests.

*Results.*—Intimal thickening in the grafts stored in UWs was similar to that noted in control grafts, whereas grafts stored in NS and AWB had significantly increased intimal thickening (Fig 3). In all 4 groups, scanning electron microscopy revealed an intact endothelial cell monolayer that stained positively for factor VIII. On isometric tension studies, maximum contraction and sensitivity to norepinephrine was significantly lower than control levels for grafts stored in AWB, but not for those stored in UWs or NS. There were no significant differences in maximum relaxation produced by acetylcholine, although vessels preserved in AWB were more

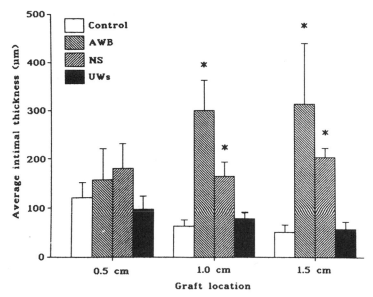

FIGURE 3.—Bar graphs of initial thickness according to graft location in specimens from control grafts and vein grafts stored in AWB, NS, and UWs. Autogenous vein grafts stored in AWB and NS exhibit marked intimal proliferation at 1.0 and 1.5 cm from the proximal anastomosis. Data are expressed as mean ± standard error of the mean from 11 observations (* *RP*< 0.05 vs control and UWs). *Abbreviations: AWB,* autologous whole blood; *NS,* normal saline; *UWs,* University of Wisconsin solution. (Courtesy of Cavallari N, Abebe W, Hunter WJ III, et al: University of Wisconsin solution effects on intimal proliferation in canine autogenous vein grafts. *J Surg Res* 59:433–440, 1995.)

sensitive than those preserved in UWs. All 4 groups had similar responses to sodium nitroprusside.

*Conclusions.*—University of Wisconsin solution appears to be superior to AWB and NS for storage of autogenous vein grafts. Graft morphology and the functional integrity of the smooth muscle and endothelium are better preserved with UWs.

▶ I am not quite sure what to make of this study. Dog veins stored in UWs for 24 hours at 4°C and reimplanted into dogs showed less intimal hyperplasia than veins stored in either NS or AWB for the same time but no less than control veins reimplanted immediately after harvest. Although interesting, I cannot conceive of a situation in which a vascular surgeon would store an autogenous vein for 24 hours before reimplantation. Perhaps these data will have some relevance in certain transplant applications.

## Inhibition of Intimal Hyperplasia in Balloon Injured Arteries With Adjunctive Phthalocyanine Sensitised Photodynamic Therapy

Nyamekye I, Buonaccorsi G, McEwan J, et al (Univ College London; Hatter Inst for Cardiovascular Studies, London; Middlesex Hosp, London)
*Eur J Vasc Endovasc Surg* 11:19–28, 1996                          1–40

*Introduction.*—Percutaneous transluminal angioplasty (PTA) offers promise as a safer and less costly means of treating selected patients with arterial disease, but early follow-up studies report a high rate of recurrence or restenosis. An important component of the process of restenosis is the formation of fibrocellular intimal hyperplasia (FCIH). No drugs have been able to prevent or reduce the FCIH response to angioplasty. An animal study investigated the effects of photodynamic therapy (PDT) on FCIH.

*Methods.*—All experiments used adult male Wistar rats. The photosensitizer used in PDT was aluminum disulphonated phthalocyanine ($AlS_2Pc$), an agent with good fluorescence properties. Four groups of rats were sensitized with $AlS_2Pc$ at different doses: 0.5, 1.0, 2.5, and 5 mg/kg, then killed at intervals ranging from 5 minutes to 24 hours after sensitization, and the arteries were prepared for analysis of the distribution of $AlS_2Pc$ in the normal carotid artery. Sensitized rats that underwent carotid artery laser irradiation were assessed after 3 and 14 days and 1–6 months in an examination of PDT of normal arteries. In the final investigation, rats underwent standard carotid artery balloon injury immediately before PDT. Arteries were evaluated at 2 to 26 weeks, together with laser, $AlS_2Pc$, and untreated controls.

*Results.*—The intensity of $AlS_2Pc$ fluorescence increased with increasing dosage. Maximal fluorescence was noted in the arterial media at 30 minutes. Medial cell depletion persisting for 6 months was produced by PDT at 3 days. At 2 and 4 weeks, PDT completely inhibited FCIH. This effect was partial at 2 to 26 weeks, reaching 51% of the level in untreated arteries. At all times in the study, inhibition of FCIH was significantly greater in the PDT group than in any of the control groups. None of the treated arteries showed thrombosis or aneurysm formation.

*Conclusion.*—Preliminary fluorescence studies showed that $AlS_2Pc$ preferentially accumulated in the media of the vessel wall and that normal arteries could be effectively sensitized. Experimental intimal hyperplasia was inhibited by adjunctive $AlS_2Pc$-sensitized PDT, thus suggesting a new approach to the problem of angioplasty restenosis caused by FCIH.

▶ I have never been able to generate much enthusiasm for PDT in the control of intimal hyperplasia. This modality has been hanging out on the edges of vascular research for the past decade. I predict little or no clinical application for this arcane technology, despite its offensively regular appearances in the literature.

### Inhibition of Matrix Metalloproteinase Activity Inhibits Smooth Muscle Cell Migration But Not Neointimal Thickening After Arterial Injury

Bendeck MP, Irvin C, Reidy MA (Univ of Washington, Seattle)
*Circ Res* 78:38–43, 1996                              1–41

*Background.*—Normal rat carotid artery does not contain smooth muscle cells (SMC), but after balloon catheter injury, a neointima forms, consisting of SMCs that have migrated to the site. This migration requires degradation of basement membrane and extracellular matrix. The SMCs produce enzymes, such as matrix-degrading metalloproteinases (MMPs), which can degrade these extracellular proteins to permit migration to the site of injury. To examine the role of these MMPs in intimal lesion development after injury to the carotid artery, a rat model and an MMP inhibitor, GM 6001, were used.

*Methods.*—Male Sprague Dawley rats received either GM 6001 or placebo prior to balloon catheter injury to the common carotid artery. Rats then continued to receive inhibitor or placebo daily until they were killed at day 2, 4, 7, 10, or 14 after injury.

*Results.*—Inhibition of MMP activity with GM 6001 was associated with a 97% decrease in SMC at the injury site at 4 days. Lesion growth was slowed by the continued inhibitor treatment up to 10 days, compared with placebo treated rats. The SMC replication rates were not affected by treatment with GM 6001. By 2 weeks after injury, the initimal area in the treated rats was the same size as that in the control rats, due to a significantly increased rate of SMC replication.

*Conclusions.*—Rats with balloon catheter injury to the common carotid artery were treated with the metalloproteinase inhibitor, GM 6001. Treatment with this inhibitor resulted in a decrease in the migration of SMCs into the injury site for at least 10 days after injury. At longer time periods, the lesions in the treated rats increased to the same size as those in the control rats due to increased SMC replication. These results indicate that MMPs are important mediators of SMC migration into injured artery intima, but inhibition of these enzymes is insufficient to completely inhibit lesion growth.

▶ These clever investigators note that SMCs elaborate MMP enzymes to assist in their migration through the basement membrane during the course of intimal hyperplasia. The MMP inhibitor in this study reduced early postinjury intimal hyperplasia, but interestingly, at 10 days, the inhibited SMCs proliferated at a prodigious rate and "caught up" with the control group. Although this substance is probably not adequate to achieve any significant clinical effect alone, it may point the way to a future productive area of investigation.

## Intra-Arterial Beta Irradiation Prevents Neointimal Hyperplasia in a Hypercholesterolemic Rabbit Restenosis Model

Verin V, Popowski Y, Urban P, et al (Univ Hosp, Geneva; Schneider (Europe) AG, Bülach, Switzerland)

*Circulation* 92:2284–2290, 1995                                          1–42

*Background.*—Arterial restenosis after percutaneous transluminal coronary angioplasty continues to be problematic. The use of intraluminal beta-irradiation with 90-yttrium ($^{90}$Y) at different dose schedules to decrease neointimal hyperplasia was studied.

*Methods.*—Anesthetized, hypercholesterolemic rabbits underwent balloon denuding of portions of carotid and iliac arteries. A titanium-coated wire of $^{90}$Y was then inserted through a catheter with a series of 4 balloons in its wall, to center the wire in the artery. Three doses of radiation were used, 6 Gy, 12 Gy, and 18 Gy. At 8 days and 6 weeks, groups of rabbits were killed and the arteries were harvested and examined for neointimal growth. Bromodeoxyuridine (BrdU) staining permitted identification of smooth muscle cells (SMC) in the S-phase of mitosis.

*Results.*—At 8 days, both total SMC and BrdU-positive SMC per centimeter were significantly fewer than in control vessels for all radiation doses. The 18 Gy dose was significantly more effective in inhibiting neointimal growth than the other 2 doses. Medial SMC growth was not inhibited at any dose, compared with control arteries. At 6 weeks, only arteries exposed to 18 Gy showed significant reduction in histologic percent-area stenosis and number of neointimal layers, compared with controls. At 18 Gy, neointimal growth was significantly more inhibited at the middle of the lesions, compared with intima at the ends of the catheter balloons.

*Conclusion.*—Intra-arterial beta-irradiation with $^{90}$Y at a dose of 18 Gy is effective in limiting neointimal growth for up to 6 weeks after angioplasty.

▶ Slowly accumulating information continues to indicate that irradiation at the site of arterial injury may indeed inhibit intimal hyperplasia. I suspect this is a "shotgun" effect, basically derived from cellular injury. In this way, it may be akin to hyperdose steroid, which will achieve the same thing, and possibly for the same reason. As I expressed in the 1995 YEAR BOOK OF VASCULAR SURGERY,[1] I continue to be concerned with the potential of this therapy to do harm. I doubt this will ever find a major niche in the treatment of human disease. See also Abstract 1–43.

*Reference*

1. 1995 YEAR BOOK OF VASCULAR SURGERY, p 92.

## The Effects of Low-Dose Radiation on Neointimal Hyperplasia

Sarac TP, Riggs PN, Williams JP, et al (Univ of Rochester, NY)
*J Vasc Surg* 22:17–24, 1995                                       1–43

*Introduction.*—Low-dose radiation has proved safe and effective in controlling a variety of nonmalignant neoproliferative disorders. An animal study was designed to determine whether single low-dose radiation could prevent neointimal hyperplasia (NIH) after arterial injury, a significant cause of bypass graft and angioplasty failure.

*Methods.*—Twenty-eight male Sprague-Dawley rats underwent balloon injury to the common carotid artery (CCA). Before skin closure, the 3 treatment groups received high-dose rate brachytherapy (HDRB) radiation to the segment of the injured vessel. Radiation doses were 5 Gy (5 animals), 10 Gy (10 animals), and 15 Gy (5 animals); 8 rats served as controls and received no radiation. Vessels were harvested 3 weeks later and compartment areas measured on fixed specimens. The effects of HDRB on endothelial regeneration were studied by scanning and transmission electron microscopy, together with Evans blue dye uptake into injured vessels.

*Results.*—Radiation treatment did not appear to cause skin sensitivity or focal irritation. All untreated controls exhibited NIH in the CCA subjected to balloon injury, whereas contralateral untreated CCAs showed no abnormalities. In contrast, only 1 of 20 rats in the HDRB treatment groups exhibited NIH. None of the treated animals had evidence of aneurysmal degeneration, media necrosis, or decreases in the lumen size of treated vessels. Endothelial regeneration was significantly greater in the radiation-treated groups than in controls, and treated animals had no signs of fibrosis or hemorrhage.

*Conclusion.*—None of the interventions used to limit NIH formations in animal models has proved effective in humans. In the present experiment, 19 of 20 rats treated at 3 different radiation doses demonstrated suppression of NIH. Possible causes of this effect are a rapid regeneration of endothelium, a reduction in smooth muscle cell activity, and a reduced sensitivity to a variety of growth factors. Low-dose radiation appears to offer promise as a method of improving the success rate of vascular grafting.

▶ Previous studies have evaluated the effect of radiation therapy on NIH and have reached different conclusions, likely due to differences in the animal models, the type of radiation, and the dose used. In this study, the Rochester group has selected brachytherapy, in which small doses of irradiation can be delivered locally via a hollow-core catheter, as used clinically for tumor treatment. The potential advantage of this technique is that it would be applicable to endovascular treatment, such as balloon angioplasty. In the rat carotid artery balloon injury model, the authors found a dramatic reduction in intimal hyperplasia with low-dose brachytherapy. The authors point out that endothelial cells appear less sensitive to radiation injury than smooth muscle cells, potentially allowing endothelial regeneration at the site of injury while preventing smooth muscle cell proliferation. Before we become too enthusiastic, however, it is important to recall that nearly every agent that has been evaluated to reduce intimal hyperplasia (e.g. heparin, dexamethasone, angiotension-converting enzyme inhibitors, antiplatelet antibodies, etc.) has been successful in the rat model, but none have been successful in humans or primates. Furthermore, whereas endothelial regeneration in rats after arterial injury appears to inhibit intimal hyperplasia, this is not true in humans. Thus, although the rat model may be appropriate for the initial screening of new techniques, primate studies would be a better predictor of the expected results in humans. This has not prevented at least 1 group of radiologists in Germany from trying this technique in humans, unfortunately in an uncontrolled study. The search for the magic bullet to prevent NIH continues.

**J. Cronenwett, M.D.**

# Homocysteine

## Prevalence of Moderate Hyperhomocysteinemia in Patients With Early-Onset Venous and Arterial Occlusive Disease

Fermo I, Vigano S, Paroni R, et al (Istituto Scientifico H S Raffaele, Milan, Italy)
*Ann Intern Med* 123:747–753, 1995 1–44

*Objective.*—Hyperhomocysteinemia is suspected of playing a role in the development of premature vascular disease, including thrombophilia (defined as increased tendency to thrombosis), a genetic disorder. The prevalence of moderate hyperhomocysteinemia and established disorders of inherited thrombophilia in patients with early onset venous or arterial occlusive disease was evaluated.

*Methods.*—Between November 1992 and October 1994, plasma homocysteine, antithrombin III, protein C, protein S, activated protein C resistance, plasminogen, and heparin cofactor II levels were determined for 3 months in 107 patients (47 men) with early onset venous thromboembolic disease, 50 patients (24 men) with early onset arterial occlusive disease, and 60 healthy controls. Family members of patients with abnormalities were studied when possible. Total plasma homocysteine levels were determined in 87 patients 8 hours after methionine administration.

*Results.*—Homocysteine levels after methionine loading were twice as high as fasting levels in both patient groups for an overall moderate hyperhomocysteinemia prevalence of 13.1% in patients with venous thromboembolic disease and 18.0% in patients with arterial occlusive disease. Inherited defects of thrombophilia observed only in patients with venous thromboembolic disease included poor coagulation response to activated protein C in 11.2 %, protein S deficiency in 4.7%, protein C deficiency in 1.9%, and plasminogen deficiency in 0.9%. In patients with defects, 49% had a family history of thrombosis. The disease recurrence rate was 40% in patients with defects and 25% in patients without defects.

The difference was significant. The presence of defects, predisposing risk factors, and family history of thrombosis had a significant impact on event-free survival. Relative to controls, patients with defects had a relative risk of an occlusive event of 1.7. Compared with controls, patients with a family history and predisposing risk factors had a relative risk of 1.25. Patients with defects experienced thromboembolic events at a significantly younger age than patients without defects. Patients with mild hyperhomocysteinemia were more than twice as likely to have a recurrence than patients without defects.

*Conclusion.*—Significant numbers of patients with early onset venous and arterial occlusive disease were found to have moderate hypercysteinemia and inherited thrombophilia disorders. Measurement of homocysteine levels should be included in the clinical evaluation of thrombophilia.

▶ These investigators found that a moderate but significant percentage of patients with venous thromboembolic disease or arterial occlusive disease have elevations of plasma homocysteine, and homocysteine may be additive with inherited hypercoagulable defects. They conclude that homocysteine should be included when screening patients for hypercoagulability. I believe their recommendation to be premature. I hope we will be able to carefully define basic relationships between homocysteine and vascular injury before considering widespread recommendations for treatment.

---

**Is Hyperhomocysteinaemia a Risk Factor for Recurrent Venous Thrombosis?**
den Heijer M, Blom HJ, Gerrits WBJ, et al (Municipal Hosp Leyenburg, The Hague, The Netherlands; Univ Hosp, Nijmegen, The Netherlands; Univ Hosp Leiden, The Netherlands)
*Lancet* 345:882–885, 1995                                   1–45

---

*Background.*—Several researchers have reported a relationship between hyperhomocysteinemia and arterial vascular disease. Because hyperhomocysteinemia is easily corrected by vitamin supplementation, its association with venous thrombosis could be important clinically.

*Methods.*—One hundred eighty-five patients with a history of recurrent venous thrombosis and 220 control subjects from the general population were studied. Homocysteine levels were determined before and 6 hours after oral methionine loading. Hyperhomocysteinemia was defined as a homocysteine concentration exceeding the fasting or postmethionine value at the 90th percentile among control subjects.

*Findings.*—Twenty-five percent of the patients with recurrent thrombosis had fasting homocysteine levels higher than the 90th percentile. The odds ratio was 2.0 after adjustment for age, sex, and menopausal status. The adjusted odds ratio for the postmethionine value was 2.6 (Table 1).

TABLE 1.—Homocysteine Concentrations and Risk of Recurrent Venous Thrombosis

| | Cases n=105 | Controls n=220 | Odds ratio |
|---|---|---|---|
| Fasting homocysteine concentrations | | | |
| >90th percentile (18·6 µmol/L) | 46 | 21 | |
| <90th percentile (18·6 µmol/L) | 130 | 199 | 3·1 (1·8–5·5) |
| Post-methionine homocysteine concentrations | | | |
| >90th percentile (58·8 µmol/L) | 44 | 20 | |
| <90th percentile (58·8 µmol/L) | 141 | 200 | 3·1 (1·7–5·5) |

(Courtesy of den Heijer M, Blom HJ, Gerrits WBJ, et al: Is hyperhomocysteinaemia a risk factor for recurrent venous thrombosis? *Lancet* 345:882–885, copyright by The Lancet Ltd. 1995.)

*Conclusions.*—Hyperhomocysteinemia is a common risk factor for recurrent venous thrombosis. In the current study, it was associated with a two- to three-fold increase in risk.

▶ Although the potential relationship between hyperhomocysteinemia and venous thrombosis has been reported previously[1], it has attracted little attention. These authors studied 185 patients with recurrent venous thrombosis and found that 25% had significant homocysteine elevations. They conclude that hyperhomocysteinemia is a well-defined risk factor for deep vein thrombosis, resulting in a two- to threefold risk increase, compared with individuals without hyperhomocysteinemia. See also Abstracts 1–44 and 1–46.

*Reference:*

1. Falcon CR, Cattaneo M, Panzeri D, et al: High prevalence of hyperhomocyst(e)inemia in patients with juvenile venous thrombosis. *Arterioscler Thromb* 14:1080–1083, 1994.

---

**Hyperhomocysteinemia as a Risk Factor for Deep-Vein Thrombosis**
den Heijer M, Koster T, Blom HJ, et al (Municipal Hosp Leyenburg, The Hague, The Netherlands; Univ Hosp, Leiden, The Netherlands; Univ Hosp, Nijmegen, The Netherlands)
*N Engl J Med* 334:759–762, 1996                                    1–46

*Background.*—Hyperhomocysteinemia is a possible risk factor for venous thrombosis. This association was tested by comparing plasma homocysteine levels in patients with their first episode of deep vein thrombosis vs. normal controls.

*Methods.*—The study included 269 patients with their first, objectively diagnosed episode of deep vein thrombosis and 296 age- and sex-matched healthy controls. Patients whose plasma homocysteine level exceeded 18.5 µmol/L—the 95th percentile in the control group—were considered to have hyperhomocysteinemia.

*Results.*—Ten percent of patients vs. 5% of controls had hyperhomocysteinemia, for a matched odds ratio of 2.5 with a 95% confidence interval of 1.2 to 5.2. Women showed a stronger relationship between high homocysteine levels and age, and the association increased with age. The risk associated with hyperhomocysteinemia was not significantly influenced by exclusion of subjects with other known risk factors for thrombosis, such as protein C, protein S, or antithrombin deficiency; activated protein C resistance; pregnancy or recent childbirth; or oral contraceptive use.

*Conclusions.*—Individuals with elevated plasma homocysteine levels appear to be at increased risk for deep vein thrombosis. Further studies are needed to see if interventions to lower homocysteine levels, such as folic acid, vitamin $B_6$, or vitamin $B_{12}$, can help prevent recurrent venous thrombosis.

▶ In this study, 269 patients undergoing a first, objectively diagnosed episode of deep vein thrombosis, as well as age- and sex-matched controls, were examined for hyperhomocysteinemia. Ten percent of the patients had hyperhomocysteinemia, twice as many as the controls. These authors conclude, just as did the authors of the previous paper (Abstract, 1–45), that high plasma homocysteine levels represent a risk factor for venous thrombosis. It should be remembered that it is also a risk factor for arterial thrombosis. The obvious question posed by this information is whether lowering homocysteine by using such drugs as folic acid or the B vitamins will reduce the risk of venous thrombosis. Further data are eagerly awaited. See also Abstract 1–44.

---

## Higher Plasma Homocyst(e)ine and Increased Susceptibility to Adverse Effects of Low Folate in Early Familial Coronary Artery Disease

Hopkins PN, Wu II, Hunt SC, et al (Univ of Utah, Salt Lake City)
*Arterioscler Thromb Vasc Biol* 15:1314–1320, 1995                    1–47

---

*Background.*—Plasma homocysteine (H[c]) levels are determined in part by genetic, plasma creatine, and nutritional factors, such as vitamin B6, B12, and folate levels. Previous studies have demonstrated an increased prevalence of coronary artery disease (CAD), peripheral and cerebrovascular disease, and carotid stenosis in individuals with elevated H(c). The graded risk of H(c) levels on CAD was examined and an attempt was made to determine whether this risk was independent of other influences, such as vitamin status.

*Patients and Methods.*—Patients with early familial CAD were identified as surviving a myocardial infarction, or undergoing percutaneous transluminal angioplasty or coronary artery bypass grafting before age 55 for men or before age 65 for women, and having another sibling with early CAD. One hundred twenty men and 42 women with early familial CAD were compared to 85 men and 70 women selected from a random population or who were spouses of patients with hypertension. Their H(c) levels were measured by high-pressure liquid chromatography after overnight fasting

*Results.*—Increasing H(c) levels above 9 µmol/L were associated with an increased risk of CAD. Relative odds for CAD were significantly higher in men and women, 13.8 and 12.8, respectively, with an H(c) level of 19 µmol/L or less, compared with those with levels below 9 µmol/L. After adjustment for age, sex, body mass index, cigarette smoking, hypertension, diabetes, total cholesterol, low-density lipoprotein, high-density lipoprotein, triglycerides, and vitamin levels, plasma H(c) levels were shown to have an independent, statistically significant relationship to CAD. These adjustments demonstrated that a 10 µmol/L increase in plasma H(c) levels yielded an 8.1-fold increased risk of CAD (95% CI, 3.2–20.4). Those patients with familial CAD who had depressed folate levels were also found to have greater elevations of H(c) levels, suggesting a greater sensitivity to low folate levels in these patients.

*Conclusion.*—Plasma H(c) levels are an independent, graded risk factor in CAD development.

▶ These investigators found, not surprisingly, that hyperhomocysteinemia is a risk factor for CAD. It is obvious that many factors may result in hyperhomocysteinemia. Some of these include deficiency of folic acid, deficiency of vitamins $B_6$ and $B_{12}$, advancing age, renal disease, hepatic disease, and, importantly, inherited deficiencies of 1 or more of a number of enzymes important in the metabolism of methionine and homocysteine. At present, we do not know which of these multiple causes is most important in the production of hyperhomocysteinemia, although considerable epidemiologic research suggests that the American public in general is substantially deficient in the B vitamins and folic acid. In fact, the public health suggestion has been made that certain American foods, such as bread, should be supplemented with folic acid. This has not yet been implemented, but it is being discussed. This article concludes that the hyperhomocysteine-CAD relationship is enhanced in patients who are deficient in folate. I suspect this is correct.

**Hyperhomocysteinemia and Low Pyridoxal Phosphate: Common and Independent Reversible Risk Factors for Coronary Artery Disease**

Robinson K, Mayer EL, Miller DP, et al (Cleveland Clinic Found, Ohio; Tufts Univ, Boston)

*Circulation* 92:2825–2830, 1995                                        1–48

*Objective.*—The levels of homocysteine associated with increased risk for coronary artery disease in women and the elderly were examined.

*Background.*—Coronary artery disease is a major health problem in Western countries. Increased plasma homocysteine concentration may be associated with arterial disease. The exact level of plasma homocysteine associated with increased coronary risk is unknown, and this risk in women and the elderly has not been investigated. Low levels of B vitamins increase homocysteine, but the association between coronary disease and these vitamins is unknown.

*Methods.*—In 304 patients (103 women) with coronary artery disease, risk factors and plasma concentrations of homocysteine, folate, vitamin B12, and pyridoxal 5'-phosphate were analyzed and compared with findings from control subjects.

*Results.*—With a homocysteine concentration of 14 µmol/L, an odds ratio of 4.8 was seen. With 5 µmol/L increments across the range of homocysteine, an odds ratio of 2.4 was seen. Women had an odds ratio of 3.5, and patients 65 years or older had an odds ratio of 2.9. There was a negative correlation between homocysteine and all vitamins. Low pyridoxal 5'-phosphate was noted in 10% of patients with coronary disease and 2% of control subjects. After adjusting for all risk factors, including high homocysteine, the odds ratio for coronary disease was 4.3.

*Conclusions.*—High concentrations of homocysteine and low concentrations of pyridoxal 5'-phosphate are independent risk factors for coronary artery disease. This risk increases with higher levels of plasma homocysteine regardless of age or gender and has no threshold.

▶ These authors conclude that low levels of vitamin B6 (pyridoxal phosphate) constitute an independent risk factor for coronary disease exclusive of its effect in increasing homocysteine. Although I am certain their statistical calculations are correct, I wonder if low B6 is really an independent risk factor exclusive of its relationship to hyperhomocysteinemia. Perhaps. See also Abstract 1–47.

---

**Hyperhomocysteinemia-Induced Vascular Damage in the Minipig: Captopril-Hydrochlorothiazide Combination Prevents Elastic Alterations**
Rolland PH, Friggi A, Barlatier A, et al (INSERM, Paris; Hosp La Timone, Marseilles, France; Rhône-Poulenc-Rorer/Theraplix Lab, Paris)
*Circulation* 91:1161–1174, 1995                                                      1–49

---

*Background.*—The relationship between homocysteine and vascular disease in patients with hyperhomocysteinemia remains inconclusive as relevant animal models are not available. Methionine is the metabolic precursor of homocysteine. Previous studies have shown that minipigs fed a methionine-rich caseinate-based diet will develop hypermethioninemia. Investigators attempted to determine whether this hypermethioninemia will induce hyperhomocysteinemia and mimic the vascular alterations seen in humans. The therapeutic effects of captopril-hydrochlorothiazide (Cp) administration were also examined.

*Methods.*—Thirty-two minipigs were randomized into 4 equal groups of control diet-fed (C), C plus Cp-treated (C+CP), methionine-rich diet-fed (M), and M+Cp animals. Hemodynamics and vascular reactivity were studied by noninvasive and invasive assessment of arterial flow conditions

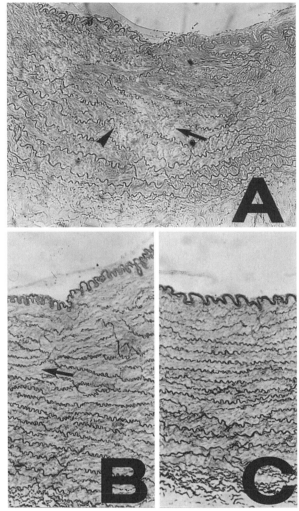

FIGURE 5.—Photomicrographs show the typical histologic appearance of the carotid bifurcation in minipigs in the hyperhomocysteinemic (M) and captopril-hydrochlorothiazide-treated hyperhomocysteinemic (M + Cp) groups, illustrating **A**, the thinning and fragmentation of elastic laminae (*arrowhead*) and smooth muscle cell hypertrophy (*arrow*) in animals of the M group (Masson's trichrome; magnification, × 200) and **B**, the occurrence of smooth muscle cell hypertrophy and cell reorientation and migration (*arrow*) (Darrow orcein staining; magnification, × 150), providing evidence **C** that the stacking up of the elastic laminae was preserved and cellular hypertrophy and reorientation were prevented, at least in part, in the carotid bifurcation in animals of the M + Cp group (Darrow orcein staining; magnification, × 140) (note the similarities between histologic features of abdominal aorta and carotid bifurcation). (Courtesy of Rolland PH, Friggi A, Barlatier A, et al: Hyperhomocysteinemia-induced vascular damage in the minipig: Captopril-hydrochlorothiazide combination prevents elastic alterations. *Circulation* 1995; 91:1161–1174. Reproduced with permission *Circulation*. Copyright 1995 American Heart Association.)

in the hind-limb arteries and by examining the histopathology of the arterial tree. The dietary regimens were maintained for 4 months.

*Findings.*—Minipigs in the M group developed systolic-diastolic hypertension, extended hyperemia, and a mega-artery syndrome in hyperpulsatile arteries. At histologic examination, hypertrophic endothelial cells covering a thickened subendothelial space were found in their arterial tree (Fig 5). Major elastic lamina dislocations, hypertrophy, and reorientation of smooth muscle cells were also observed. Treatment with Cp prevented diastolic hypertension and also improved and prevented the disappearance of the vascular elastic structures and intrinsic elastic component. However, treatment with Cp did not prevent systolic hypertension and did not normalize the hyperhomocysteinemia.

*Conclusions.*—A methionine-rich caseinate-based diet can induce hyperhomocysteinemia and induce vascular alterations in minipigs that mimic those seen in humans with the disorder. Treatment with Cp has therapeutic effects on the vascular wall.

▶ Early experiments with hyperhomocysteinemia in laboratory animals suggested profound vascular toxicity. Attempts to duplicate these experiments have been substantially unsuccessful. Thus, this is an important study, in that the induction of hyperhomocysteinemia in laboratory animals did produce major morphologic changes in the arterial system. The observation that angiotensin-converting enzyme inhibition minimized these abnormalities is interesting, although the importance of this observation is unclear. It is interesting to note that this appears to be the first report of experimental hyperhomocysteinemia having clear pathologic relevance. This article is recommended for anyone wanting more detailed information on the effects of hyperhomocysteinemia on the arterial wall.

---

**Induction of Cyclin A Gene Expression by Homocysteine in Vascular Smooth Muscle Cells**

Tsai J-C, Wang H, Perrella MA, et al (Harvard School of Public Health, Boston; Harvard Med School, Boston; Brigham and Women's Hosp, Boston)
*J Clin Invest* 97:146–153, 1996                                                        1–50

---

*Introduction.*—Recent studies identify elevated levels of homocysteine as an important and independent risk factor for arteriosclerosis. Increased levels of this intermediate metabolite of methionine can be caused by enzyme or vitamin deficiencies, drugs, and perhaps other factors. The mechanisms by which arteriosclerosis is induced by hyperhomocysteinemia are not well understood. A study using human and rat aortic smooth muscle cells (RASMCs) demonstrated that homocysteine and serum increase DNA synthesis and cyclin A mRNA synergistically.

*Findings.*—Cyclin A mRNA levels were increased eightfold when quiescent RASMCs were treated with 1 mM homocysteine for 36 hours; the increase was 14-fold when 2% calf serum was the treatment. The effect of homocysteine plus serum indicated a synergistic induction of cyclin A mRNA, which was increased 40-fold in this treatment protocol. The half-life of cyclin A mRNA (2.9 hours) was not increased by homocysteine, but the transcriptional rate of the cyclin A gene was increased in nuclear run-on experiments. The finding that homocysteine increased cyclin A promoter activity and ATF-binding protein levels in RASMCs supports a positive effect of homocysteine on cyclin A gene transcription. Cyclin A protein levels and cyclin A-associated kinase activity were increased threefold by 1 mM homocysteine.

*Discussion.*—There is considerable epidemiologic evidence that elevated homocysteine is a risk factor for arteriosclerosis, yet the molecular basis for relationship has not been well understood. These investigations demonstrate that homocysteine increases levels of cyclin A mRNA, and this effect is markedly increased by serum. Cyclin A was selected because it is known to be required in more than 1 phase of the cell cycle. Because homocysteine-induced increases in cyclin mRNA levels are associated with increases in cyclin A protein and cyclin A-associated kinase activity, homocysteine-induced cyclin A gene expression may play an important part in the vascular smooth muscle cell proliferation observed in arteriosclerosis.

▶ This study attempts to address the molecular mechanisms involved in the action of homocysteine on the vascular wall. These investigators purport to show that homocysteine induces vascular smooth muscle proliferation and that it, in conjunction with serum, markedly enhances the expression of the cyclin A gene and also increases cyclin A mRNA levels, a substance important in cell cycle proliferation. This may prove to be a pivotal action of homocysteine in the induction of vascular pathology.

## Epidemiology

**Survival After the Age of 80 in the United States, Sweden, France, England, and Japan**
Manton KG, Vaupel JW (Sanford Inst of Public Policy, Durham, NC; Duke Univ, Durham, NC; Odense Univ, Denmark)
*N Engl J Med* 333:1232–1235, 1995                                    1–51

*Background.*—Mortality among young Americans is greater than among residents of many European countries and Japan. These differences lessen in the 65- to 80-year-old age group. New data are now available for mortality comparisons among individuals aged 80 to 100 years.

*Methods.*—Extinct-cohort methods were used to determine death rates among those born between 1880 and 1894 in United States, Japan, Sweden, France, and England, including Wales. Only white Americans were included in the United States analysis. Extinct-cohort methods use continuously collected data from death certificates rather than census data, which are less reliable.

*Findings.*—Life expectancy at the age of 80 years and survival between 80 and 100 years of age in the United States significantly exceeded life expectancy in the other countries investigated (Fig 1). Cross-sectional data for 1987 were used to confirm this finding. In the United States, the mean

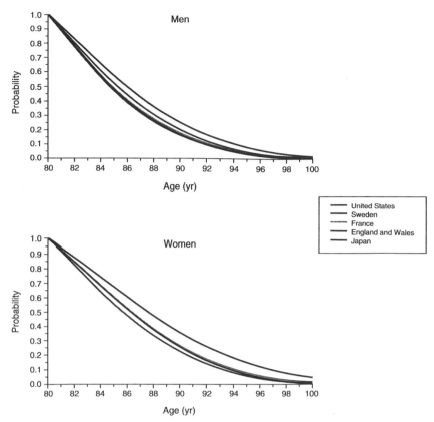

FIGURE 1.—Probability of survival after the age of 80 among whites in the United States and Japanese, Swedish, French, and English and Welsh people born from 1885 to 1889. (Reprinted by permission of *The New England Journal of Medicine.* Manton KG, Vaupel JW: Survival after the age of 80 in the United States, Sweden, France, England, and Japan. *N Engl J Med* 333:1232–1235. Copyright 1995, Massachusetts Medical Society.)

life expectancy for an 80-year-old white woman is 9.1 years and for an 80-year-old white man, 7 years.

*Conclusions.*—Life expectancy for Americans between the ages of 80 and 100 years is higher than for the Swedish, French, English, or Japanese. The possible explanations for this include current American health policies and conditions as well as lingering cohort effects.

▶ There could be a marginal benefit from being elderly, white, and female if you live in the United States, but you will have survived a greater challenge getting there and may well have buried your neighbors. Overall, the Japanese are still in the lead as far as life expectancy from birth is concerned. Furthermore, their population enjoys more universal access to this benefit than is the case in the United States or Europe, where the populations are much more heterogenous. The evidence linking health care expenditure to longevity is not yet as convincing as we might wish.

**A.E.B. Giddings, M.D.**

---

### Aspirin and the Risk of Colorectal Cancer in Women

Giovannucci E, Egan KM, Hunter DJ, et al (Harvard Med School, Boston)
*N Engl J Med* 333:609–614, 1995                                           1–52

---

*Introduction.*—Research undertaken to study the effect of aspirin use and the risk of colorectal cancer has been inconsistent. An attempt was made to establish a correlation between colon and rectal cancers and aspirin usage.

*Methods.*—Almost 90,000 women in the Nurses' Health Study, with no diagnosis nor any family history of colorectal cancer, completed a baseline questionnaire on medication usage and diet. This was followed up every 2 years with another questionnaire on aspirin and other nonsteroidal anti-inflammatory drug usage. Cases of adenomatous polyps in both participants and their next of kin were documented. The association between aspirin use and the occurrence of a new colon or rectal cancer during a 12-year period was then analyzed.

*Results.*—During the 8-year period of this study, 331 cases of colorectal cancer not previously reported were documented among women in the Nurses' Health Study. Individuals who in the initial questionnaire reported themselves as being regular aspirin users (those who took at least 2 aspirins per week for a 4-year period) had a lower risk of cancer development than did nonusers. A drop in risk was observed for women who used aspirin regularly for at least 10 years, and this decrease became significant at 20 years of regular aspirin usage. After controlling for other risk factors, women who on 3 consecutive questionnaires (which were filled out every 2 years) reported regular aspirin use were 38% less likely to have colorectal cancer develop. A significant inverse relationship was shown between the intake of 4 to 6 aspirins a week and the risk of development of colorectal cancer. These results are even more impressive inasmuch as, during the course of the study, women who did take aspirin had a higher rate of endoscopy.

*Discussion.*—Results show that for women, long-term use of aspirin (10 years or more) at a rate of 4 to 6 tablets per week decreases the risk of colorectal cancer. Possible mechanisms for the action of aspirin include the inhibition of cyclo-oxygenase and subsequent inhibition of prostaglandin action or the inhibition of phospholipase activity. Also, it has been documented that aspirin can modulate levels of prostaglandin in the rectal epithelium. This work requires further research, especially because low-dose aspirin has been shown to decrease the incidence of cardiovascular disease.

▶ Increasing evidence indicates that the regular use of aspirin substantially reduces the risk of colorectal cancer in our aging patients. This particular study addresses the risk in women, but other studies have addressed both genders.[1] Overwhelming evidence suggests that in the absence of the rare but potentially fatal aspirin allergy and/or bleeding diathesis, we should recommend that all of our vascular patients take aspirin daily. I believe the optimal dose is 1 tablet per day, and I doubt if it makes much difference whether it is 80 mg or 320 mg.

*Reference*

1. 1993 YEAR BOOK OF VASCULAR SURGERY, p 6.

---

### Alcohol Consumption and Mortality Among Women
Fuchs CS, Stampfer MJ, Colditz GA, et al (Harvard Med School, Boston; Dana-Farber Cancer Inst, Boston)
*N Engl J Med* 332:1245–1250, 1995                                    1–53

---

*Objective.*—Whereas light-to-moderate alcohol drinking in men is associated with a lower risk of mortality from coronary heart disease, studies in women are less clear. The prospective relationship between light-to-moderate alcohol drinking in women and mortality and the risk of coronary heart disease is reported.

*Methods.*—A total of 85,709 female nurses, aged 34 to 59, were followed up every 2 years, from 1980 to 1992, to assess risks for coronary heart disease and cancer and the amount and type of alcoholic beverages consumed. Deaths were recorded.

*Results.*—In 1980, approximately 30% of women reported that they did not drink; only 1% reported heavy drinking (more than 50 g/day of alcohol). During the follow-up period, 2,658 women died: 503 of cardiovascular causes, 1,495 of cancer (including 350 of breast cancer), 203 of injury, 52 of cirrhosis of the liver, and 405 of other causes. Light-to-moderate drinkers had a significantly lower risk of death than did nondrinkers or heavy drinkers, primarily due to a lower risk of cardiovascular disease. The increased risk for heavy drinkers was due primarily to breast cancer and cirrhosis. Controlling for other risks for breast cancer did not affect the results. Age and mortality were significantly related for women older than age 50. There was a significant benefit from light-to-moderate alcohol consumption for women with 1 or more risk factors for coronary heart disease. Former heavy drinkers who had achieved abstinence were excluded from the study. When analyzed separately, this group had an age- and smoking-adjusted risk of death from cardiovascular causes of 1.49.

*Conclusion.*—Light-to-moderate alcohol consumption in women reduces mortality particularly in those who have multiple risks for coronary heart disease.

► It is important to note that the overall survival benefit ascribed to alcohol is only present at low-to-moderate intake (the equivalent of 1–3 drinks per week). Heavy alcohol consumption, although probably still showing benefit in the reduction in death from cardiovascular disease, increases death from other causes, including breast cancer and cirrhosis, so that the overall death risk is increased. In summary, overwhelming evidence indicates that light-to-moderate alcohol consumption has a favorable effect upon survival due to reduction in cardiovascular risk. I wonder how the Baptists feel about this?

## Vascular Biology

### Retroviral Vector-Mediated Transfer and Expression of Human Tissue Plasminogen Activator Gene in Human Endothelial and Vascular Smooth Muscle Cells

Ekhterae D, Stanley JC (Univ of Michigan, Ann Arbor)
*J Vasc Surg* 21:953–962, 1995                                               1–54

*Purpose.*—Reduction of the luminal thrombogenicity of diseased arteries and veins and of synthetic grafts by altering the balance between the production of tissue plasminogen activator (tPA) and plasminogen activator inhibitor-1 (PAI-1) in endothelial cells (EC) would be a valuable clinical technique. The effect of the retroviral-mediated transfer of the human tPA gene into human EC and vascular smooth muscle cells (SMC) on the fibrinolytic activity of these cells and on PAI-1 secretion was assessed.

*Methods.*—Segments of human saphenous vein and iliac artery were used to harvest EC and SMC by standard enzymatic techniques. These cells were transduced with a murine leukemia retroviral vector (MFG) containing the human tPA gene. The control cells were also exposed to the lacZ gene or the media alone. Fourteen and 28 days after transduction, the secreted tPA and PAI-1 antigen levels were determined by enzyme-linked immunosorbent assay (ELISA), and human tPA activity was measured with a spectrolyse tPA/PAI kit. The DNA and RNA extracted from the EC after 14 and 28 days of culture were examined by autoradiography after Northern and Southern blot analysis.

*Results.*—Retroviral-mediated gene transfer was shown for the first time to enhance the fibrinolytic activity of adult human EC. Transduced EC had significantly higher levels and about a fivefold increase in activity of tPA antigen than nontransduced control EC at 14 and 28 days of culture. Transduced SMC also had significantly higher levels of tPA antigen than control SMC, but there was no significant increase in tPA activity of transduced SMC. In addition, the level of endogenous PAI-1 antigen was significantly reduced compared with control levels in transduced EC but not in transduced SMC. Integration and transcription of the tPA gene in both EC and SMC were documented by Northern and Southern blot analyses. The changes in PAI-1 in transduced EC were probably due to posttranslational events because PAI-1 mRNA was unchanged following transduction.

*Conclusions.*—Murine leukemia retroviral vector-mediated tPA gene transfer into human EC causes a significant increase in tPA activity. This enhancement of human EC fibrinolytic activity may be useful in the prevention of thrombotic complications of vascular disease.

▶ This sophisticated study concludes that cultured human EC can be transduced with an MFG containing the human tPA gene. The differential effect on EC vs. SMC is interesting, and the lack of production of increased amounts of PAI is noteworthy. One area that has always caused me concern, however, is the control of the transduced substance. Certainly, in vivo, a remarkable system of feedback controls invariably exists for almost every cellular product. If we simply induce the product without the requisite control, I can envision the continuous inappropriate elaboration of the transduced product to the detriment of the organism. I suspect that induction of the requisite controls will be far more complicated than induction of the product itself.

---

**Unfractionated Heparin and Low Molecular Weight Heparin Do Not Inhibit the Growth of Proliferating Human Arterial Smooth Muscle Cells in Culture**
Stavenow L, Lindblad B, Xu C-B (Univ Hosp of Malmö, Sweden; Univ of Lund, Sweden)
*Eur J Vasc Endovasc Surg* 10:215–219, 1995                                    1–55

---

*Background.*—Heparin has been shown to reduce intimal thickening after arterial injury in animals, but it does not prevent myointimal hyperplasia in vein grafts or restenosis after angioplasty in humans. Most studies that have shown heparin inhibits smooth muscle cell (SMC) proliferation, used SMCs that were growth arrested before stimulation. The effects of unfractionated heparin (UH) and low molecular weight heparin (LMWH) on growth of both proliferating and growth-arrested human SMCs in vitro were investigated.

*Methods.*—Human arterial tissue for the SMC cultures was obtained during vascular surgery and organ transplantation. Proliferating SMCs were exposed to different concentrations of UH and LMWH, and the effects on proliferation and on collagen secretion were assessed. Also, the effect of UH on proliferation was measured after growth-arrested SMCs (grown in serum-free minimal essential medium for 24 hours) were stimulated with serum. $^3$H-thymidine incorporation was used to measure DNA synthesis. Newly synthesized $^3$H-labeled collagen was measured after pepsin digestion.

*Results.*—In proliferating SMCs, both UH and LMWH (1 or 10 IU/mL) significantly increased total cellular DNA; however, DNA synthesis was not influenced. The increased total cellular DNA seemed to be caused by reduced cell death, not increased proliferation. High concentrations (10 IU/mL) of UH and LMWH increased collagen secretion. Synthesis of DNA was decreased in stimulated SMCs that had been growth arrested before exposure to UH.

*Conclusions.*—The effects of UH and LMWH on human SMC proliferation depend on whether the SMCs have been growth arrested before stimulation. In vitro, both UH and LMWH seem to reduce cell death of proliferating SMCs and to support collagen secretion. These findings may be helpful in the development of pharmacologic agents to control SMC proliferation.

▶ This short report has an important message that has not always been considered in previous studies: When analyzing the effect of glycosaminoglycans on SMCs, the proliferative state of the cells must be defined. Although not stated in the study, I presume that the units are Xal units and one may wonder what happens with LMWH if it is given in IIal units. One important methodologic question is how SMCs were identified in the study.

**D. Bergqvist, M.D., Ph.D.**

---

### Oxidized Low Density Lipoprotein Stimulates Collagen Production in Cultured Arterial Smooth Muscle Cells

Jimi S, Saku K, Uesugi N, et al (Fukuoka Univ, Japan)
*Atherosclerosis* 116:15–26, 1995                                    1–56

---

*Background.*—Oxidatively modified low-density lipoprotein (LDL) appears to have an important role in the development of atherosclerotic disease, particularly the formation of foam cells. Collagenolysis is a key aspect of human atherosclerosis, but the mechanisms underlying fibrogenesis remain uncertain. Oxidized LDL influences the cellular secretion of many cytokines. Ascorbic acid, an antioxidant, stimulates collagen production.

*Objective and Methods.*—The interactive effects of oxidized LDL and ascorbic acid on collagen production were studied in cultured smooth muscle cells from porcine aorta. The cells were incubated with 50 to 200 µg/mL of human LDL with and without cupric ion for 24 hours, and collagen production was quantified by analyzing pepsin digestion of collagenous protein labeled with triated proline. Low-density lipoprotein oxidation was estimated by electrophoresis and by quantifying thiobarbituric acid-reactive substances.

*Results.*—Exposure to ascorbic acid inhibited the oxidation of LDL in the presence of cupric ion by about half. Comparable collagen production was noted in the presence of ascorbic acid whether or not cupric ion was present but, without ascorbic acid, LDL with cupric ion increased collagen production as much as sixfold in a dose-dependent manner. No such effect was seen with native LDL. Adding butylated hydroxytoluene to the LDL/Cu combination suppressed oxidation by nearly 90% and significantly decreased collagen production.

*Conclusion.*—Oxidized LDL may promote collagenosis in atherosclerotic disease by stimulating the production of collagen in arterial smooth muscle cells.

▶ Another piece of evidence indicates that oxidized LDL may be the central harmful substance in the pathogenesis of atherosclerosis. The differential effects of oxidized LDL vs. native LDL in stimulating collagen production in smooth muscle cells appear noteworthy. An increasingly impressive body of evidence indicates that the deposition of oxidized LDL may be a pivotally important initial event in the development of the atherosclerotic lesion. See also Abstract 1–3.

---

**Progesterone Receptor Expression in Human Saphenous Veins**
Perrot-Applanat M, Cohen-Solal K, Milgrom E, et al (INSERM U 135, Arcueil, France)
*Circulation* 92:2975–2983, 1995                                    1–57

---

*Background.*—The predominance of varicose veins in women and the occurrence of venous stasis during sex hormone therapy, the luteal phase of the menstrual cycle, and pregnancy suggest that this venous abnormality depends on sex hormones. Whether these effects are due to a direct hormonal action on the saphenous vein was investigated.

*Methods and Findings.*—Fifteen premenopausal women, 10 postmenopausal women, and 5 men undergoing stripping removal of varicose saphenous veins were studied. Biopsy samples were obtained. Ninety percent of the biopsy samples were progesterone receptor (PR) positive on enzyme immunoassay (EIA). Progesterone receptor staining occurred in the cell nuclei of the tunica media and the subendothelial layer. There was no significant variation in the PR content of different regions in the same saphenous vein. However, EIA detected no or very low levels of estrogen receptors (ER) in 25 of 30 biopsy samples. Reverse transcription-polymerase chain reaction (RT-PCR) was used to analyze PR and ER mRNAs in PR positive/ER negative samples. An RT-PCR product of the expected size was detected with primers to the hormone-binding region encoded by PR mRNA. Its identity was confirmed by Southern blot by a PR cDNA probe. There were no RT-PCR products detected by use of primers to the DNA-binding domain, the hinge region, and the ligand-binding domain encoded by ER mRNA (Table 2).

*Conclusions.*—Human saphenous veins from men as well as women express PR. Progesterone apparently acts directly on these veins through a classic receptor-mediated pathway.

TABLE 2.—ER and PR Status of Human Varicose Veins According to Sex and Menopausal Status

|  | Number of PR-Positive Patients* | Number of ER-Positive Patients† |
|---|---|---|
| Premenopausal women (*n* = 15) | 15(100%) | 3 (20%) |
| Postmenopausal women (*n* = 10) | 8 (80%) | 1 (10%) |
| Men (*n* = 5) | 4 (80%) | 1 (20%) |

ER and PR were analyzed by EIA. The limit of detection was 5 fmol/mg cytosol protein.
* Range, 5–53 fmol of PR per mg cytosol protein.
† Most biopsy samples contained no ER (<5 fmol/mg cytosol protein). Five samples contained 6–9 fmol of ER per mg cytosol protein.
*Abbreviations: ER,* estrogen receptors; *PR,* progesteron receptors; *EIA,* enzyme immunoassay.
(Courtesy of Perrot-Applanat M, Cohen-Solal, Milgrom E, et al: Progesterone receptor expression in human saphenous veins. *Circulation* 1995; 92:2975–2983. Reproduced with permission *Circulation.* Copyright 1995 American Heart Association.)

▶ To my knowledge, this article is the first report of estrogen and progesterone receptor activity in human saphenous veins. Using varicose vein specimens, the authors found that most saphenous veins, from both men and women, express a low level of PR activity on the nuclei of smooth muscle cells, whereas ERs were seldom present. This is comparable to previous reports of ER and PR expression in human arteries. Because progesterone has a relaxing effect on uterine smooth muscle cells, a similar effect on the saphenous vein might lead to venodilation, and possibly varicose changes. Whether physiologic levels of progesterone, however, even during pregnancy, actually cause venodilation is not known. Furthermore, it is a long leap from venodilation to varicose veins. Thus, while this article may establish the presence of PRs in human venous smooth muscle cells, the functional significance of these receptors is unknown, and I will be surprised if they have any significant relation to varicose vein formation. Nonetheless, this report should stimulate research to determine the functional significance of venous PRs at physiologic progesterone levels, which might contribute to gender-related differences in venous (and perhaps arterial) tissue. See also Abstract 1–67.

**J. Cronenwett, M.D.**

## Morphologic Change in Rabbit Femoral Arteries Induced by Storage at Four Degrees Celsius and by Subsequent Reperfusion

Crowe D, O'Loughlin K, Knox L, et al (St Vincent's Hosp, Melbourne)
*J Vasc Surg* 22:769–779, 1995                                     1–58

*Background.*—Because an autologous graft is not always available for replantation surgery, the discovery of a viable alternative prosthesis would have great clinical value. The possibility of cold-stored small arteries serving this function was investigated with the histologic, electron microscopic, tissue culture, and immunohistochemical study of cold-stored rabbit arterial grafts.

*Methods.*—Rabbit femoral artery grafts were harvested and stored at 4°C for 24 hours; 1, 4, or 10 weeks; or 6 months. Grafts from each group plus grafts freshly harvested (controls) were examined histologically, with electron microscopy, and immunohistochemically. The immunohistochemical examination included staining with antibodies for α smooth muscle actin (SMA-α), vimentin, immunoglobulin G, and nitroblue tetrazolium (NBT) (as a test for cell viability). The medial wall thickness was measured in each graft. Grafts from each group were also brought to room temperature and anastomosed to femoral artery segments in other rabbits, reperfused, and examined in the same fashion after 24 hours.

*Results.*—There were no differences in suture ease or anastomosis leakage between the fresh and the cold-stored grafts. There was a uniform staining for α-SMC actin throughout the SMC cytoplasm, but not in the extracellular spaces. All cells showed the presence of vimentin, with especially intense staining in the fibroblasts and extracellular spaces. Cell viability, as detected by NBT staining, decreased with increasing storage time, with more rapid decreases in the reperfused vessels. There were no viable cells by 6 months in the cold-stored grafts and by 10 weeks in the cold-stored and reperfused grafts. Examination with electron microscopy demonstrated that white blood cell infiltration attended the accelerated breakdown and removal of necrotic cells in reperfused vessels and confirmed the lack of change in the extracellular framework of the vessels. The medial wall thickness increased during the first 24 hours of cold storage, from both swelling of SMC and extracellular edema, then decreased progressively, with more accelerated shrinkage in the reperfused vessels.

*Conclusions.*—Cold storage results in acellular grafts (despite the continued presence of microfilaments) with unaltered connective tissue structure. Therefore, cold-stored arteries may provide a reliable, but noncontractile vascular prosthesis with reduced antigenicity. These findings warrant further study.

▶ This study concludes exactly what one would predict. Namely, after 4 weeks or so of cold storage, all viable cells are gone and we are left with the extracellular framework and elastic lamellae. Presumably, this will decrease the antigenic burden if and when these acellular grafts are subsequently reimplanted. Unfortunately, to date, cold-stored vein grafts have most assuredly not functioned satisfactorily in clinical use, and I don't think they ever will.

### Interstitial Collagenase (MMP-1) Expression in Human Carotid Atherosclerosis

Nikkari ST, O'Brien KD, Ferguson M, et al (Univ of Washington, Seattle; Washington Univ, St Louis, Mo; Univ of Tampere, Finland)
*Circulation* 92:1393–1398, 1995                    1–59

*Background.*—Matrix metalloproteinase-1 (MMP-1) is a proteolytic enzyme that degrades types I and III collagen found in human atherosclerotic plaque. Compromise of atherosclerotic plaque can lead to adverse clinical events. The purpose of this study was to identify the cellular source and location of MMP-1 in human carotid atherosclerotic plaque and examine its role in plaque expansion, rupture, hemorrhage, or other evidence of plaque instability.

*Methods.*—Carotid endarterectomy specimens were obtained from 14 men and 6 women with a mean age of 71 years who were operated on for occlusive carotid disease. All patients had more than 75% occlusion of the common carotid artery. Six nonatherosclerotic carotid arteries from organ donors were used as controls. All specimens were examined by in situ hybridization and immunohistochemistry.

*Results.*—All atherosclerotic carotid endarterectomy specimens had fibrous caps overlying lipid cores containing old, intraplaque hemorrhage ranging from 2% to 73% of lipid core volume. Lipid core size varied from 1 mm$^3$ to 28mm$^3$. In situ hybridization and immunohistochemistry revealed intense expression of MMP-1 mRNA and protein in a subset of plaque macrophages located at the lipid core borders adjacent to fibrous caps. Evidence of some MMP-1 expression was also found in subsets of plaque smooth muscle cells and endothelial cells. There was a direct linear correlation between the percentage of lipid core occupied by hemorrhage and the percentage of lipid core perimeter positive for MMP-1. No MMP-1 was found in any of the nonatherosclerotic human carotid specimens.

*Conclusions.*—Matrix metalloproteinase-1 mRNA and protein are expressed by several cell types but primarily by a subset of plaque macrophages located in areas that are critical to plaque integrity. The strong association between MMP-1 expression and hemorrhage suggests that MMP-1 is an important contributing factor to plaque instability and the resulting adverse clinical events.

▶ This is another study focusing on the mechanism of plaque rupture as the event largely responsible for clinical complications of atherosclerosis. As seen in Abstracts 1–7 and 1–26, things are undoubtedly not that simple. Nonetheless, these authors conclude that the finding of MMP-1 enzyme in human carotid atherosclerosis correlates with histopathologic evidence of plaque instability. They circuitously conclude that this substance may be important in plaque rupture. Perhaps.

### In Situ Localization and Quantification of Seventy-Two-Kilodalton Type IV Collagenase in Aneurysmal, Occlusive, and Normal Aorta

McMillan WD, Patterson BK, Keen RR, et al (Northwestern Univ, Chicago)
*J Vasc Surg* 22:295–305, 1995                                        1–60

*Purpose.*—Previous studies have shown that 72-kilodalton (kd) type IV collagenase (MMP-2) is present in inflammatory disease states. Because MMP-2 is a potent collagenase and elastase, it has been postulated that alterations in MMP-2 expression or its inhibitor, tissue inhibitor of metalloproteinases type 2 (TIMP-2), could have an important role in the collagen and elastin destruction found in aneurysmal disease. An attempt was made to clarify the role of MMP-2 in aneurysmal and occlusive aortic disease.

*Methods.*—Infrarenal aortic specimens were obtained from patients undergoing abdominal aortic aneurysm resection or aortobifemoral bypass for occlusive disease, and from 11 autopsied normal controls. Total RNA

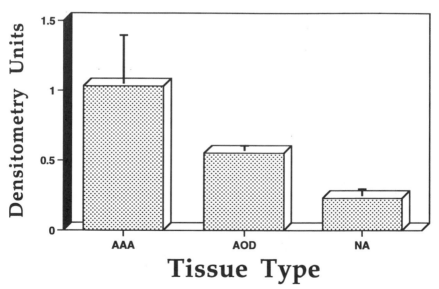

**FIGURE 2.**—Seventy-two kilodalton type IV collagenase messenger RNA in abdominal aortic aneurysms, occlusive aortoiliac tissue, and normal infrarenal aorta. All signals were normalized to α-tubulin to control for loading differences in total RNA and were expressed as mean ± SD. The MMP-2mRNA levels were increased significantly in aneurysmal tissue when compared with occlusive ($P$ <0.02) and normal aorta ($P$ <0.002). No significant differences between MMP-2 occlusive and normal tissue mRNA levels were identified. *Abbreviations: MMP-2 mRNA,* 72-kilodalton type IV collagenase messenger RNA; *AAA,* abdominal aortic aneurysm; *AOD,* occlusive aortoiliac tissue; *NA,* normal infrarenal aorta. (Courtesy of McMillan WD, Patterson BK, Keen RR, et al: In situ localization and quantification of seventy-two-kilodalton type IV collagenase in aneurysmal, occlusive, and normal aorta. *J Vas Surg* 22:295–305, 1995.)

was extracted from the specimens and subjected to Northern analysis and measurement of relative tissue levels of MMP-2 and TIMP-2 mRNA. In addition, aneurysmal and normal vascular smooth muscle cells (VSMCs) were cultured, passaged, and grown to confluence before RNA extraction and Northern analysis.

*Results.*—Both MMP-2 and TIM-2 were expressed in aneurysmal, occlusive, and normal aortic tissue samples. However, the mean MMP-2 RNA level in aneurysmal tissue was almost 2 times higher than that in the occlusive aortic tissue samples, and 5 times higher than that in normal aortic tissue (Fig 2). The differences between the groups were statistically significant ($P<0.005$). However, tissue extraction experiments did not demonstrate statistically significant differences in TIMP-2 mRNA levels between the 3 tissue types ($P=0.34$). Normal and aneurysmal aortic cultured VSMCs constitutively expressed MMP-2 and TIMP-2 mRNA. Both MMP-2 and TIMP-2 were expressed by macrophages and VSMCs within diseased aorta, but the patterns of expression in the 2 disorders differed. Whereas MMP-2 and TIMP-1 expression in occlusive disease was localized primarily to the atherosclerotic plaque, in aneurysmal disease it was found in the adventitia.

*Conclusions.*—Seventy-two kd type IV collagenase expression in aneurysmal tissue samples is significantly greater than it is in either occlusive or normal aortic tissue. Cultured aneurysmal and normal VSMCs constitutively express both MMP-2 and TIMP-2. The finding that the increased MMP-2 levels are localized to VSMCs and macrophages in the adventitia of aortic aneurysms suggests that this enzyme has an important role in the collagen and elastin destruction that characterizes aneurysmal disease.

▶ The search continues to document enzyme abnormalities as the cause of aneurysms. I continue to believe that attempts to reach sophisticated molecular conclusions by studying aneurysms is akin to studying garbage to determine the composition of the garbage can. Many aneurysms, in my experience, consist of a bag of necrotic tissue surrounded by a thin veneer of viable tissue. I continue to believe that attempts at sophisticated vascular biological studies of mature aneurysms will always be consigned to the dustbin of biological uncertainty because of the impossibility of knowing if the observed changes were the cause or the effect of the aneurysm. The legitimate models for study are immature aneurysms in the 3–5 cm range, which contain neither large quantities of intraluminal thrombus nor vascular wall necrosis. I will have considerably greater confidence in data derived from the studies of this tissue as compared to the mature aneurysm. If we confine our analysis to large aneurysms, I fear we will always be dealing with garbage in–garbage out.

## Inhibition of Aortic Aneurysm Development in Blotchy Mice by Beta Adrenergic Blockade Independent of Altered Lysyl Oxidase Activity

Moursi MM, Beebe HG, Messina LM, et al (Univ of Michigan, Ann Arbor; Toledo Hosp, Ohio)
*J Vasc Surg* 21:792–800, 1995                                    1–61

*Purpose.*—The blotchy mouse is an animal model of spontaneous aortic aneurysmal disease. Aneurysm formation in these animals has been attributed to a decrease in lysyl oxidase (LO) activity, an enzyme responsible for elastin and collagen cross-linking. β-Adrenergic blockers retard the development of aortic aneurysms. The mechanism responsible for this protective effect was examined.

*Methods.*—Aortic LO activity and hemodynamic responses associated with β-blocker administration were compared in 3 groups of mice: untreated normal male litter mates of blotchy mice (normal controls, group I), untreated blotchy mice (blotchy controls, group II), and blotchy mice treated with propranolol, atenolol, or nadolol (treated animals, group III). All measurements were obtained when the mice were 4 months of age. The LO activity in the aorta was measured by bioassay.

*Results.*—By 4 months of age, aneurysms were found in the aortic arch of all blotchy controls, but not in the aortic arch of normal controls or

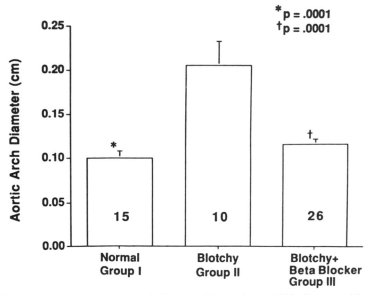

FIGURE 1.—Comparison of aortic arch diameters. Untreated group II blotchy mice exhibited arch diameters ($0.21 \pm 0.03$ cm) significantly greater than either group I normal litter mates ($0.10 \pm 0.01$, $p = 0.0001$) or group III blotchy mice receiving β blockers ($0.11 \pm 0.01$ cm, $p = 0.0001$). Number within *bar* of this and all subsequent figures represents number of animals or specimens analyzed in that specific group. (Courtesy of Moursi MM, Beebe HG, Messina LM, et al: Inhibition of aortic aneurysm development in blotchy mice by beta adrenergic blockade independent of altered lysyl oxidase activity. *J Vasc Surg* 21:792–800, 1995.)

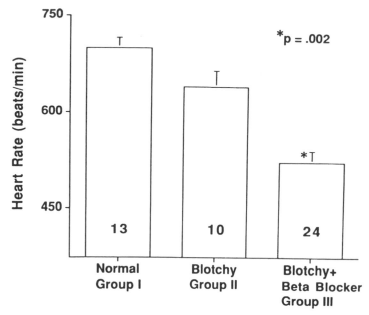

**FIGURE 5.**—Comparison of heart rates. No statistically significant difference was detected between group II blotchy (638 ± 25 beats/min) and group I normal mice (699 ± 16 beats/min). Group III blotchy mice treated with β-blockers exhibited a statistically significant reduction in heart rate (521 ± 17 beats/min) compared with both blotchy and normal groups ($p = 0.002$). (Courtesy of Moursi MM, Beebe HG, Messina LM, et al: Inhibition of aortic aneurysm development in blotchy mice by beta adrenergic blockade independent of altered lysyl oxidase activity. *J Vasc Surg* 21:792–800, 1995.)

β-blocker-treated animals (Fig 1). The LO activity in aortic tissue from blotchy controls was about half of that in tissue from normal controls. Aortic LO activity in treated blotchy mice was not increased, compared with untreated blotchy controls, but was significantly less than that in normal controls. However, treated animals had a 25% reduction in heart rate compared with normal controls or untreated controls (Fig 5). All 3 β-blockers produced the same reduction in heart rate, supporting the view that LO was not involved in the reduction in heart rate, and that β-blockers do not act by a direct effect on collagen or elastin cross-linking. There was no significant difference in systolic blood pressure between the 3 groups.

*Conclusions.*—The effect of β-blockade on the inhibition of aneurysm development in blotchy mice appears to be related to hemodynamic alterations, rather than to alterations in aortic LO activity.

▶ The real question is, should patients with small aneurysms be given β-blocker to reduce the rate of aneurysm development and/or enlargement? Certainly in this highly structured mouse model, β-blockers appeared effective in the short haul. It will be interesting to see if the recently proposed multicenter trial to evaluate this in patients is funded.

## Increased Turnover of Collagen in Abdominal Aortic Aneurysms, Demonstrated by Measuring the Concentration of the Aminoterminal Propeptide of Type III Procollagen in Peripheral and Aortal Blood Samples

Satta J, Juvonen T, Haukipuro K, et al (Univ of Oulu, Finland)
*J Vasc Surg* 22:155–160, 1995      1–62

*Purpose.*—The pathogenesis of abdominal aortic aneurysm (AAA) is still unclear, but elastin degradation in the abdominal wall is thought to be associated with the initial aneurysmal dilation. The major collagens in the aortic wall are types I and III, with collagen type III largely responsible for the tensile strength of the aortic wall. It has been suggested that changes in collagen structure predispose the AAA to rupture. The question of whether changes in serum levels of a biologically relevant marker of type III collagen turnover are involved in AAA was examined.

*Methods.*—The study was done in 87 patients with a mean age of 69.9 years, who were hospitalized with a diagnosis of AAA. Twenty-nine patients with femorodistal arteriosclerotic disease (FDD) and 61 patients with aortoiliac occlusive disease (AOD) served as controls. Concentrations of the aminoterminal propeptide of type III procollagen (PIIINP) and the carboxyterminal propeptide of type I collagen in peripheral venous blood were measured by radioimmunoassay. Aortic blood samples were obtained from above and below the aneurysm in 13 patients who had elective surgery and also in 13 age- and sex-matched controls with AOD who had aortography. The abdominal aorta was visualized by B-mode ultrasound.

*Results.*—The mean serum PIIINP concentration in patients with AAA was higher than that in the control groups. There was a slight positive correlation between serum PIIINP values and the diameter of the AAA, and a more distinct positive correlation between serum PIIINP values and the maximum thickness of the intraluminal thrombus. There was a statistically significant difference between the mean gradient of the PIIINP concentrations at the upper and lower ends of the abdominal aorta in AAA patients and that in the 13 controls with AOD who underwent aortography and aortic blood sampling. The overall PIIINP levels in both control groups were in line with previously established values for normal populations.

*Conclusions.*—Turnover of type III collagen is increased in patients with AAA as demonstrated by increased PIIINP levels in peripheral venous blood. These findings further support the view that AAA rupture is preceded by changes in collagen structure.

▶ I suspect these authors are correct that there is indeed increased turnover of type III collagen in patients with AAAs. The evidence is consistent that tissue from aneurysm contains numerous proteases and collagenases. However, as mentioned in the comment to Abstract 1–60, it is unclear whether the detected changes are the cause or the effect of the aneurysm.

I do not believe we will ever accurately assess the relationship of the cart to the horse from studies upon mature aneurysms.

---

**Graft Smooth Muscle Cells Specifically Synthesize Increased Collagen**
Mesh CL, Majors A, Mistele D, et al (Case Western Reserve Univ, Cleveland, Ohio; Cleveland Clinic Research Inst, Ohio)
J Vasc Surg 22:142–149, 1995                                           1–63

---

*Purpose.*—The healing process in arterial grafts after bypass surgery involves the migration and proliferation of smooth muscle cells (SMC) and the deposition of extracellular matrix components such as collagen and elastin. However, ultimately 80% of the volume of the mature intimal lesion consists of extracellular matrix, mostly collagen. The role of cellular collagen synthesis in healing arteries was examined in an experimental canine study.

*Methods.*—Thoracoabdominal bypass grafts were implanted by standard surgical methodology in female beagles. Twenty weeks after operation, the graft and adjacent native artery were excised; the graft was carefully separated from the native artery at the anastomosis. Vascular SMCs were harvested from anastomotic graft segments and adjacent na-

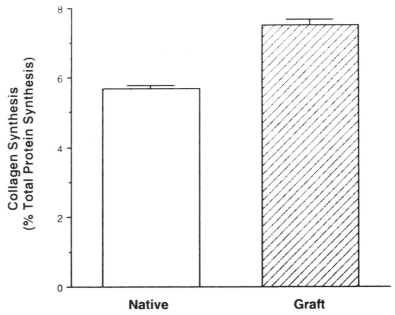

FIGURE 3.—Collagen synthesis as percentage of total protein synthesis in graft anastomotic and adjacent native aortic SMCs. Graft anastomotic SMCs produced significantly more collagen as percentage of total protein synthesis than did adjacent native aortic SMC (mean ± standard error; $n = 6$; $P = 0.001$). *Abbreviations*: SMC, smooth muscle cell. (Courtesy of Mesh CL, Majors A, Mistele D, et al: Graft smooth muscle cells specifically synthesize increased collagen. *J Vasc Surg* 22:142–149, 1995.)

tive artery segments, grown in cell culture to near confluence, and assayed for collagen synthesis and total protein synthesis.

*Results.*—The SMCs harvested from grafts reached confluence faster than SMCs harvested from adjacent native artery. Total collagen synthesis in anastomotic graft SMCs was significantly increased compared with that in adjacent native artery SMCs. Total protein synthesis varied between animals, but there was no significant difference between total protein synthesis in grafts and that in native artery. However, collagen synthesis as a percentage of total protein synthesis in graft SMCs was increased by a mean of 23%, compared with that in native SMCs (Fig 3). Graft SMCs showed modest increases in type I α-1 procollagen mRNA levels as compared to native artery, but the difference did not reach statistical significance.

*Conclusions.*—Smooth muscle cells harvested from canine bypass graft anastomotic segments produce more collagen, both per cell and as a percentage of total protein synthesis, than SMCs from adjacent native artery.

▶ Because intimal hyperplasia is largely composed of matrix protein derived from SMCs, it is gratifying to see more attention devoted to this subject. In the present study, the authors ask whether SMCs from areas of anastomotic intimal hyperplasia in dogs behave differently than SMCs in adjacent normal artery. To do this, however, the authors have explanted these cells and compared their behavior in culture, which itself significantly modifies SMC behavior and may diminish the expected differences between the proliferating, synthetic phenotype of SMCs found in intimal hyperplasia and the quiescent, contractile SMCs found in normal artery. The results of this study are confusing inasmuch as the authors report that anastomotic SMCs reached confluence more rapidly than normal arterial SMCs, but showed no difference in thymidine incorporation (and thus proliferation). I cannot explain this discrepancy, and neither did the authors. Their finding that anastomotic SMCs showed increased collagen synthesis is not surprising, given that collagen is the principal component of this hyperplastic matrix, and it is derived from SMCs. It is not clear whether this represents a unique behavior of SMCs in this setting or is a nonspecific response to any SMC stimulation. To address these questions in vivo, there are a variety of techniques, such as in situ hybridization, that hopefully will allow the authors to better define differences between anastomotic SMCs and normal SMCs in future studies. As the authors are aware, matrix deposition depends on the balance between protein production and proteinase production, both of which are derived from SMCs. A better understanding of the genetic regulation of both of these SMC products in vivo will be necessary to understand the regulation of matrix deposition during intimal hyperplasia.

**J. Cronenwett, M.D.**

### Fluid Shear Stress Stimulates Mitogen-Activated Protein Kinase in Endothelial Cells

Tseng H, Peterson TE, Berk BC (Univ of Washington, Seattle)
*Circ Res* 77:869–878, 1995                                              1–64

*Background.*—Endothelial cell function is governed by local changes in the hemodynamic environment. However, little is known about the signal transduction mechanisms affecting this process. Physical forces are known to activate mitogen-activated protein (MAP) kinases. The signal events occurring in the endothelial cell response to fluid shear stress were studied by measuring the phosphorylation and enzyme activity of MAP kinase.

*Methods and Results.*—In studies of cultured endothelial cells from bovine aorta, physiologic shear stress flows of 3.5 to 117 dyne/cm$^2$ activated MAP kinases of 42 and 44 kD. This response was inhibited by the nonhydrolyzable GDP analog GDP-βS, suggesting that MAP kinase activation required activation of a G protein. Experiments with protein kinase C (PKC) inhibition suggested that PKC inhibition was necessary as well. Flow increased both $Ca^{2+}$-dependent and $Ca^{2+}$-independent PKC activity, as measured by translocation and substrate phosphorylation. Chelation of $Ca^{2+}$ did not cause an inhibitory effect, suggesting that MAP kinase activation did not require $Ca^{2+}$ mobilization.

*Conclusions.*—The role played by fluid shear stress in the activation of MAP kinase in endothelial cells is examined. Two signal transduction pathways appear to be involved in this process. Phospholipase C activation and increased intracellular $Ca^{2+}$ are involved in 1 pathway, which is $Ca^{2+}$-dependent. The other pathway, which is $CA^{2+}$-independent, involves G protein activation and increased PKC and MAP kinase activity.

▶ I have been absolutely fascinated over the years by the unequivocal demonstration that vascular endothelium possesses shear stress receptors, and that activation of these receptors has significant effects. This remarkable study concludes that blood flow activates at least 2 distinct signal transduction pathways in endothelial cells, 1 calcium-dependent, involving the activation of phospholipase C, and a new pathway, calcium-independent, involving G protein and increases in PKC and MAP kinase activity. The tendency of the artery to maintain normal shear stress by either vascular dilatation or, as suggested by the University of Chicago group, by intraluminal atherosclerotic deposition, is possibly related to the signal transduction pathway now being described for the first time.

## Failure of Heparin to Inhibit Intimal Hyperplasia in Injured Baboon Arteries: The Role of Heparin-Sensitive and -Insensitive Pathways in the Stimulation of Smooth Muscle Cell Migration and Proliferation

Geary RL, Koyama N, Wang TW, et al (Univ of Washington, Seattle; Wake Forest Univ, Winston-Salem, NC)
*Circulation* 91:2972–2981, 1995                                                1–65

*Background.*—In vitro and in vivo studies in animal models have shown that heparin is a potent inhibitor of smooth muscle cell (SMC) hyperplasia. This has been demonstrated by heparin's inhibition of intimal hyperplasia in rat carotid arteries after vascular injury. Although heparin has been shown to inhibit SMC hyperplasia in humans in vitro, results of in vivo experiments in humans have been negative.

*Objective.*—The objective of this study, conducted by the University of Washington (Seattle) and Wake Forest Schools of Medicine, was to assess the effects of low molecular weight heparin (LMWH) on SMC proliferation and migration in baboon arteries that had been subjected to vascular injury.

*Methods.*—The saphenous arteries of 12 male baboons were subjected to catheter-induced intimal denudation. The animals were then randomly assigned to receive continuous infusions of either LMWH or saline. Plasma levels of LMWH and coagulation profiles were obtained at 7 and 28 days. After 28 days, bromodeoxyuridine was injected intramuscularly to label the nuclei and permit counting of proliferating SMCs. The saphenous arteries were removed and examined histologically. To determine whether heparin inhibition of SMC proliferation varied depending on the mitogen used, cell cultures were taken from the intima of the aorta, internal jugular vein, and peripheral arteries of 3 baboons. The stimulating mitogens used were normal serum and platelet-derived growth factor. Smooth muscle cell migration was assayed by a modification of the Boyden method.

*Results.*—At 28 days, all balloon-injured arteries, regardless of the infusion used, had re-endothelialized. Low–molecular-weight heparin failed to inhibit intimal thickening or SMC proliferation. Uninjured arteries showed no evidence of significant SMC proliferation or intimal thickening. In cultures, LMWH and, to a lesser degree, standard heparin, both inhibited serum-stimulated SMC proliferation, but neither LMWH nor standard heparin inhibited SMC proliferation induced by platelet-derived growth factor. These data are presented in Table 3.

*Conclusions.*—Low–molecular-weight heparin failed to inhibit intimal hyperplasia that had been induced in baboon arteries by balloon catheterization. Additionally, LMWH inhibited serum-induced SMC proliferation in culture but failed to inhibit SMC migration and proliferation that had been induced by platelet-derived growth factor. This suggests that both heparin-sensitive and -insensitive pathways exist for SMC stimulation. The relative importance of each pathway may vary between species and explain species differences in the response to heparin.

TABLE 3.—Heparin Inhibition of Smooth Muscle Cell Proliferation in Culture

| | Percent of Serum Stimulation | Percent of PDGF-BB Stimulation |
|---|---|---|
| Inhibition by standard heparin ($n = 3$ animals) | | |
| Saphenous artery | 25.5±7.5 | 126.5±30.8 |
| Aorta | 46.4±17.6 | 69.4±5.5 |
| Jugular vein | 16.3±3.8 | 77.0±7.1 |
| Mean of all sites | 29.4±8.2* | 91.0±14.4 |
| Inhibition by low-molecular-weight heparin ($n = 2$ animals) | | |
| Saphenous artery | 65.7±6.6 | 145.5±11.1 |
| Aorta | 54.5±10.5 | 93.2±4.8 |
| Jugular vein | 61.3±4.8 | 114.3±19.2 |
| Mean of all sites | 60.5±4.0* | 117.7±11.3 |

(Courtesy of Geary RL, Koyama N, Wang TW, et al: Failure of heparin to inhibit intimal hyperplasia in injured baboon arteries: The role of heparin-sensitive and -insensitive pathways in the stimulation of smooth muscle cell migration and proliferation. *Circulation* 1995; 91:2972–2981. Reproduced with permission *Circulation*. Copyright 1995 American Heart Association.)

▶ In this study, the Clowes' laboratory continues its indefatigable assault on intimal hyperplasia. These investigators have previously demonstrated that heparin (and nearly everything else) will inhibit intimal hyperplasia after rat carotid artery injury, but that these same agents have little effect in baboons. This suggests an important species-specific effect that likely explains the failure to inhibit intimal hyperplasia in a variety of clinical trials. In the present study, the authors discovered that LMWH is also ineffective for preventing intimal hyperplasia in baboons. Beyond this negative result, they also investigated details of heparin inhibition of SMC proliferation and found that heparin will inhibit SMC proliferation in serum but not when stimulated by platelet-derived growth factor. Thus, they conclude that there are both heparin-sensitive and -insensitive mechanisms for SMC proliferation (and intimal hyperplasia development). This is another way of saying that many factors likely contribute to the development of intimal hyperplasia and that no single inhibitory technique is likely to be successful. Inasmuch as they incriminated a heparin-insensitive, platelet-associated pathway, I am sure they are already investigating the combination of heparin and aspirin in their baboon model. Importantly, in this ongoing series of investigations, the authors have demonstrated the irrelevance of results in the rat carotid injury model for predicting the potential therapeutic success of agents to inhibit intimal hyperplasia in humans.

**J. Cronenwett, M.D.**

### Doxycycline Inhibition of Aneurysmal Degeneration in an Elastase-Induced Rat Model of Abdominal Aortic Aneurysm: Preservation of Aortic Elastin Associated With Suppressed Production of 92 kD Gelatinase

Petrinec D, Liao S, Holmes DR, et al (Washington Univ, St Louis, Mo)
*J Vasc Surg* 23:336–346, 1996                                                    1–66

*Background.*—Increased local production of matrix metalloproteinases (MMPs) may contribute to structural protein deterioration in abdominal aortic aneurysms (AAA). Pharmacologic treatment with an MMP-inhibitor tetracycline could prohibit the occurrence of experimental AAA in vivo, and this hypothesis was tested using an elastase-induced rodent model.

*Methods.*—A 2-hour perfusion of the abdominal aorta was done in 48 Wistar rats using 50 U of porcine pancreatic elastase. Twenty-four of the animals subsequently were treated with 25 mg of doxycycline, administered subcutaneously on a daily basis, whereas 24 received saline solution vehicle. Measurements of aortic diameter were obtained before and after elastase perfusion and before animals were sacrificed at 0, 2, 7, or 14 days. Abdominal aortic aneurysms were considered as an increase in aortic diameter that was more than twice that noted before perfusion. Aortic tissues were perfusion-fixed for histologic assessment or extracted for substrate zymographic assessment at the time of death.

*Results.*—No between-group differences in aortic diameter were noted at 0 or 2 days. At both 7 and 14 days, however, aortic diameters in the doxycycline-treated animals were significantly less than those in the untreated animals. The occurrence of AAA was decreased from 83% (10 of 12 control animals) to 8% (1 of 12 doxycycline-treated animals) after day 2. Doxycycline blocked the structural degradation of aortic elastin without reducing the influx of inflammatory cells. An increase in aortic wall production of 92 kD gelatinase was noted in the saline solution control group. In comparison, production was notably suppressed in the doxycycline-treated animals.

*Conclusions.*—The occurrence of experimental AAA in vivo is suppressed by treatment with an MMP-inhibiting tetracycline. This inhibition may be the result of selective blockage of elastolytic MMP expression in infiltrating inflammatory cells. Further studies are needed to fully clarify this process.

▶ In rats, the inhibition of MMP enzymes, in this case by tetracycline, limits the development of the aneurysms induced by aortic perfusion with elastase. This forces one to conclude that elastase does not directly cause aneurysm development, but does so only through the recruitment of inflammatory cells, which in turn elaborate MMP. The authors' suggestion that MMP inhibition may be a potential target for the pharmacotherapy of small aneurysms appears a bit of a stretch.

### Differential-Display Polymerase Chain Reaction Identifies Nucleophosmin as an Estrogen-Regulated Gene in Human Vascular Smooth Muscle Cells

Koike H, Karas RH, Baur WE, et al (Tufts Univ, Boston)

*J Vasc Surg* 23:477–482, 1996

1–67

*Introduction.*—The leading cause of morbidity and death in American women is atherosclerotic disease of the coronary and peripheral vessels. After menopause, the incidence of cardiovascular disease increases sharply in women, suggesting that estrogen exerts a protective effect on the development of atherosclerosis. Whereas it has been shown that estrogen can regulate vascular cell function directly, the molecular mechanisms responsible for such effects are not clear. A highly sensitive screening method, differential-display polymerase chain reaction, was used to identify altered gene expression in human vascular smooth muscle cells whose expression was altered by estrogen exposure.

*Methods.*—Using 10% fetal bovine serum in the absence or presence of $10^{-8}$ mol/L estrogen, human vascular smooth muscle cells were stimulated and total cellular RNA was harvested. On each RNA sample, differential-display polymerase chain reaction was performed 3 times and the differentially expressed candidate genes were isolated. Dot blotting confirmed differential expression of candidate genes. Sequence analysis identified positive bands. Immunoblotting was used to investigate estrogen-mediated regulation at the protein level.

*Results.*—A 462 bp gene product, EAo8, was identified as a candidate estrogen-regulated gene from RNA harvested from aortic vascular smooth muscle cells using differential-display polymerase chain reaction. In response to estrogen treatment, there was a $5.8 \pm 3.9$-fold increase in EAo8 expression, which was demonstrated using dot blotting with probes derived from 4 independent vascular smooth muscle cells. Using sequence analysis, EAo8 was identified as nucleophosmin, a nuclear phosphoprotein that regulates cell growth and synthesizes protein. Immunoblotting in the saphenous vein and the mammary artery vascular smooth muscle cells showed estrogen-induced expression of nucleophosmin protein.

*Conclusion.*—In human vascular smooth muscle cells, estrogen induces nucleophosmin expression. Estrogen-regulated gene expression in vascular smooth muscle cells can be effectively studied using differential-display polymerase chain reaction. This study represents the first step in demonstrating the molecular mechanisms by which estrogen can regulate vascular cell function.

▶ The Tufts group has been interested for a considerable time in the effects of the female sex hormones on the vascular wall. Earlier, they demonstrated the presence of a functional estrogen receptor on human vascular smooth muscle cells. Activation of the estrogen receptor results in many vascular smooth muscle effects, such as nitric oxide production, stimulation of endothelial cell migration, and proliferation of vascular smooth muscle. Herein, the authors conduct a sophisticated series of experiments in an effort to identify estrogen-regulated genes. Their results suggest that such an estrogen-regulated gene product may be nucleophosmin, a protein implicated in the regulation of cell growth and protein synthesis. The potential relationships of observations such as this to the relative protection from atherosclerosis enjoyed by premenopausal women remains to be discovered. This certainly appears to be a fruitful area of inquiry. See also Abstract 1–57.

# 2 Endovascular

## Endovascular Grafts

### Endovascular Repair of Abdominal Aortic Aneurysms and Other Arterial Lesions

Parodi JC (Instituto Cardiovascular de Buenos Aires, Argentina)
J Vasc Surg 21:549–557, 1995
2–1

*Background.*—Elective replacement with a synthetic graft has long been the accepted method to prevent rupture of abdominal aortic aneurysm (AAA). The increasing number of older patients with severe comorbid medical conditions has led to a search for a simpler and less invasive treatment of this lesion. After a series of experiments in dogs, endovascular graft treatment of AAAs was introduced in the clinical setting. This procedure, which has now been performed on 50 patients with AAAs or aortoiliac aneurysms, is described here and its application reported for 7 patients with other arterial lesions.

*Methods.*—Forty-five men and 5 women with an average age of 73 years were treated between September 1990 and April 1994. In all but 3 cases the diameter of the aneurysms was larger than 5 cm; none had ruptured. Other arterial lesions treated included 5 posttraumatic arteriovenous fistulas, 1 infected femoral false aneurysm, and 1 false aneurysm of the right common carotid artery. Associated pathologic conditions were common in the patient group, with 25 having severe, chronic heart disease and 20 severe pulmonary insufficiency. Devices used in endovascular graft treatment consisted of either a Dacron or an autogenous vein graft sutured to a balloon-expandable stent. The stented grafts were placed through remote arteriotomies, advanced under fluoroscopic guidance to predetermined sites, then secured into position.

*Results.*—Forty (80%) of the procedures for AAA or aortoiliac exclusion were judged successful, based upon complete exclusion of the aneurysm and restoration of normal blood flow. Although 4 patients required a second covered stent to repair an initial leak, recovery after successful graft repair was rapid. Ten AAA procedures were failures, associated with procedural death in 5 cases and leaks in 5. All 7 patients with arteriovenous fistulas or false aneurysms had a successful outcome. With a mean follow-up of 17 months, the ultimate outcome has been satisfactory in those surviving the procedure.

*Conclusion.*—Based upon these preliminary data and short-term follow-up, endovascular stented graft procedures appear to be feasible for treating AAAs and other arterial lesions. A number of technical problems related to the procedure and the stented graft devices are yet to be resolved, however, as well as the complication of microembolization that led to death in 3 of 4 cases.

▶ Dr. Parodi describes experience with 50 patients treated with endografts for AAAs, and 7 patients for other indications. He forthrightly presents the problems encountered, including difficulty with precise measurement of the diameter and length of the involved artery, access problem through stenotic and tortuous iliac arteries, absence of a distal aortic cuff, stent migration, and finally, microembolism, which he considers to be the most important unsolved problem with endovascular grafts for aneurysm treatment. Dr. Parodi concludes, presciently, that much work remains to be done to solve these problems. On balance, this is a thoughtful and sobering appraisal of the field by its innovator. We should all pay careful attention to these comments.

---

**Transfemoral Endovascular Repair of Abdominal Aortic Aneurysm: Results of the North American EVT Phase 1 Trial**
Moore WS, for the EVT Investigators (Emory Univ, Atlanta, Ga; Henry Ford Hosp, Detroit; Massachusetts Gen Hosp, Boston; et al)
*J Vasc Surg* 23:543–553, 1996                                                    2–2

---

*Background.*—Only 1 device—the endovascular grafting system (EGS) designed by Lazarus—has been approved for clinical trial in the United States for endovascular repair of abdominal aortic aneurysm (AAA). The EGS was studied in a phase 1 trial of transfemoral repair of AAA (Fig 1).

*Methods.*—The trial included 46 patients treated at 13 centers in the United States. The AAAs ranged from 3.8 to 7.1 cm in diameter. Fifteen

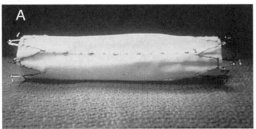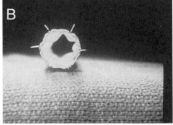

FIGURE 1.—**A,** opened-out appearance of endograft, a lightweight woven-Dacron graft. Radiopaque markers have been sewn in longitudinal axis. Both proximal and distal attachment systems are fully expanded. **B,** end-on view of endograft. Attachment system is fully expanded; 6 radially arranged pins are designed to engage wall of aorta and are seated with expandable balloon. (Courtesy of Moore WS, for the EVT Investigators: Transfemoral endovascular repair of abdominal aortic aneurysm: Results of the North American EVT phase 1 trial. *J Vasc Surg* 23:543–553, 1996.)

patients underwent repair with the original device (EGS-I) and 31 with a revised over-the-wire device (EGS-II). The patients were followed up with contrast-enhanced CT scans, color-flow duplex scans, and plain abdominal radiographs to assess the stability of the prosthesis, any vascular communication with or entry of blood into the aneurysmal sac, or any change in aneurysmal size.

*Results.*—The implants were successfully placed in 85% of patients in an average of 194 minutes. The remaining 7 attempts were converted to open repairs, including one third of cases using the EGS-I. Most conversions were necessitated by iliac stenosis. There were no deaths within 1 month after surgery. The most common complication was transient unexplained fever in 9 patients, followed by iliofemoral arterial injury and need for transfusion in 8 patients each, wound infection in 7 patients, minor emboli with foot petechiae in 2 patients, and myocardial infarction in 1 patient. None of the patients required amputation nor experienced major emboli or mesenteric ischemia. At first, 17 grafts showed contrast enhancement outside the graft but contained within the aneurysmal sac; 53% of these leaks resolved on their own. Eight patients showed persistent leakage into the aneurysmal sac, although 6 had no signs of aneurysm enlargement in up to 26 months' follow-up. Transluminal balloon angioplasty and surgical removal of the graft were required in 1 patient each.

The patients stayed in the hospital for an average of 4 days. One patient died of respiratory failure, unrelated to EGS placement, at 6 months. The metallic attachment system fractured in 23% of cases. One of these implants had to be removed, but the other 8 continued to function normally. This source of device-related malfunction led to suspension of the study protocol.

*Conclusions.*—The safety and efficacy of endovascular repair of AAA are demonstrated in this phase I trial. Fracture of the attachment system has been a problem, the long-term consequences of which remain to be determined. There is also concern about the long-term effects of leakage into the aneurysmal sac. The defect in the attachment system has been corrected, and approval to proceed with the phase 2 portion of the implant study has been granted.

▶ At present, this form of aneurysm repair appears appropriate for only about 15% of screened AAA patients. A number of patients with attempted endograft require conversion to conventional surgery. Of considerable concern is the presence of persistent leak into the aneurysm sac in 18% of patients at 1 year. I suspect that as the infrarenal aorta dilates with time, the number that develop a leak ultimately will be considerably higher than this. It is important from time to time for us to drop back to review clearly just what we are trying to accomplish by the endovascular grafting of infrarenal aneurysms. Currently, there is no indication that morbidity or mortality is any different from operative surgery. Initial indications suggest there will be no substantial difference in cost, compared with conventional operative surgery. I still believe the only real benefit will be a somewhat more rapid period of recovery, the significance of which does not appear overwhelming. I continue to have significant reservations about the future of endovascular grafts. I suppose, as so often happens in vascular surgery, the procedure will eventually sort itself out as being appropriate for a few highly selected patients. I doubt its widespread applicability.

### Surgical Management of Complications Following Endoluminal Grafting of Abdominal Aortic Aneurysms

May J, White GH, Yu W, et al (Royal Prince Alfred Hosp, Australia; Univ of Sydney, Australia)

*Eur J Vasc Endovasc Surg* 10:51–59, 1995                                    2–3

*Background.*—Although endoluminal repair of abdominal aortic aneurysms (AAA) has been shown to be a feasible procedure, the associated risks and long-term outcomes are unknown. The outcomes and complications of endoluminal grafting of AAA are reported.

*Methods.*—The experience included 53 patients who underwent endoluminal repair of AAA during a 2-year period. All of the operations were performed on an elective basis, and all patients were prepared for open surgery in case the endoluminal repair failed. Tubular endografts were used in 36 cases, tapered aortoiliac/aortofemoral grafts in 12, and bifurcated grafts in 5. All grafts were placed in the aorta under radiographic guidance via a delivery sheath through the femoral or iliac arteries.

*Results.*—Eighty-one percent of patients had successful endoluminal repair. In the rest, the endoluminal procedure was converted to an open repair. The rate of local or vascular complications was 32%, and the rate of systemic or remote complications was 25%. When the complications of successful endoluminal repairs were added to those leading to failure of the endoluminal procedure, the total complication rate was 75%. There were 2 procedure-related cardiac deaths within 30 days, and 4 late deaths that were unrelated to the aneurysm repair procedure. Three of the 4 late deaths occurred in patients with completed endoluminal repairs.

*Conclusions.*—Endoluminal repair of AAA can be carried out successfully in most patients with a low risk of perioperative death. However, there are many complications. The complications leading to failure of endoluminal repair must be added to the systemic or remote and local or vascular complications of successful endoluminal repair when the morbidity of this procedure is considered.

▶ The mortality and morbidity reported herein is clearly not one bit better than what one would expect with conventional surgery for infrarenal aneurysm. In fact, a rather remarkable morbidity of 75% is reported. With time, we are acquiring a more accurate understanding of the complications of this procedure. The procedure is both novel and fascinating. I just wish it worked better.

## Initial Experience With Transluminally Placed Endovascular Grafts for the Treatment of Complex Vascular Lesions

Marin ML, Veith FJ, Cynamon J, et al (Montefiore Med Ctr/Albert Einstein College of Medicine, New York)
*Ann Surg* 222:449–469, 1995                                                    2–4

*Background.*—In patients with other severe medical or surgical problems, it may be impossible to manage complex occlusive, traumatic, and aneurysmal lesions of the arteries by standard surgical techniques. Transluminally placed endovascular grafts may be an option in these situations (Fig 1). An experience with endovascular grafting of arterial lesions is reported.

*Methods.*—A total of 100 arterial lesions in 92 patients were treated with a total of 96 endovascular graft procedures. Forty-eight patients had a total of 53 multilevel limb-threatening aortoiliac and/or femoropopliteal occlusive lesions, 33 patients had a total of 36 large aneurysms of the aorta and/or peripheral artery, and 11 patients had traumatic injuries of the arteries. The latter category included patients with false aneurysms and arteriovenous fistulas. In each case, a remote arteriotomy was used for the placement of endovascular grafts. Epidural anesthesia was used for 43% of operations, general anesthesia for 40%, and local anesthesia for 17%.

*Results.*—The rate of technical and clinical success was 91% for patients with aneurysms, 91% for those with occlusive lesions, and 100% for those

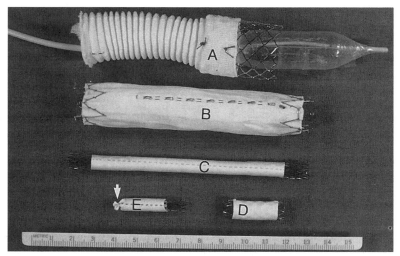

FIGURE 1.—Endovascular grafts used for the repair of aortic and peripheral artery aneurysms, arterial occlusions, and traumatic vascular injuries. **A,** balloon expandable (Parodi) endovascular device; **B,** Endovascular Technologies endograft; **C,** PTFE endovascular graft used for the treatment of peripheral artery aneurysms and arterial occlusive disease; **D,** PTFE-covered Palmaz balloon expandable stent used for the treatment of traumatic arterial injuries; **E,** an occluding PTFE-covered Palmaz stent (1 end of this device is closed with a purse-string suture [*arrow*]). *Abbreviation: PTFE,* polytetrafluoroethylene. (Courtesy of Marin ML, Veith FJ, Cynamon J, et al: Initial experience with transluminally placed endovascular grafts for the treatment of complex vascular lesions. *Ann Surg* 222:449–469, 1995.)

with traumatic arterial lesions. Mean follow-up was 13 months. The 18-month primary patency rate for aortoiliac occlusions was 77%, with a secondary patency rate of 95%. The limb salvage rate at the same interval was 98%. Perigraft channels were detected immediately after excision of aortic aneurysms in one third of cases. Three of the 6 channels closed within 8 weeks. Major complications occurred in 10% of endovascular stented graft procedures and minor complications in 14%. The 30-day mortality in the series as a whole was 6%.

*Conclusions.*—Good results are reported with endovascular grafting of complex arterial lesions. The results warrant further investigation of endovascular graft techniques for major arterial reconstruction.

▶ The initial experience of the Montefiore Group includes a veritable pot-pourri of diseases. Unfortunately, these are all anecdotal cases not performed as part of a precisely defined clinical protocol. Clearly the authors are enthusiastic about the results, but insofar as no 2 cases were either the same or treated the same, it is difficult for the rest of us to take away any hard data from this experience. IDE protocols produce data–anecdotes don't.

## Human Transluminally Placed Endovascular Stented Grafts: Preliminary Histopathologic Analysis of Healing Grafts in Aortoiliac and Femoral Artery Occlusive Disease

Marin ML, Veith FJ, Cynamon J, et al (Montefiore Med Ctr/Albert Einstein College, New York; Instituto Cardiovascular de Buenos Aires, Argentina)
*J Vasc Surg* 21:595–604, 1995                                    2–5

*Objective.*—The healing of transluminally placed endovascular stented grafts (TPEGs), used to treat occlusive disease, has not been studied. The preliminary histopathologic analysis of explanted human TPEGs is reported.

*Methods.*—A total of 26 polyfluoroethylene stent grafts were placed in 21 patients with limb-threatening ischemia. During the follow-up period, 2 patients died of heart disease, and graft stenosis developed in 5. The 7 grafts were recovered, fixed in formalin, embedded in paraffin, and sectioned. Sections were stained with hematoxylin, eosin, and trichrome and with antigens to PC-10, alpha smooth muscle actin, MAC-387, Ulex-Europeaus, and factor VIII.

*Results.*—After 3 weeks, organizing thrombus encased both surfaces; at 6 weeks, a neointima was present near the anastomosis, and at 3 months, a neointima was present 1 to 3 cm from the anastomotic site. Factor-VIII positive cells were seen at 8 cm from the anastomotic site in 1 specimen explanted at 5 months. Grafts that contained an external wrap or were placed intra-adventitially demonstrated a foreign body reaction typified by mononuclear and multinucleated giant cells. Medially inserted grafts had a less pronounced reaction and were surrounded by antialpha smooth muscle positive cells. Little PC-10 labeling was observed in plaque tissues.

*Conclusion.*—Endovascular stented grafts used to treat extensive atherosclerotic occlusive vascular disease appear to have a healing advantage over conventional grafts. Failure as a result of the occurrence of neointimal hyperplasia and progressive atherosclerotic disease in outflow vessels is still a problem.

▶ Histopathology on 7 recovered endovascular grafts from humans reveals about the findings one would expect. Did anyone really expect the histopathology to differ substantially from that of grafts conventionally placed?

## Delayed Rupture of Aortic Aneurysms Following Endovascular Stent Grafting

Lumsden AB, Allen RC, Chaikof EL, et al (Emory Univ, Atlanta, Ga; Morristown Mem Hosp, NJ; Columbia Univ, NY)
*Am J Surg* 170:174–178, 1995                        2–6

*Background.*—For patients with abdominal aortic aneurysms, endovascular stent graft placement via the transfemoral route avoids the need for an abdominal incision and aortic cross-clamping, offers the potential for regional anesthesia, and reduces hospital stay. However, there are continuing questions about the ability of these devices to exclude the aneurysm completely and prevent aneurysmal rupture, as well as concerns about their long-term integrity. There are also important questions about what training is necessary to perform these procedures. Two patients with delayed rupture of aortic aneurysms after endoluminal aortic stent graft placement are reported.

*Patients.*—Both patients had Dacron endovascular grafts placed for the treatment of infrarenal abdominal aortic aneurysms. The grafts were anchored proximally and distally by Palmaz stents. One patient lacked a distal cuff and so should not have been treated by endovascular graft stenting—the graft did not reach the level of the aortic bifurcation. The patient died as a result of aneurysmal rupture 4 months after graft deployment.

The other patient did have appropriate vascular anatomy for endovascular stent grafting but experienced persistent perigraft leakage at the distal anastomosis. Two weeks later, the aneurysm ruptured. Emergency aneurysm repair was successful, although the patient experienced acute renal failure.

*Discussion.*—Complications of transfemoral endovascular stent grafting may be avoided by appropriate patient selection, especially preoperative evaluation of the aortic anatomy. Patients without a distal cuff of at least 1 cm should not undergo this procedure. In addition, when perigraft leakage is present, the endograft will not prevent aneurysmal rupture. All patients undergoing endovascular graft stenting must be evaluated by vascular surgeons before the operation. When complications occur, vascular surgeons must be involved in their evaluation and management.

▶ This is the chilling report that we have all been fearing. Two patients with perigraft leaks after abdominal aortic aneurysm endograft deployment presented with aneurysm rupture, 14 days and 4 months after surgery, respectively, with death occurring in 1 of the patients. Clearly a perigraft leak represents a threat to life. We now know that about 20% of patients have perigraft leakage at 12 months, and it is likely that more will develop as time passes because of the inevitable dilatation of the infrarenal aorta with disattachment of the proximal anchoring stent. This may well represent the fatal flaw in the concept.

## Stents

### Hydrophilic Surface Modification of Metallic Endoluminal Stents
Seeger JM, Ingegno MD, Bigatan E, et al (Univ of Florida, Gainesville)
*J Vasc Surg* 22:327–336, 1995                                           2–7

*Objective.*—The use of metallic stents after balloon dilatation seals intimal dissections, decreases arterial recoil, and may improve long-term patency, but metallic stents are inherently thrombogenic. Coating the surface of the stent with a polymer could improve hemocompatibility. Results of a study of a hydrophilic coating on the stent surface to minimize platelet reactivity are presented.

*Methods.*—Stainless steel stents and slabs were coated with hydrophilic N-vinylpyrrolidone (neutral [NVP]) and potassium sulfopropyl acrylate (highly anionic [KSPA]) monomers using the plasma-γ technique. Surfaces were scanned with an electron microscope and x-ray photoelectron spectrometry. In vivo and in vitro platelet reactivity were determined as [111]Indium-labeled accumulation.

*Results.*—Contact angle measurements and spectral examinations showed a significant increase in surface hydrophilicity after coating. Adhesion of [111]Indium-labeled platelets and of endothelial cells was significantly decreased by the coating (Fig 4). Albumin adsorption was significantly higher and fibrinogen adsorption was significantly lower on the coated slabs. Microscopic and spectroscopic scans demonstrated that monomer coating smoothed the stainless steel surfaces.

*Conclusion.*—Because hydrophilic polymer coating of stainless steel stents smooths the surface and decreases platelet adhesion, it may lower the thrombogenic potential associated with these stents.

▶ Perhaps chemical surface modification of stainless steel stents will decrease platelet accumulation and the associated risk of vessel thrombosis. On balance, I suspect any improvements resulting from this will be minimal and not likely to alter the big picture.

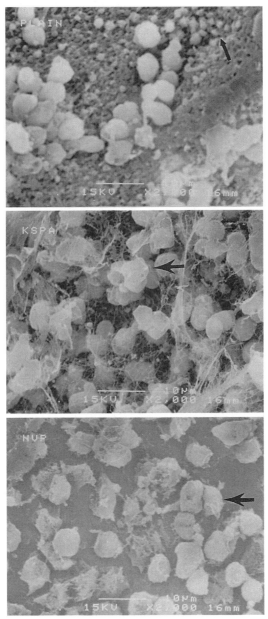

FIGURE 4.—Scanning electron micrographs of plain (**top**), poly-KSPA modified (**middle**), and poly-NVP modified (**bottom**) Palmaz stainless steel stents after 1 hour of blood flow exposure in canine arteriovenous shunt. Significant platelet accumulation (*small arrow*) is seen on surface of plain stent (**top**), whereas red blood cells, white blood cells, and some fibrin (*large arrows*) but few platelets are seen on surface of modified stents (*middle and bottom*). *Abbreviations:* NVP, N-vinylpyrrolidone; KSPA, potassium sulfopropyl acrylate. (Courtesy of Seeger JM, Ingegno MD, Bigatan E, et al: Hydrophilic surface modification of metallic endoluminal stents. *J Vasc Surg* 22:327–336, 1995.)

## Pure β-Particle-Emitting Stents Inhibit Neointima Formation in Rabbits

Hehrlein C, Stintz M, Kinscherf R, et al (Univ of Heidelberg, Germany)
*Circulation* 93:641–645, 1996                                          2–8

*Background.*—Several experimental studies indicate that radiation therapy after balloon angioplasty or stent implantation markedly reduces neointimal hyperplasia in treated arteries. In contrast to γ-radiation, β-particle radiation is absorbed in tissue within a shorter distance away from the source and may be more suitable for localized vessel irradiation. A method to implant β-particle-emitting radioisotope ($^{32}$P; half-life, 14.3 days) into metallic stents was described.

*Methods.*—$^{32}$P activity was produced by neutron irradiation of red amorphous phosphorus ($^{31}$P). $^{32}$P and $^{31}$P were kept separated in a mass separator and the $^{32}$P ions were implanted into Palmaz-Schatz stents (7.5 mm in length). The radioisotope was tightly fixed to the stents, and the ion implantation process did not alter the surface texture. Stent activity levels of 4 and 13 μCi were chosen for the study. Conventional stents and radioisotope stents with activity levels of 4 or 13 μCi were placed in rabbit iliac arteries. Vascular injury and neointima formation were studied by histomorphometry 4 and 12 weeks after stent placement. Immunostaining for smooth muscle cell (SMC) α-actin was performed to determine SMC cellularity in the neointima, and the density of α-actin immunoreactive SMC was measured by computer-assisted counting. Endothelialization of the stents was evaluated by immunostaining for endothelial cell von Willebrand factor.

*Results.*—The extent of vessel wall injury did not differ with conventional and $^{32}$P-implanted stents. At 4 weeks, neointima formation was markedly inhibited in arteries with 4- and 13-mCI radioisotope stents, compared with arteries treated with conventional stents. However, at 12 weeks, neointima formation was potently inhibited only with 13-mCI radioisotope stents. The SMC density in the neointima decreased in a dose-dependent fashion in the $^{32}$P-implanted stents compared with conventional stents. Radioactive stents were endothelialized after 4 weeks, but endothelialization was less dense than in conventional stents.

*Discussion.*—A β-particle-emitting stent incorporating the radioisotope $^{32}$P is very effective in inhibiting neointima formation after angioplasty in rabbits. There is dose-dependent reduction in neointima formation in this type of radioactive stent, indicating that a threshold radiation dose must be delivered to inhibit neointima formation after stent placement over the long term.

▶ The Europeans appear absolutely hung up on the use of radiation to attenuate intimal hyperplasia. I fear this may be akin to burning the house to kill the cockroaches. Nonetheless, these investigators have made a stent radioactive as a delivery system. I think we know that β emitters properly applied will acutely diminish intimal hyperplasia, but I continue to have great concern over the real utility of this methodology. Clearly there is major potential to do harm. See also Abstracts 1–42 and 1–43.

## Lower Extremity Angioplasty

### Efficacy of Balloon Angioplasty of the Superficial Femoral Artery and Popliteal Artery in the Relief of Leg Ischemia

Stanley B, Teague B, Raptis S, et al (Univ of Adelaide, Australia)
*J Vasc Surg* 23:679–685, 1996                                            2–9

*Background.*—Because it is minimally invasive, percutaneous transluminal angioplasty (PTA) is often used to treat leg ischemia. However, its long-term efficacy has not been studied. The short- and long-term efficacy of PTA in treating severe ischemia or claudication due to disease of the superficial femoral and popliteal arteries was studied.

*Methods.*—All patients undergoing PTA of the superficial femoral artery or popliteal artery during a 57-month period were re-evaluated at 1, 3, and 6 months after the procedure and every 6 months thereafter, for symptoms and signs of recurrent disease. Duplex ultrasonography and arteriography were performed if indicated.

*Results.*—During the study period, 176 patients undergoing 200 angioplasties entered the study and were followed up for a median of 25 months. Although 93% of procedures were technically successful, only 73% were still successful at 24 hours. Short occlusions and those with

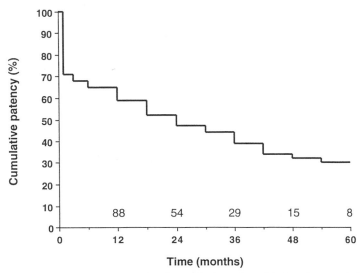

**FIGURE 1.**—Cumulative patency rates for all angioplasties performed during a 5-year period. Primary patency was 58% (SE, 4.0) at 1 year, 46% (SE, 4.7) at 2 years, 38% (SE, 5.8) at 3 years, 30% (SE, 6.8) at 4 years, and 26% (SE, 8.3) at 5 years. (Courtesy of Stanley B, Teague B, Raptis, et al: *J Vasc Surg* 23:679–685, 1996.)

good distal runoff were significantly more likely to be initial successes. There were 51 complications (25%) in 45 procedures. The early success rate was 69% at 1 month. The late success rate was 58% at 1 year and 46% at 2 years, declining to 26% at 5 years (Fig 1). Ten patients required amputation within 6 months after PTA, and 1 at 63 months. Limb survival was 95% at 24 months, with significant predictors being good runoff and presentation with claudication instead of critical ischemia. Overall patient survival was 91% at 2 years, but those presenting with claudication had significantly greater survival than those presenting with severe ischemia.

Conclusion.—The use of PTA for claudication is not recommended, because the 2-year success rate is 49%, and the lesions most likely to remain patent are those that would be expected to do well with conservative management.

▶ Carefully consider the results reported herein. Sixty percent of these patients had stenoses and 74% were undertaken for relief of claudication. The cumulative patency at 24 months for all patients was 46%. The authors appropriately conclude that superficial femoral artery and popliteal angioplasty occasionally works, but is associated with a high initial failure rate and very poor patency at 24 months. They go on to note specifically that, in their opinion, infrainguinal balloon angioplasty should not be used for treatment of claudication. Amen, Amen, and Amen!

---

**The Cost-Effectiveness of Treatment of Short Occlusive Lesions in the Femoropopliteal Artery: Balloon Angioplasty Versus Endarterectomy**
Vroegindeweij D, Idu M, Buth J, et al (Catharina Hosp, Eindhoven, The Netherlands)
*Eur J Vasc Endovasc Surg* 10:40–50, 1995                    2–10

---

*Introduction.*—Long-term patency rates for balloon angioplasty (BA) are typically lower than for thromboendarterectomy (EA) in the treatment of segmental occlusive disease of the superficial femoral artery. Reports of lower costs for endovascular techniques have influenced the increased use of BA and decreased use of EA. The late costs incurred by the need for redo procedures may actually offset any savings of choosing BA over EA. The actual costs of in- and out-of-hospital investigations, treatment, follow-up by clinical and noninvasive examinations, and expenses for revision and redo procedures were correlated with the duration of the arterial patency in patients who underwent EA and those for whom BA was performed.

*Methods.*—Clinical data on 39 patients (41 lower limbs) who underwent EA procedures from 1980–1988 were reviewed retrospectively. Data were collected prospectively from 1988–1993 concerning 62 patients who underwent BA. Information was collected in 2 different time periods, so total costs were calculated accordingly. Patency was assessed by clinical

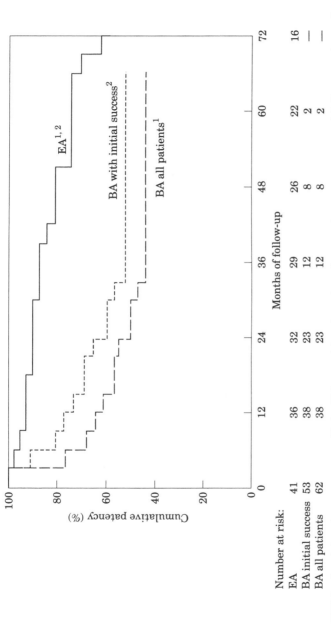

FIGURE 1.—Cumulative primary patency rates (Kaplan-Meier curves) in patients who underwent endarterectomy, patients with balloon angioplasty with initial success, and all patients with balloon angioplasty (including early failures). Numbers at risk represent patients at risk as indicated time points. *[1]p = 0.0024 †[2]p = 0.0064 *Abbreviations: EA,* endarterectomy; *BA,* balloon angioplasty. (Reprinted from *European Journal of Vascular and Endovascular Surgery* 10. Vroegindeweij D, Idu M, Buth J, et al: The cost-effectiveness of treatment of short occlusive lesions in the femoropopliteal artery: Balloon angioplasty versus endarterectomy, pp 40–50, 1995 by permission of the publisher Academic Press Limited London.)

follow-up using color-Duplex scanning and intra-arterial digital subtraction angiography.

*Results.*—Patient groups were similar in age, clinical characteristics, and risk factors of peripheral arterial occlusive disease. Patients in the EA group tended to have more severe symptoms at initial evaluation. The most common complication was early occlusion or failed recanalization in 9 (15%) patients who underwent BA. After the primary procedure, the 3-year patency rate was 87% and 44% in patients with EA and BA, respectively (Fig 1). To maintain a patent femoropopliteal artery, secondary procedures were required in 7 and 24 patients with EA and BA, respectively. In redo procedures, the tertiary 3-year patency for patients undergoing EA and BA, respectively, was 94% and 74%. The mean cost for initial investigation, admission, and treatment in patients undergoing EA was significantly higher, compared with patients undergoing BA. However, initial BA failure resulted in a higher cost than EA because of the cost of 2 procedures and prolonged admission. The initial higher cost of the EA was closely offset by secondary treatment costs of BA.

*Conclusion.*—The costs per month of primary patency in patients with EA were comparable to the overall costs of performing BA, when costs are expressed in a cost-to-patency ratio. It is important when making claims about favorable cost-effectiveness that an unbiased assessment be performed.

▶ In this series from the Netherlands, surgical patency of superficial femoral artery lesions was twice that of angioplasty patency at 3 years. When these authors calculated cost-effectiveness, they concluded that if the costs are expressed as a cost-to-patency ratio, there is no substantial difference between the cost of surgical treatment and endovascular treatment. This has been noted by others. Clearly, mortality, morbidity, and cost are similiar between endovascular procedures and operative surgery. Patency is almost always much better in the surgical group. I continue to conclude that the only clear benefit in favor of endovascular is a somewhat shorter recovery period, the significance of which is not immediately apparent, considering 90% of vascular patients are retired.

---

**Comparison of Effects of High-Dose and Low-Dose Aspirin on Restenosis After Femoropopliteal Percutaneous Transluminal Angioplasty**
Minar E, Ahmadi A, Koppensteiner R, et al (Univ Clinic, Vienna)
*Circulation* 91:2167–2173, 1995                                           2–11

---

*Introduction.*—Patients with large-vessel peripheral arterial disease are at high risk of death from cardiovascular causes. The most important complication after percutaneous transluminal angioplasty (PTA) is late restenosis. Patients with peripheral arterial diseases often require long-term treatment with aspirin to reduce the risk of cardiovascular events. The effects of high dose aspirin (1000 mg/day) and low-dose aspirin (100

CUMULATIVE PATENCY (Kaplan-Meier)

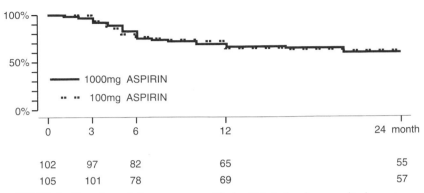

FIGURE 1.—Plot of cumulative patency rate (Kaplan-Meier) after femoropopliteal percutaneous transluminal angioplasty, according to assigned treatment. Numbers below the figure indicate the number of patients at risk. (Courtesy of Minar E, Ahmadi A, Koppensteiner R, et al: Comparison of effects of high-dose and low-dose aspirin on restenosis after femoropopliteal percutaneous transluminal angioplasty. *Circulation* 1995; 91:2167–2173. Reproduced with permission *Circulation*. Copyright 1995 American Heart Association.)

mg/day) were compared during long-term follow-up of 24-months after femoropopliteal PTA.

*Methods.*—A total of 216 patients who were treated successfully by PTA for femoropopliteal lesions were randomly assigned to either a high- or low-dose aspirin group. Patients underwent history, clinical examination, laboratory assessment, and color flow duplex sonography of the femoropopliteal segment at 24-month follow-up.

*Results.*—Complete follow-up information was available for 207 patients. At 2-year follow-up, 36 patients in the high-dose aspirin group and 36 patients in the low-dose group showed angiographically confirmed reobstruction within the recanalized segment. Intention-to-treat analysis revealed that cumulative patency rates were 62.5% and 62.6% in the high- and low-dose aspirin groups at 24-month follow-up. The cumulative survival rate was 86.6% and 87.7% in the high- and low dose groups, respectively. Thirty patients in the high-dose group and 11 patients in the low-dose aspirin group terminated aspirin therapy. Four patients in the low-dose group and 20 patients in the high-dose group discontinued aspirin use because of gastrointestinal symptoms.

*Conclusion.*—There is no reason to recommend aspirin doses of more than 100 mg/day to prevent restenosis after fermorpopliteal PTA. Patients are less likely to discontinue treatment with low-dose aspirin therapy.

▶ Cardiologists dilating coronary arteries have long agonized over the usefulness of concomitant medications, including aspirin, anticoagulants, thrombolytics, omega-3 fatty acids, etc. These same intellects are now asking the haunting question of the importance of concomitant medication in femoropopliteal angioplasty. Remarkably, they conclude that 100 mg of aspirin is no worse than 1,000 mg of aspirin and has predictably fewer side effects. It is always gratifying to see confirmation of the obvious. For this outstanding example of intellectual virtuosity it is only appropriate to present these authors with the Honorable Mention Camel Dung Award.

---

### Should Percutaneous Transluminal Angioplasty Be Recommended for Treatment of Infrageniculate Popliteal Artery or Tibioperoneal Trunk Stenosis?

Treiman GS, Treiman RL, Ichikawa L, et al (Cedars-Sinai Med Ctr, Los Angeles)
*J Vasc Surg* 22:457–465, 1995                                              2–12

---

*Introduction.*—The success rate of percutaneous transluminal angioplasty (PTA) of the infrageniculate popliteal artery and tibioperoneal trunk (IGPA) has improved to the point where some authors recommend PTA over arterial reconstruction in patients with localized stenosis in this area. The results of PTA for patients with stenosis of the IGPA were reviewed.

*Methods.*—Twenty-five such patients were treated during a 10-year period. During the mean follow-up period of 44 months, the patients were monitored by clinical examination, ankle-brachial index, duplex scanning, and arteriography. Outcomes were compared against the patients' demographic variables and cardiovascular risk factors.

*Results.*—The clinical and hemodynamic success rate, as calculated by the life-table method, was 59% at 1 year, 32% at 2 years, and 20% at 3 years (Fig 1). Recurrences developed at an average of 17 months. Another procedure was required in 16 patients—8 had arterial bypass, 6 had repeat PTA followed by bypass, and 2 had repeat PTA only. Repeat PTA offered a mean of 8 more months before recurrence. Of 14 patients who under-

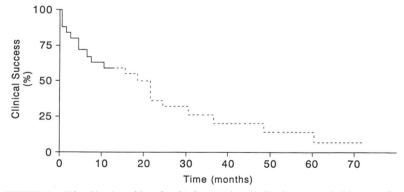

**FIGURE 1.**—Life-table plot of benefit of infrageniculate popliteal artery and tibioperoneal trunk percutaneous transluminal angioplasty. (Courtesy of Treiman GS, Treiman RL, Ichikawa L, et al: Should percutaneous transluminal angioplasty be recommended for treatment of infrageniculate popliteal artery or tibioperoneal trunk stenosis? *J Vasc Surg* 22:457–465, 1995.)

went arterial bypass, 11 were asymptomatic with patent grafts at a mean follow-up of 52 months. None of the risk factors evaluated was able to predict successful PTA.

*Conclusions.*—For most patients with localized stenosis of the IGPA, PTA is an expensive procedure of only short-lived effectiveness. When PTA of the IGPA is performed for limb salvage, operative intervention will very likely be required later on.

▶ In this study directed specifically at the efficacy of balloon angioplasty of the below-knee popliteal artery and tibioperoneal trunk, these authors conclude that the 59%, 32%, and 20% patencies at 1, 2, and 3 years is not very impressive. I applaud their conclusion that balloon angioplasty of the popliteal artery is "an expensive temporizing measure with a high rate of recurrence requiring subsequent intervention." Well said! They got it right.

---

**Retrograde Aortic Dissection After Bilateral Iliac Artery Stenting: A Case Report and Review of the Literature**
Cisek PL, McKittrick JE, (Santa Barbara Cottage Hosp, Calif)
*Ann Vasc Surg* 9:280–284, 1995                                               2–13

---

*Background.*—Only rarely does abdominal aortic dissection occur with retrograde extension into the thoracic aorta. A patient with retrograde dissection of the abdominal aorta developing after bilateral iliac artery and stent placement is reported.

*Case.*—Woman, 36, with peripheral vascular disease and claudication underwent aortography with distal runoff. Her localized stenoses and good distal runoff made her a good candidate for percutaneous transluminal angioplasty. The patient underwent balloon angioplasty for bilateral lesions of the common iliac arteries, followed by vascular stenting. This was followed immediately by dyspnea and chest and back pain. Not until 24 hours later was she found to have an acute aortic dissection extending from just distal to the left subclavian artery and extending to the aortic bifurcation. A 2-day follow-up scan revealed differences in opacification of the true and false lumens, with slower flow in the false lumen (Fig 5).

*Discussion.*—This is the first reported case of retrograde aortic dissection occurring after bilateral iliac artery angioplasty. The initial symptom of this complication, which occurred in a patient with hypertension and chronic steroid use, was chest pain immediately after stent placement.

▶ I am fascinated by the occurrence of a complete retrograde aortic dissection incident to iliac artery stent placement. As far as any of us can tell, this is the first report of such an occurrence after iliac angioplasty.

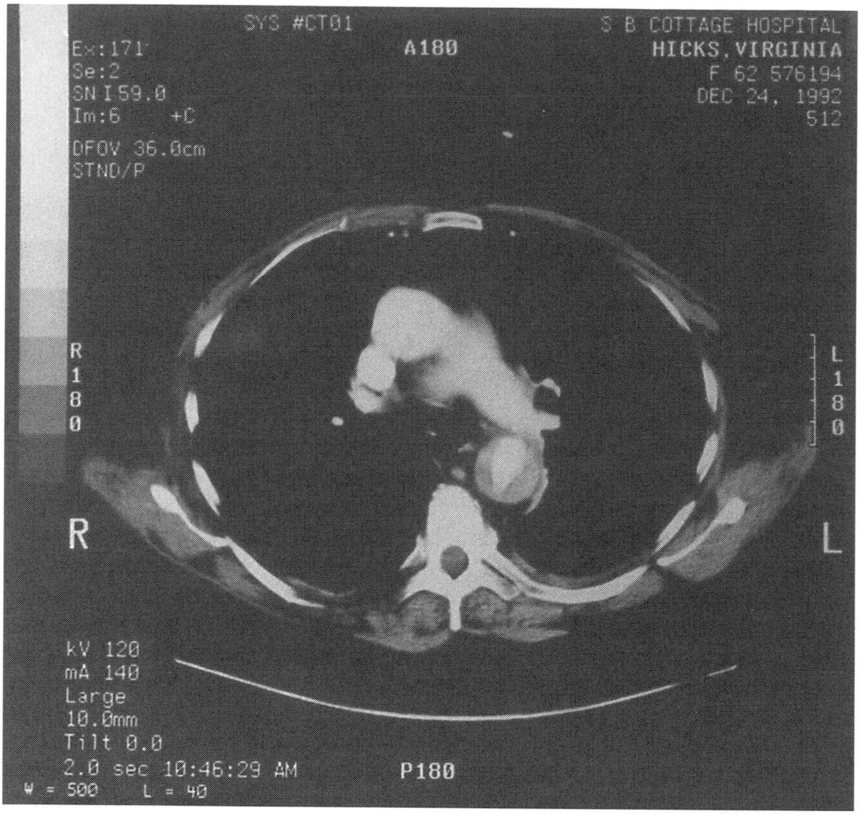

FIGURE 5.—Computed tomography scan 2 days after stent placement showing differentiation of true and false lumens. (Reprinted from Cisek PL, McKittrick JE: Retrograde aortic dissection after bilateral iliac artery stenting: A case report and review of the literatures. *Annals of Vascular Surgery* 9:280–284, 1995.)

---

## Iliac Artery Stenoses After Percutaneous Transluminal Angioplasty: Follow-Up With Duplex Ultrasonography

Spijkerboer AM, Nass PC, de Valois JC, et al (Univ Hosp, Utrecht, The Netherlands; St Antonius Hosp, Nieuwegein, The Netherlands)
*J Vasc Surg* 23:691–697, 1996                                                    2–14

---

*Background.*—The natural history of residual iliac artery stenosis after percutaneous transluminal angioplasty (PTA) is not clear. A 1-year study was conducted, using duplex ultrasound, to determine the recurrence rate of stenosis after PTA and to link ultrasound results to patients' clinical status.

*Methods.*—Duplex ultrasound studies were performed on 61 patients with 70 iliac artery lesions before and 1 day, 3 months, and 1 year after PTA. Peak systolic velocity (PSV) was determined at the stenotic site and in a region of normal flow proximal or distal to the lesion to calculate a

PSV ratio between flows at the 2 sites. Clinical symptoms were scored at each examination.

*Results.*—Of the 70 stenoses studied, 45 segments (64.3%) had a good result, 15 (21.4%) still had residual stenosis, and 10 (14.3%) developed recurrent stenosis. Overall, the segments showed significant improvement in PSV ratio at 1 year, but segments with recurrent stenosis did not, when considered separately. Residual stenoses, considered separately, also showed significant improvement in PSV ratio at 1 year. The clinical score of the group with a good result was significantly better at 1 year than the group with recurrent stenoses but was not significantly different from the score of the group with residual stenosis.

*Conclusion.*—After PTA for iliac artery stenosis, the majority of stenotic sites still show good results at 1 year. Residual stenoses improve significantly as well.

▶ These authors have reached some rather remarkable conclusions. Some of these include the observation that by duplex ultrasound velocity criteria, only 64% of these best-case iliac artery angioplasties had good objective results after 1 year. Their most remarkable conclusion was the observation that the clinical outcome of patients with objectively defined residual stenoses did not differ from patients with good ultrasound results. The substantial lack of relationship between clinical outcome and sonographic outcome in this well-presented study is most interesting. On balance, don't you all feel that vascular surgery has been substantially duped by angioplasty? Angioplasty for even the very best of indications produces objectively lousy results.

## Carotid Angioplasty

**Results of Balloon Angioplasty in the Carotid Arteries**
Kachel R (Inst of Diagnostic Radiology, Erfurt, Germany)
*J Endovasc Surg* 3:22–30, 1996                                    2–15

*Objectives.*—The results of percutaneous transluminal angioplasty of the carotid artery were reported, and a new coaxial dilatation system with temporary balloon occlusion to avoid cerebral embolization was described.

*Background.*—For many years, percutaneous transluminal angioplasty of the carotid arteries was controversial because the risk of embolization to the brain was overestimated. Percutaneous transluminal angioplasty was first proposed in 1977 as treatment for lesions of the proximal aortic arch vessel. Since then, it has been demonstrated that this procedure is feasible in the brachiocephalic arteries without unjustified risk.

*Methods.*—In 220 patients with 245 stenosed or occluded supra-aortic arteries, percutaneous transluminal angioplasty was performed. There were 74 carotid stenoses in the proximal common, distal common, internal, and external carotid arteries. Before and after angioplasty, duplex and B-mode ultrasonography, CT, MRI, single photon emission computed tomography, indium 111-labeled platelet scintigraphy, and angiography were performed. Intravascular ultrasound imaging was also used to monitor results.

> *Technique.*—A guide catheter is inserted with a deflated occlusion balloon at the top in the common carotid artery. The dilating portion of the angioplasty catheter is placed across the carotid stenosis. The stenosis is dilated while the common carotid artery is simultaneously occluded with the balloon. The dilatation catheter is then deflated and removed, and blood and possible detached plaque material are aspirated. Finally, the occlusion balloon is deflated, and results are documented by angiography.

*Results.*—All patients except 1 had cerebrovascular insufficiency. In 69 of the 74 carotid stenoses, angioplasty was successful. There was 1 major and 2 minor complications. During the following 70 months, stenosis did not recur in any treated artery. A review of more than 500 patients revealed a very low complication rate for carotid angioplasty similar to that for carotid endarterectomy.

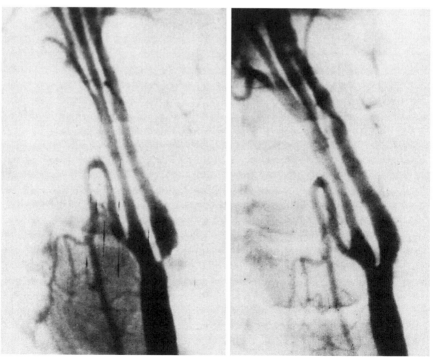

FIGURE 5.—A high-grade internal carotid artery stenosis before (*left*) and after (*right*) angioplasty. (Courtesy of Kachel R: Results of balloon angioplasty in the carotid arteries. *J Endovasc Surg* 3:22–30, 1996.)

*Conclusions.*—Percutaneous transluminal angioplasty of the carotid artery is an effective alternative to vascular surgery in patients with symptomatic carotid and supra-aortic stenoses. Indications for percutaneous transluminal angioplasty and vascular surgery are the same: only high-grade stenoses of the internal carotid artery with signs of cerebrovascular insufficiency (Fig 5).

▶ This ex cathedra report is by a single author who has already published 7 other papers on the subject. Looking at the short, smooth-contoured stenosis illustrated in Figure 5 and the excellent radiologic result achieved, we can understand why radiologists might covet these lesions, even if stable and symptomless. Surgeons who are used to seeing long, irregular strictures with loose insoluble debris in patients with previous cerebral damage would like to know more. For example, what were the precise indications for angioplasty and by whom were they assessed? Would the same success be achieved in more complex strictures? Is vessel repture or thrombosis a possibility, and are flaps and dissections generally satisfactorily controlled by stenting? To protect the brain, the author suggests a 9F catheter system, leaving the sheath in place for 24 hours after the procedure while giving heparin. How often was that useful and for what, and is that never associated with complications? How can the author be sure that further angioplasty for recurrent stricture is so valuable if it occurs so seldom? The author was unable to catheterize 7.7% of internal carotid artery lesions. Are these to be the future surgical rump?

As Rothwell and Warlow have said, "The reliability of assessment by the clinician who performed a procedure is open to question."[1] It is time for a controlled and independent assessment of this technique to match the extensive canon of independently validated surgical data if publication bias is to be avoided. In Table 1 in the article, the author collects 1,971 cases of supra-aortic angioplasty, quoting a 94.6% success rate, no mortality, a morbidity rate of 0.9% and a minor complication rate of 4.2%. Symptomatic patients would like this to be true. However, as surgeons with an independently validated track record, we should demand proof beyond all reasonable doubt, and budget managers should seek reassurance that the claimed cost benefits are not offset by more liberal indications for treatment. At present, useful debate is frustrated by the lack of independently validated evidence.

**A.E.B. Giddings, M.D.**

*Reference:*

1. Rothwell P, Warlow: *Lancet* 346:1623, 1995.

▶ Right on.

**J.M. Porter, M.D.**

## European Carotid Angioplasty Trial

Sivaguru A, Venables GS, Beard JD, et al (Royal Hallamshire Hosp, Sheffield, England)

*J Endovasc Surg* 3:16–20, 1996                                                2–16

*Introduction.*—The Carotid and Vertebral Artery Transluminal Angioplasty Study is an international, multicenter trial. Its goals are to determine risks and benefits of carotid and vertebral artery transluminal angioplasty and to compare these to carotid endarterectomy or best medical treatment.

*Rationale and Design.*—Initial experience with carotid and vertebral angioplasty indicated that the risk of stroke might be similar to that of carotid endarterectomy. This led to the development of a trial to compare these procedures. Patients with symptomatic stenoses (30% or more luminal diameter reduction) of the carotid or vertebral arteries are randomized to angioplasty, or surgery, or best medical treatment. The benefits of carotid endarterectomy to patients with 30% to 69% stenosis are still being investigated in other studies. Therefore, most patients enrolled in the Carotid and Vertebral Artery Transluminal Angioplasty Study have 70% or greater carotid artery stenosis.

*Patients.*—In all, 36 patients have been treated; 16 with transient ischemic attack, 17 with amaurosis fugax, 13 with mild stroke, and 1 with central retinal artery occlusion. All had 70% or greater carotid artery stenosis, most often in the proximal internal carotid artery. Before angioplasty, all patients were receiving best medical treatment, usually aspirin. Bilateral femoral catheterization allows postdilation angiographic evaluation of the treated region with a second catheter without losing access to the guidewire from the initial femoral artery.

*Results.*—Technical outcome has been very satisfactory. All intended procedures were completed with no perioperative deaths. At 30 days, 2 patients had a disabling stroke. Only 1 patient has had recurrent symptoms. Follow-up is ongoing.

*Discussion.*—Investigation of cognitive changes before and after angioplasty and endarterectomy is also ongoing. This trial will offer valuable information on the use of carotid angioplasty. The low complication rates for carotid endarterectomy were achieved after many years of refinement. The comparable rates for carotid angioplasty are very encouraging because this procedure should also evolve with time.

▶ This is another preliminary report of a carotid angioplasty series. This method of treatment is acquiring momentum. The proponents are now clamoring for a prospective, randomized comparison with endarterectomy. In my opinion, this would be unethical without publication of a great deal more carotid angioplasty results with much longer follow-up. It is not appropriate to subject patients to a dangerous randomized trial unless there is a genuine state of equipoise, which in my opinion most assuredly is not present. See also Abstract 2–15.

## Miscellaneous Topics

### Laparoscopic Vascular Surgery: Four Case Reports

Berens ES, Herde JR (St Joseph's Hosp, Tucson; Tucson Med Ctr, Ariz)
*J Vasc Surg* 22:73–79, 1995                                         2–17

*Background.*—Progress has been slow in applying the principles of laparoscopic surgery to vascular surgery. Four laparoscopic vascular surgical procedures—performed by a new technique that avoids gas insufflation of the peritoneal cavity—are reported.

*Methods.*—The gasless laparoscopic technique, developed in swine, used a mechanical arm to elevate the abdominal wall, thus creating a working cavity (Fig 2). The procedures performed were 2 iliofemoral bypasses, 1 aortobifemoral bypass, and 1 aortoiliac endarterectomy. The operating surgeons used conventional vascular instruments in combination with laparoscopic instruments through a total of 5 to 7 ports: 4 to 6 ports measuring 0.5 to 1.5 cm and 1 incision measuring 4.0 cm. Roticulating fan retractors and laparotomy sponges were used to maintain exposure, and all graft anastomoses were performed by end-to-side technique. Cross-clamp time for these anastomoses ranged from 40 to 70 minutes. An open femoral incision was used to make distal anastomoses.

*Results.*—The iliac procedures took about 5 hours and the aortic procedures about 7 hours. Within 24 hours and 48 hours, respectively, the patients were ambulating and eating a regular diet. All were discharged home on the second or third day after surgery and resumed their normal activities within 1 week. There were no complications and no need for blood transfusion. Recovery was faster with the laparoscopic procedures than it would have been with the standard open approach. Pain was reduced, as were the risks of wound herniation, dehiscence, and infection. The gasless procedure minimized the use of disposable instruments and eliminated the risk of $CO_2$ embolism.

*Conclusions.*—The feasibility of laparoscopic iliac and aortic vascular bypass procedures is demonstrated. The gasless technique described permits the recognized advantages of laparoscopy to be extended to vascular surgery patients.

▶ With the use of 7 ports through the abdominal wall, a variety of highly specialized instruments, and 7 hours of diligent effort, these authors were able to perform a laparoscopic aortic procedure satisfactorily in a few patients. The outcome was excellent and the authors conclude, I suspect correctly, that these patients enjoyed a faster postoperative recovery and appeared to have less postoperative pain. From a cost standpoint, however, one would have to be concerned about the consumption of expensive equipment, as well as the monumental 7 hours of operating time.

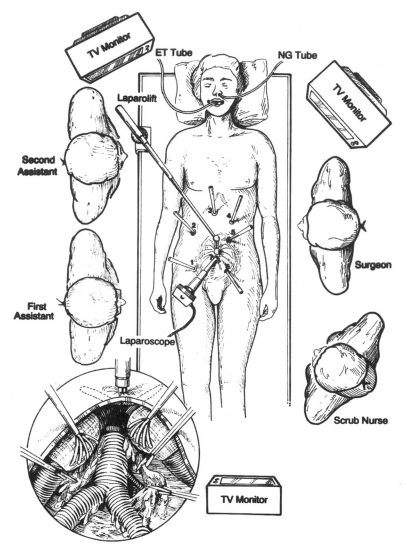

**FIGURE 2.**—Basic operating room setup. Laparolift positioned to right of patient's upper torso in this case. Two television monitors are at head and 1 at foot. Port numbers 1 to 4 and number 6 are 0.5 to 1.5 cm in length. Port number 5 is 4 cm in length. Laparoscope is usually positioned with a laparolift in port number 7 for aortic dissection and in port number 3 for pelvic dissection. Laparoscopic fan retractors in port numbers 2 and 4 and vascular clamps in port numbers 3 and 6. Inset shows retroperitoneal dissection with lower abdominal wall cut out. (Courtesy of Berens ES, Herde JR: Laparoscopic vascular surgery: Four case reports. *J Vasc Surg* 22:73–79, 1995.)

## Should Percutaneous Transluminal Renal Artery Angioplasty Be Applied to Ostial Renal Artery Atherosclerosis?

Eldrup-Jorgensen J, Harvey HR, Sampson LN, et al (Maine Med Ctr, Portland)
*J Vasc Surg* 21:909–915, 1995                                        2–18

*Background.*—Atherosclerosis of the renal artery can be either ostial or nonostial. In initial studies of percutaneous transluminal renal artery angioplasty (PTRA), the anatomic and functional results were poor in patients with ostial lesions. Differences in outcome between ostial and nonostial lesions were assessed as part of a retrospective study of the results of PTRA.

*Methods.*—Fifty-two patients underwent attempted PTRA for renal artery atherosclerosis in a total of 60 arteries during a 5-year period. The patients' mean age was 68 years, and 81% had generalized atherosclerosis. The reason for PTRA was an attempt to salvage the functional renal parenchyma in 81% of patients. Eight patients were undergoing dialysis when the angioplasty attempt was made.

*Results.*—Dilation was unsuccessful in 8% of cases. Within 1 month after PTRA, 1 patient died of cardiac causes and 2 had arterial complications requiring surgery. Follow-up angiography showed anatomic improvement above a threshold of 1 stenotic group—i.e., a 30% to 40% improvement in diameter—in 35% of patients. These patients had less than 50% residual stenosis. Hypertension improved in half the patients who had this problem preoperatively. Creatinine levels were unchanged by PTRA, although half the patients who had been undergoing dialysis were able to discontinue it. Surgical bypass was required during follow-up in 11% and chronic dialysis was required in 14%. The results were not significantly different for ostial vs. nonostial lesions (Table 4).

*Conclusions.*—In patients with severe atherosclerosis of the renal artery, PTRA offers modest success rates at low risk. The results appear equal in ostial and nonostial lesions.

▶ The preliminary report with incomplete follow-up concludes that patients with ostial renal lesions undergoing angioplasty do as well as those with

TABLE 4.—Anatomic Results: Mean Stenosis Scores of Arteries With Successful PTRA (*n* = 51 in 48 patients)*

|  | Before | After | Average Δ | P Value | No. of Arteries |
|---|---|---|---|---|---|
| Ostial | 3.54 | 2.40 | 1.14 | 0.007 | 14 |
| Nonostial | 3.20 | 1.90 | 1.30 | 0.001 | 31 |
| Indeterminate | 3.67 | 2.50 | 1.17 | 0.012 | 6 |
| Totals | 3.44 | 2.22 | 1.19 | <0.001 | 51 |

*Excluded 5 arteries in 4 patients in whom the wire or catheter could not be passed and 4 arteries in 4 patients whose arteriograms were not available for review.

(Courtesy of Eldrup-Jorgenson J, Harvey HR, Sampson LN, et al: Should percutaneous transluminal renal artery angioplasty be applied to ostial renal artery atherosclerosis? *J Vasc Surg* 21:909–915, 1995.)

nonostial lesions. Perhaps, but I am not convinced. I urge caution in interpreting this retrospective study.

## Thrombolysis of Lower Extremity Embolic Occlusions: A Study of the Results of the STAR Registry

Huettl EA, Soulen MC (Univ of Pennsylvania, Philadelphia)
*Radiology* 197:141–145, 1995                                                        2–19

*Background.*—Although intra-arterial thrombolysis has long been used for the treatment of acute thrombosis, there are few data on its usefulness for arterial emboli. Thrombolysis was retrospectively evaluated as a primary therapy for embolic occlusions of the lower extremity.

*Methods.*—Three hundred six consecutive urokinase-treated cases of arterial occlusion of the lower extremity were identified from the Transluminal Angioplasty and Revascularization Registry of the Society of Cardiovascular and Interventional Radiology. Of these, 45 cases were believed to result from emboli, based on clinical and angiographic findings.

*Results.*—Half the patients had comorbid atrial fibrillation. Forty percent had had a previous myocardial infarction, and 35% had had a cerebrovascular event. The limb was considered viable in 71% of cases, threatened in 27% of cases, and irreversibly ischemic in 1 case. The symptoms had been present for a mean of 9 days.

The occlusions averaged 17 cm in length. The lesion location was femoropopliteal in 65% of cases, tibial in 24%, graft in 7%, and aortoiliac in 4%. The major complication rate was 18%. Thrombolysis had a technical success rate and a 1- and 2-year primary patency rate of 55%.

*Conclusions.*—In most patients with arterial emboli of the lower extremity, intra-arterial thrombolysis is a successful treatment. The results appear comparable to those reported for surgical embolectomy in terms of limb salvage and survival.

▶ Forty-five patients with lower extremity embolic occlusions underwent lytic therapy as primary treatment with major complications in 18%, and a 1- and 2-year patency of 55%. Although better than a poke in the eye with a sharp stick, this is not the stuff dreams are made of. Let's face it, across vascular surgery in general, thrombolytic therapy remains an accident looking for a place to happen. You would think after 30 years of clinical use, clear indications would have been long since identified. Because they have not, I can reach only 1 conclusion.

# 3 Vascular Laboratory and Imaging

## Magnetic Resonance Imaging

### Magnetic Resonance Angiography in the Preoperative Evaluation of Abdominal Aortic Aneurysms

Petersen MJ, Cambria RP, Kaufman JA, et al (Harvard Med School, Boston)
*J Vasc Surg* 21:891–899, 1995                    3–1

*Introduction.*—Preoperative contrast arteriography (CA) in patients with abdominal aortic aneurysm (AAA) provides crucial anatomic information that facilitates performance and improves outcome of repair. However, the potential risk and cost of this invasive procedure have raised concerns. The use of magnetic resonance arteriography (MRA) as a preoperative planning tool in AAA repair was examined.

*Methods.*—In a prospective study, 38 patients with AAA underwent both standard CA and MRA with a gadolinium-enhanced technique. The imaging studies were independently evaluated by blinded radiologists for

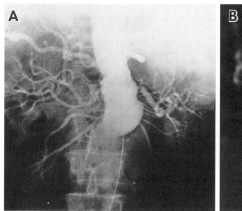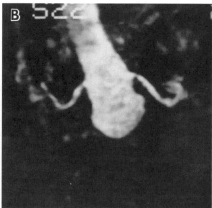

FIGURE 1.—**A,** contrast arteriogram notes bilateral high-grade renal artery stenosis; **B,** MRA of same patient also noting high-grade bilateral renal artery stenosis. *Abbreviations: MRA,* magnetic resonance arteriography. (Courtesy of Petersen MJ, Cambria RP, Kaufman JA, et al: Magnetic resonance angiography in the preoperative evaluation of abdominal aortic aneurysms. *J Vasc Surg* 21:891–899, 1995.)

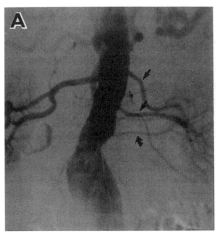
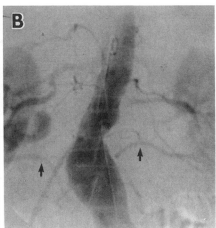
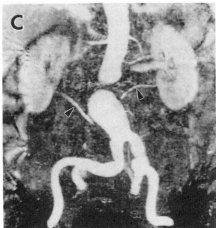

FIGURE 2.—A, B, digital subtraction contrast arteriograms noting 4 left and 2 right renal arteries (*arrows*); C, MRA of same patient noting 4 left and 2 right renal arteries. *Arrows*, lower pole accessory arteries. *Abbreviaions: MRA, magnetic resonance arteriography.* (Courtesy of Petersen MJ, Cambria RP, Kaufman JA, et al: Magnetic resonance angiography in the preoperative evaluation of abdominal aortic aneurysms. *J Vasc Surg* 21:891–899, 1995.)

anatomical findings, using CA as the standard. Furthermore, imaging studies were independently evaluated by blinded vascular surgeons; surgical plans derived from both CA and MRA were compared with the surgical repair.

*Results.*—Compared with CA and intraoperative findings, MRA was highly accurate in the determination of multiple key anatomical elements. The proximal extent of aneurysmal disease was correctly predicted in 87% of patients with MRA and 92% with CA. Six patients had significant iliofemoral occlusive disease, and MRA correctly identified the lesion in 83%. Iliac or femoral aneurysms were detected with MRA with a sensitivity of 79% and a specificity of 86%; sensitivity was 100% and specificity was 88% with CA. Significant renal artery stenosis was detected with a relatively low sensitivity of 71% but high specificity of 99% when compared with CA (Fig 1). In addition, MRA correctly visualized 12 of 17 accessory renal arteries for a sensitivity of 71% (Fig 2). Compared with the actual conduct of the operation, surgical evaluators correctly predicted the proximal clamp site in 87% using MRA and in 92% with CA; and proximal anastomotic sites were predicted in 95% with MRA and 97% with CA. Overall, renal artery revascularization was predicted by MRA with a sensitivity of 91% and specificity of 100%. With CA, surgical evaluators predicted the revascularization with a sensitivity of 100% and specificity of 97%. Both CA (81%) and MRA (75%) were equivalent in predicting the use of bifurcated aortic prostheses. Both procedures were performed without complications, but the average total examination charge was twice as much with CA than MRA.

*Conclusion.*—For preoperative imaging before AAA repair, RA provides equivalent anatomical information as CA that is important to surgical planning, except for inferior mesenteric anatomy. With its favorable cost and improved accuracy, MRA should be increasingly used for preoperative evaluation of AAA.

▶ Overall, I am not particularly impressed by the performance of MRA as described in this publication, despite the enthusiasm of the authors. Magnetic resonance angiography seems to be about 15% off the mark in every category examined. It was especially poor in the detection of high-grade renal artery stenosis (sensitivity only 71%). Interestingly, MRA and CT apparently cost about the same at this institution. I suspect angiography was considerably more expensive. At the present time, I continue to believe angiography is the best imaging technique for aortic aneurysms. We will occasionally add CT, but rarely MRA. I keep waiting for the next generation of MR, with improved software and better arterial definition.

---

**Mural Thrombi in Abdominal Aortic Aneurysms: MR Imaging Characterization—Useful Before Endovascular Treatment?**
Castrucci M, Mellone R, Vanzulli A, et al (Univ Hosp, Milan, Italy)
*Radiology* 197:135–139, 1995                                              3–2

---

*Objective.*—Magnetic resonance (MR) imaging can demonstrate aortic wall dilatation and mural thrombi in abdominal aortic aneurysms (AAAs). The possible correlation between MR images and the macroscopic characteristics of mural thrombi noted at surgery in patients with AAAs was evaluated.

*Methods.*—Forty-five patients with an AAA with mural thrombus thicker than 1 cm at sonography underwent T1- and T2-weighted spin-echo MR imaging at a mean of 3 days before surgery. In a prospective qualitative analysis, the signal intensity (SI) of thrombi was classified into 3 categories: category 1 comprised thrombi with homogenously low SI on both T1- and T2-weighted images; category 2 included thrombi with high SI on T1- and T2-weighted images; and category 3 comprised thrombi with inhomogenous SI with hyperintense areas on both T1- and T2-weighted images. Based on gross characteristics at surgery, the thrombi were classified as organized when nearly all of the volume (> 90%) was homogenously firm and removed as a whole piece, unorganized when nearly all of the volume was composed of fresh blood clot and/or fluid, and

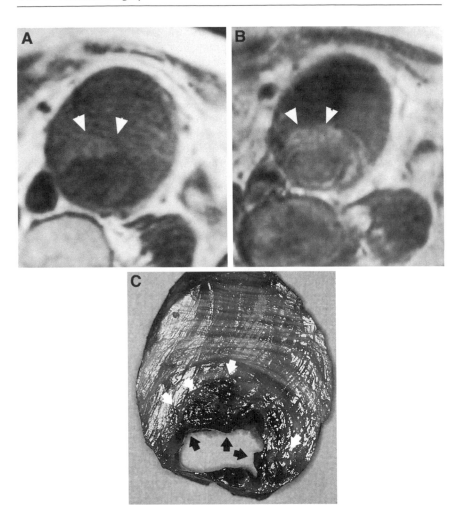

**FIGURE 1.**—Signal intensity category 1 thrombus in a 71-year-old man. **A**, T1-weighted spin-echo (500/200) and **B**, T2-weighted spin-echo (2,000/80) MR images show areas of low signal in most of the volume of thrombus and hyperintense internal bands (*arrowheads*); **C**, thrombus was removed as a whole piece from the aortic wall at surgery. Thrombus was composed of homogenous fibrotic tissue, with recent mural thrombotic deposit only in the inner layer (*arrows*). The recent thrombotic deposit corresponds to the hyperintense bands in **A** and **B**. (Courtesy of Castrucci M, Mellone R, Vanzulli A, et al: Mural thrombi in abdominal aortic aneurysms: MR imaging characterization-useful before endovascular treatment? *Radiology* 197:135–139, 1995. Radiological Society of North America.)

partially organized when the thrombi was mostly organized with portions (10% to 90% of volume) composed of fresh blood or fluid.

*Results.*—All 24 organized thrombi corresponded to thrombi classified as SI category 1 (Fig 1). All 24 organized thrombus had a thin band of recent thrombotic material on the luminal surface, but only 21 of 24 thrombi of SI category demonstrated a thin band of high SI in the inner-most layer. All 11 unorganized thrombi corresponded to category 2. In the 10 partially organized thrombi, the unorganized portions corresponded to the hyperintense areas on MR images in both sequences and the organized portions corresponded to hypointense areas on MR imaging in both sequences.

*Discussion.*—These findings illustrate the good correlation between S1 in both T1- and T2-weighted sequences and intraoperative findings of mural thrombus in patients with AAAs. In particular, hyperintensity on T1- and T2-weighted images always corresponded to an unorganized thrombus. The presence of a thin band of hyperintensity in the innermost layer of the thrombus, almost always present in even organized thrombi, should be regarded as a recent clot apposition on the luminal surface of the thrombus itself. Although the clinical relevance of these findings has yet to be assessed, evaluation of unorganized thrombi could represent an interesting preoperative exclusion criterion for endovascular aortic stent-graft prosthesis implantation.

▶ For some reason, these authors decided to determine if MR can accurately detect mural thrombi in aneurysms. They conclude, miraculously, that there is a good correlation between MR detection of mural thrombus and surgical findings. On balance, this appears to be a revelation of marginal significance. It is best to assume that all AAAs have thrombi and treat them as if they may embolize intraoperatively.

---

**Gadolinium-Enhanced Magnetic Resonance Angiography of Abdominal Aortic Aneurysms**
Prince MR, Narasimham DL, Stanley JC, et al (Univ of Michigan, Ann Arbor)
*J Vasc Surg* 21:656–669, 1995                                    3–3

---

*Introduction.*—Abdominal aorta and abdominal aortic aneurysms have been acceptably imaged using MR imaging. Additional evaluation of aortic branch vessels has been made possible with MR angiography. Gadolinium-enhanced MR angiogram has overcome some of the previous imaging problems of MR angiography, such as slow, swirling flow within aneurysms, tortuous iliac arteries, and turbulent flow in stenoses. Blood becomes distinct from surrounding tissues regardless of its flow rate or direction with gadolinium, a paramagnetic contrast agent. The usefulness of gadolinium-enhanced MR angiography was evaluated for its ability to define anatomical features relevant to performing aortic surgery for aneurysmal disease.

*Methods.*—Gadolinium-enhanced MR angiograms of abdominal aortic aneurysms were performed on 53 patients, 31 men and 21 women, ranging in age from 36 to 87 years. The gadolinium-enhanced MR angiography findings were compared with those at ultrasonography for 10 patients, angiography for 11 patients, operation for 25 patients, and CT for 11 patients. Comparisons were made on the size and character of the abdominal aortic aneurysms, the status of the celiac, mesenteric, renal, and iliac arteries.

*Results.*—In all patients, the maximum aneurysm diameter and its proximal and distal extent were defined by the gadolinium-enhanced MR angiography. Eleven suprarenal, 6 pararenal, 6 juxtarenal, and 20 infrarenal abdominal aortic aneurysms were demonstrated by the gadolinium-enhanced MR imaging sequences (Fig 1). Among 153 splanchnic, renal, or iliac branches examined, the gadolinium-enhanced MR angiography detected 33 of 35 stenosis, resulting in a sensitivity of 94% and a specificity of 98%. The status of the inferior mesenteric artery, lumbar arteries or

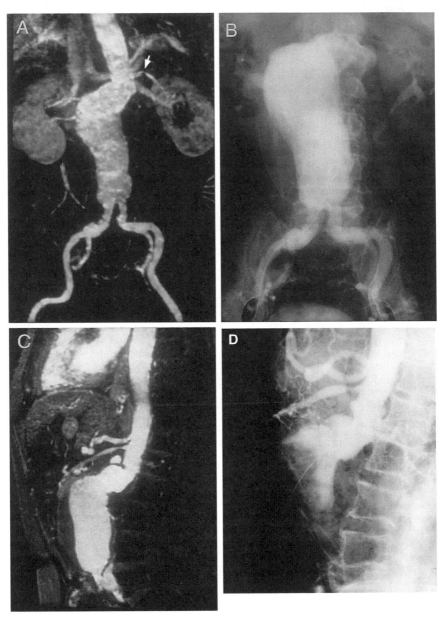

(Continued)

FIGURE 1 (cont.)

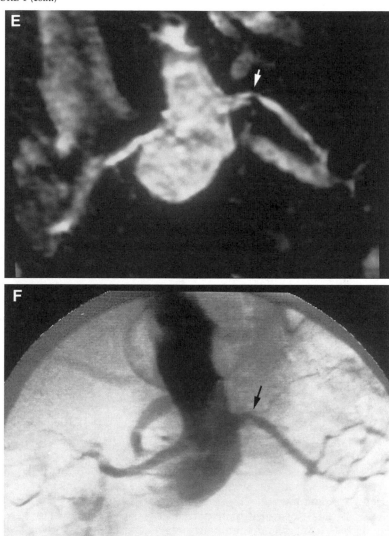

FIGURE 1.—**A**, coronal maximum intensity projection of dynamic gadolinium-enhanced 3DF MRA of abdominal aortic aneurysm. Preferential enhancement of arteries allows evaluation of iliac arteries without confounding effects of overlapping veins. However, there is moderate advancement of renal, splenic, and portal veins. Note left renal artery stenosis *(arrow)*. **B**, conventional aortogram. **C**, sagittal second time-of-flight MR angiogram after gadolinium infusion shows same abdominal aortic aneurysm with thrombus anteriorly, normal preaortic left renal vein, normal celiac trunk, and moderate stenosis of superior mesenteric artery. **D–F**, conventional lateral aortogram confirms MRA findings. **E**, oblique axial reformation shows proximal renal arteries with moderate left renal artery stenosis *(arrow)* confirmed by (**F**) conventional digital subtraction angiography. (Courtesy of Prince MR, Narasimham DL, Stanley JC, et al: Gadolinium-enhanced magnetic resonance angiography of abdominal aortic aneurysms. *J Vasc Surg* 21:656–669, 1995.)

internal iliac arteries was not reliably defined by the gadolinium-enhanced MR angiography, which also did not resolve the degree of aortic branch stenotic disease to allow for grading of its severity. The gadolinium-enhanced MR angiography helped to correctly diagnose 1 inflammatory and 1 ruptured abdominal aortic aneurysm. No complications resulted with the gadolinium-enhanced MR angiography.

*Conclusion.*—In patients with abdominal aortic aneurysm, gadolinium-enhanced MR angiography can provide anatomical information for planning aortic reconstructions. When specific questions are not adequately resolved by gadolinium-enhanced MR angiography, conventional angiography can be used for selected patients.

▶ The objective of this publication is very much the same as that of Abstract 3–1. The results, however, are significantly different in that these authors claim almost 100% sensitivity in all MR angiographic parameters examined. On balance, the findings in this paper suggest a considerably increased accuracy for MR angiography, compared with that in Abstract 3–1. However, the analytic paradigm in the first abstract was considerably stricter than in this one. On balance, available evidence has indicated to me that MR angiography is still not ready for prime time.

## Breath-Hold Gadolinium-Enhanced MR Angiography of the Abdominal Aorta and Its Major Branches

Prince MR, Narasimham DL, Stanley JC, et al (Univ of Michigan, Ann Arbor)
*Radiology* 197:785–792, 1995                                      3–4

*Objective.*—A group of patients referred for imaging of the abdominal aorta was entered into a study designed to develop and evaluate a sequence for breath-hold three-dimensional (3D) gadolinium-enhanced MR angiography. Because distal segments of renal and splanchnic arteries are often not visualized, it was hypothesized that blurring of the image is caused by respiration-induced motion of the abdominal organs and mesentery.

*Methods.*—The patients ranged in age from 22 to 87 years and had been referred for a number of reasons, but primarily suspected renovascular hypertension and suspected mesenteric ischemia. All underwent MR imaging with a 1.5-T superconducting imager, use of the body coil, and during infusion of 42 mL of a gadolinium chelate. The abdominal artery and its branches were imaged for 29, 43, or 58 seconds with breath holding. Correlation with conventional angiography was available in 19 cases. Breath holding and free breathing techniques were compared for image quality.

*Results.*—The abdominal aorta and the origins of the celiac artery, superior mesenteric artery, and renal arteries were visualized in all patients on breath-hold 3D gadolinium-enhanced MR angiograms (Fig 3). Compared with free-breathing, the breath-hold technique identified 71% more renal artery branches. Blurring in the abdominal organs occurred in 90%

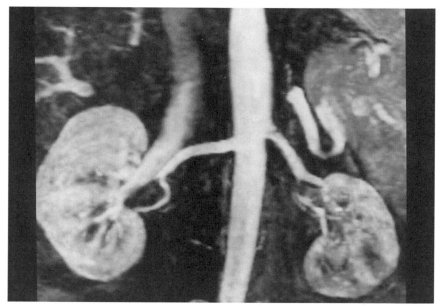

**FIGURE 3.**—Maximum intensity projection image from a 3-D gadolinium-enhanced MR angiogram obtained after balloon angioplasty shows correction of the differential enhancement. (Courtesy of Prince MR, Narasimham DL, Stanley JC, et al: Breath-hold gadolinium-enhanced MR angiography of the abdominal aorta and its major branches. *Radiology* 197:785–792, 1995 Radiological Society of North America.)

of examinations during free breathing vs. 66% of breath-hold examinations. Distal renal artery signal-to-total noise ratio was 3.1 with breath holding and 2.1 with free breathing, a significant difference.

*Conclusion.*—The technique described here attempts to eliminate respiratory motion by acquiring images in a single breath. Elimination of motion and a faster infusion of contrast material led to overall improvement in the quality of images obtained with MR angiography. Distal renal arteries and renal artery branches were seen in more patients than when free breathing was used, fewer patients had blurring of abdominal arteries, and more accessory renal arteries were identified.

▶ Gadolinium-enhanced 3D MR angiography can produce dramatic abdominal aortic images. Unfortunately, the images are badly degraded by respiratory motion. Although these authors have done 3D breath-holding MR angiography with generally good results, I note that the breath holding required is quite significant, being either for 29, 43, or 58 seconds. I wonder just how many of our patients can really hold their breath for that long? Certainly, we can expect future generations of MR technology to greatly reduce, or hopefully eliminate, requirements for prolonged breath holding.

### Fast MR Angiography of the Aortoiliac Arteries and Arteries of the Lower Extremity: Value of Bolus-Enhanced, Whole-Volume Subtraction Technique

Douek PC, Revel D, Chazel S, et al (Hôpital Cardio-Vasculaire et Pneumologique, Lyon, France)
AJR 165:431–437, 1995                                                3–5

*Objective.*—The short imaging times used in MR angiography of the abdominal aorta and lower limb arteries are not sufficient to visualize long segments of the arteries. Contrast enhancement has been suggested to improve signal intensity. The results of a preliminary study of fast acquisition of coronal sections using the bolus-enhancement technique, subtraction, and whole-volume projection display are reported.

*Methods.*—In the first phase of the study, 10 healthy volunteers (2 women), aged 44 to 78 years, were examined. In the second phase, 20 patients (15 for abdominal aortic aneurysm, 3 with vascular grafts, 1 with arteriovenous fistula, and 1 with abdominal aortic dissection) were referred for preoperative conventional angiography studied using a fast gradient-echo sequence with K-space segmentation. Two sets of coronal sections, first without and then with contrast medium, were acquired. Subtraction images were prepared, and signal intensity was measured in the aorta, interior vena cava, and background tissues. Aneurysms were categorized as infrarenal or suprarenal and as involving or not involving the iliac arteries. A graft visible at both the origin and periphery was termed patent.

*Results.*—Acquisition of the coronal data set lasted 24 seconds and of the coronal/sagittal set lasted 53 seconds. Gadolinium enhancement significantly increased the aortic signal-to-noise ratio from 25 to 232. Gadolinium enhancement did not significantly alter the sign-to-noise ratio of the inferior vena cava, muscles, and fat. Examinations were not interpretable in 2 patients. Three bypass grafts, 3 instances of graft patency, and 2 patients with occlusion were diagnosed by MR imaging and by conventional angiography. The superior mesenteric artery was observed in all patients before subtraction, and 29 renal arteries were identified before subtraction in all 15 patients having renal imaging, although in the final MR angiogram, renal arteries were usually obscured by renal veins and bowel contrast enhancement. Bolus enhancement of subtraction MR angiography visualized all lower limb arteries.

*Conclusion.*—Bolus-enhanced subtraction MR angiography appears to provide fast imaging of aortoiliac arteries and arteries of the lower extremity.

▶ This is a technical publication describing modifications of MR angiography to permit study of aortoiliac and lower extremity arteries. This combines fast acquisition of coronal sections with bolus-enhancement injection techniques, as well as subtraction and whole-volume projection display. The images are dramatic, but I have absolutely no idea whether this will prove to be a clinically useful technique. I suspect it will not.

### Iliac Artery MR Angiography: Comparison of Three-Dimensional Gadolinium-Enhanced and Two-Dimensional Time-of-Flight Techniques

Snidow JJ, Aisen AM, Harris VJ, et al (Indiana Univ, Indianapolis)
*Radiology* 196:371–378, 1995                                                                  3–6

*Background.*—Two-dimensional (2D) time-of-flight (TOF) technique is the standard method of MR angiography for patients with atherosclerotic occlusive disease of the pelvis and lower extremity, but its use has been limited by the false positive diagnoses of stenosis or occlusion in the iliac arteries. Whether 3-dimensional (3D) gadolinium-enhanced technique would improve the accuracy of MR angiography in the iliac arteries was studied.

*Methods.*—In a prospective study, 23 consecutive patients referred for preoperative evaluation of peripheral vascular disease underwent MR angiography of the iliac arteries with the standard 2D TOF technique, followed by the 3D gadolinium-enhanced technique. All but 5 patients underwent conventional arteriography, which served as the standard for diagnosis of stenosis and occlusion. Images from each examination were independently and blindly interpreted by 2 vascular interventional radiologists.

*Findings.*—For evaluation of obstructive lesions in the common and external iliac arteries, both observers provided interpretations of dynamic 3D gadolinium-enhanced MR angiograms that matched those of conventional angiograms in 67% of patients. In contrast, interpretations of 2D TOF MR angiograms agreed with those of conventional arteriograms in 33% and 39% of patients for the 2 observers, respectively. The 3D gadoliunium-enhanced images provided correct diagnoses in all 7 patients, with incorrect diagnoses on 2D TOF technique. The reverse was true in 2 patients for 1 observer and another patient for the other observer, in whom 2D TOF enabled correct diagnosis for an incorrect diagnosis with 3D gadolinium-enhanced imaging. In 1 patient, a clinically unsuspected arteriovenous fistula was identified at 3D gadolinium-enhanced MR angiography. In addition, 3D gadolinium-enhanced images demonstrated retrograde arterial flow that appeared saturated on 2D TOF images.

*Recommendations.*—These preliminary results suggest that MR angiography of the iliac arteries can be improved by complementing standard 2D TOF techniques with 3D gadolinium-enhanced acquisitions. In addition, 3D gadolinium-enhanced MR angiography is recommended when standard 2D TOF images or clinical findings suggest the presence of aneurysm, when arteriovenous fistula is suspected, or when detection of retrograde flow in native iliac arteries may be clinically important. Further studies are needed to refine and optimize the technique of 3D gadolinium-enhanced MR angiography in the iliac region.

▶ This interesting paper compares the conventional 2D TOF MR angiography technique to the 3D gadolinium-enhanced technique. I wish I knew enough engineering to understand exactly what these authors were doing. It is hardly surprising that they conclude that 3D enhanced iliac imaging provides information beyond that obtainable by the 2D TOF acquisitions. I hope the day will soon come when MR angiography is improved and standardized, and those of us who do not understand it can simply enjoy the images without devoting futile thought to their method of acquisition.

### Multicenter Trial to Evaluate Vascular Magnetic Resonance Angiography of the Lower Extremity

Baum RA, Rutter CM, Sunshine JH, et al (Univ of Pennsylvania, Philadelphia; Harvard Univ, Boston; American College of Radiology, Reston, Va; et al)
*JAMA* 274:875–880, 1995                                                          3–7

*Introduction.*—Magnetic resonance angiography (MRA) is a recent, noninvasive addition to the potential armamentarium of vascular imaging. Its application in the cerebrovascular circulation has been extensively evaluated, but its use in mapping the peripheral vasculature is limited. A prospective, blinded investigation was conducted in 6 hospitals in the United States to rigorously evaluate the value of MRA in the preoperative testing of patients with severe lower limb atherosclerotic occlusive disease. Because treatment and imaging techniques change rapidly, the study was specially designed to be completed within 15 months to assess the feasibility of rapidly conducting rigorous technology assessment.

*Methods.*—The study included 155 adult patients with signs or symptoms of severe infrainguinal peripheral vascular disease who were candidates for percutaneous or surgical intervention. Both descriptive statistics and multivariate logistic analyses were used to compare MRA with contrast arteriography (CA) for imaging 15 arterial segments of the leg and foot. Intraoperative contrast angiography (ICA) was used as the "gold standard" for assessing the accuracy of CA and MRA. In addition, the value of adding preoperative MRA to the surgical management in these patients was assessed.

*Outcome.*—Of the 1,188 vessel segments visualized by ICA, CA distinguished patent segments from completely occluded segments in 83% and MRA in 85%; both procedures had 81% specificity. For distinguishing near-normal segments that were suitable as bypass graft termini, CA was less sensitive than MRA (77% vs. 82%), but more specific (92% vs. 84%). After correcting for same-reader effects, the odds of identifying patent vessel segments were 1.6 times as great for MRA as for CA, and the odds of identifying near-normal segments were 1.5 times as great for CA as for MRA. The addition of MRA changed the revascularization plans in 15 (13%) patients, including 2 patients in whom the CA-suggested run off vessels proved to be unsuitable as indicated by MRA and actual surgery; 6 patients in whom MRA suggested an alternative run off vessel to that identified by CA; 5 patients in whom the additional MRA information resulted in a successful bypass, although CA and nonimaging studies failed to identify vessels suitable for bypass; 1 patient in whom MRA confirmed a patent vessel segment that turned out to be too diseased for grafting; and another patient in whom the CA-identified distal vessel for grafting appeared to be diseased on MRA. The revised plan was followed in 11 patients, and based on the actual surgery performed, the MRA-inclusive plan was superior in 86%.

*Conclusions.*—These findings indicate that MRA and CA are approximately equivalent in diagnostic accuracy to map the distal vasculature of the lower limb. The addition of preoperative MRA to treatment plans based only on CA and other diagnostic information clearly improves the plans. This study also demonstrates the feasibility of conducting rigorous technology assessment rapidly enough to provide results that could be applied in a timely manner, even in areas in which diagnostic and treatment techniques are rapidly changing.

▶ The evidence is conflicting about the role of MRA in the preoperative assessment of patients with infrainguinal occlusive disease. It is this reviewer's opinion that contrast arteriography remains the gold standard. However, MR technology is improving rapidly, and I predict that opinion may change. One thing is for sure—using both technologies, as suggested in this paper, is not acceptable.

**W. Abbott, M.D.**

---

**Magnetic Resonance Imaging in the Management of Diabetic Foot Infection**
Cook TA, Rahim N, Simpson HCR, et al (Royal Berkshire Hosp, London)
*Br J Surg* 83:245–248, 1996                                                        3–8

---

*Objective.*—Infection of the diabetic foot is responsible for more hospital days than other diabetic complications, major amputation, and decreased survival. Once diagnosed, accurate determination of the extent of infection is important for optimal management of the problem. The role of MRI in the identification of musculoskeletal pathology and planning of surgical intervention was evaluated prospectively.

*Methods.*—Magnetic resonance imaging was performed on 22 patients (8 women, aged 23 to 86 years) with 25 diabetic foot infections, including 12 with discharging ulcers and 8 with digital gangrene. The MRI scanning method used a head coil with the foot held in neutral position. $T_1$-weighted, $T_2$-weighted, sagittal, and axial scans were performed initially. Later, only $T_1$-weighted and short tau inversion recovery sequence sagittal and axial scans were obtained using 5-mm scans with a 1-mm gap between scans. The MRI results did not determine management. Outcome was based on operative findings or the clinical condition of the patient. Patients were followed up for an average of 9 months.

*Results.*—Operations included debridement in 6 patients, debridement plus amputation of toes in 8, toe amputation in 1, midmetatarsal amputation in 1, and below-the-knee amputation in 1. One patient died of pulmonary embolism. On 13 occasions, patients were managed conservatively, but 4 ultimately required surgery. In 13 patients, MRI scans suggested abscess formation in 10 patients, osteomyelitis in 7, and ankle effusion in 1 (Fig 2). Clinical findings identified 11 infections. The sensi-

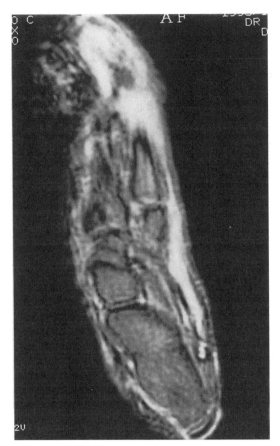

FIGURE 2.—$T_2$-weighted image of a right foot, showing extensive high-signal change in the soft tissues on the medial side of the foot, particularly around the big toe in plantar soft tissues. High-signal change is also seen in the first metatarsal and phalanges. Osteomyelitis with inflammatory change in the soft tissues was confirmed at operation. (Courtesy of Cook TA, Rahim N, Simpson HCR, et al: Magnetic resonance imaging in the management of diabetic foot infection. *Br J Surg* 83:245–248, 1996, Blackwell Science Ltd.)

tivity, specificity, positive predictive value, and negative predictive value of MRI were 91%, 77%, 77%, and 91%, respectively.

*Conclusion.*—Magnetic resonance imaging is a valuable tool for identifying and determining the extent of early infection in the diabetic foot.

▶ The use of MRI in the management of diabetic foot infections has been ricocheting around vascular surgery literature for years.[1, 2] Without question, an MRI can detect infections situated deeply in the foot. On the other hand, the experienced clinician always has a very high level of suspicion of abscess in a foot infection in a person with diabetes. Early operative debridement is clearly indicated with extension of incisions as required to fully drain all spaces affected. No matter how extensive the required debridement, if foot vascularity is adequate, a large majority of these feet will heal satisfactorily and provide a reasonable walking surface.

*References*

1. 1993 YEAR BOOK OF VASCULAR SURGERY, p 95.
2. 1994 YEAR BOOK OF VASCULAR SURGERY, p 137.

## 31P Nuclear Magnetic Resonance Spectroscopy of Acutely Ischaemic Limbs: The Extent of Changes and Progress After Reconstructive Surgery

Brotzakis PZ, Sacco P, Jones DA, et al (Univ College London)
*Cardiovasc Surg* 3:271–276, 1995                                    3–9

*Introduction.*—In reconstructive vascular surgery, there are still concerns regarding tissue viability and occurrence of reperfusion injury after surgery. Nuclear magnetic resonance (NMR) spectroscopy provides estimates of intracellular pH and relative concentrations of various phosphorous metabolites that may provide some insight into these concerns.

*Methods.*—$^{31}P$ NMR spectroscopy of the tibialis anterior muscle was performed in 8 patients with acute limb ischemia caused by acute arterial thrombosis, 13 patients with intermittent claudication, 17 patients with chronic renal failure matched for age and general levels of physical activity as those patients with acute limbs ischemia and intermittent claudication, and in 6 healthy individuals. Changes in muscle metabolites were determined in each group, and changes in muscle metabolites during 30 minutes of experimental leg ischemia were studied in normal individuals. In addition, follow-up NMR measurements were performed in 6 patients who underwent successful revascularization. Measures that would predict outcome of reconstructive surgery were studied.

*Results.*—Inorganic phosphate/phosphocreatinine ratios (Pi/PCr) were similar in normal volunteers (Fig 1, A) and in patients with claudication and chronic renal failure. In patients with acute limb ischemia, muscle Pi/PCr levels were, on average, 4 times higher than those in patients with chronic renal failure with normal limb circulation and normal volunteers. However, there was considerable variation, although the highest ratios were associated with lowest ankle:brachial pressure index values (Fig 2). In addition, Pi/PCr ratios in patients with acute limb ischemia corresponded to those seen in normal volunteers after 30-minute tourniquet ischemia. Follow-up NMR measurements showed that Pi/PCr values became normal between 3 days and 3 months after successful revascularization (Figs 1, B, C). One patient with evidence of reperfusion injury to the anterior tibial compartment showed intracellular acidosis.

*Discussion.*—Acute limb ischemia is associated with alterations in muscle metabolite levels, and there appear to be 3 levels of muscle ischemia. The first level is associated with impaired circulation that increases the Pi/PCr ratio without causing intracellular acidosis; recovery after reconstructive surgery appears to be complete and without complication. The

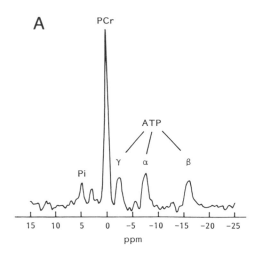

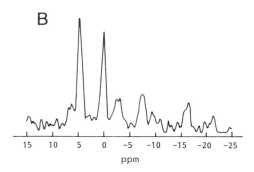

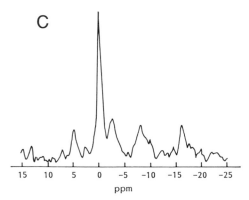

**FIGURE 1.**—[31]P spectra from tibialis anterior muscle. *A,* normal subject; *B,* patient no. 2, group I before surgery; *C,* the same patient after surgery. (Courtesy of Brotzakis PZ, Sacco P, Jones DA, et al: [31]P Nuclear magnetic resonance spectroscopy of acutely ischaemic limbs: The extent of changes and progress after reconstructive surgery. *Cardiovasc Surg* 1995; 3:271–276. Reproduced with permission Cardiovascular Surgery. Copyright 1995 American Heart Association.)

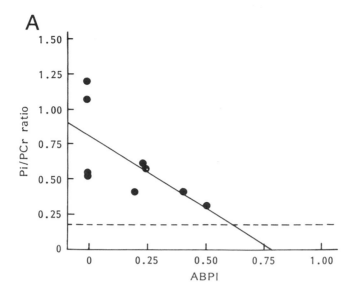

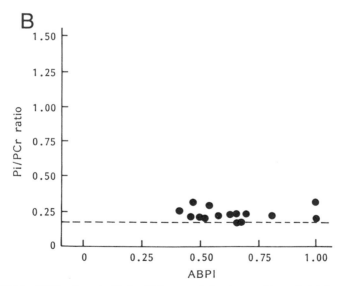

**FIGURE 2.**—Pi/PCr ratio and ankle:brachial pressure index. *A*, group I (acute limb ischaemia) patients before surgery; *B*, group II claudicants (claudicant resting) patients. *Dashed* lines, represents the mean Pi/PCr ratio of group III. *Abbreviations: Pi/PCr*, inorganic phosphate/phosphocreatinine ratio; *ABPI*, ankle:brachial pressure index. (Courtesy of Brotzakis PZ, Sacco P, Jones DA, et al: [31]P Nuclear magnetic resonance spectroscopy of acutely ischaemic limbs: The extent of changes and progress after reconstructive surgery. *Cardiovasc Surg* 1995; 3:271–276. Reproduced with permission Cardiovascular Surgery. Copyright 1995 American Heart Association.)

second level is associated with impaired circulation that leads to acidosis, and recovery after reconstruction entails the risk of reperfusion injury, but long-term viability of the tissue is maintained. It appears that acidosis is a sign of muscle changes that lead to reperfusion injury. The third level of ischemia is associated with circulatory impairment from which there is no recovery. In the future, MRI, in combination with NMR spectroscopy, may provide information about the location of ischemia and the metabolic changes in the muscle, and may predict the risk of complications after reconstructive surgery.

▶ My first reaction to this is that the Brits are tough; the normal volunteers withstood 30 minutes of above-knee tourniquet ischemia. My other reaction to this is, so what? A change in energy metabolism was found in ischemic muscle by NMR spectroscopy. Why doesn't someone look at reversible vs. irreversible ischemia and give us a test to help evaluate a tough clinical problem?

**W. Abbott, M.D.**

---

## Magnetic Resonance Angiography of the Central Chest Veins: A New Gold Standard?

Hartnell GG, Hughes LA, Finn JP, et al (Harvard Med School, Boston)
*Chest* 107:1053–1057, 1995                                                3–10

---

*Background.*—The increasing use of central venous catheters has led to a greater prevalence of acute and chronic venous thrombosis. Diagnostic imaging is needed to identify the site and severity of venous obstruction, but both contrast venography and contrast-enhanced CT have disadvantages. Venipuncture may be impossible in some patients and the injection of contrast media contraindicated. Magnetic resonance angiography (MRA) was evaluated as an alternative method of diagnosing central thoracic venous occlusion and determining sites for central venous access.

*Methods.*—Between January 1990 and April 1994, 84 patients underwent MRA on 102 occasions. Thirty-three were examined to identify possible venous access and 57 to diagnose and stage central venous occlusion. The procedures were performed using sequential, two-dimen-

TABLE 2.—Correlation With Imaging or Surgical Outcome

|                        | No.<br>(% Total) | MRA Agrees |
|------------------------|------------------|------------|
| Angiography            | 18 (18)          | 18/18      |
| Ultrasound             | 5 (5)            | 5/5        |
| CT                     | 6 (6)            | 6/6        |
| Nuclear                | 1 (1)            | 1/1        |
| Surgical line placement | 30 (30)         | 30/30*     |

* Includes 2 unsuccessful attempts at cannulation of veins predicted to be occluded by magnetic resonance angiography.
(Courtesy of Hartnell GG, Hughes LA, Finn JP, et al: Magnetic resonance angiography of the central chest veins: A new gold standard? *Chest* 107:1053–1057, 1995.)

sional, time-of-flight MRA. Selective venographic images were obtained by placing a selective presaturation pulse through the heart, thereby suppressing aortic, cardiac, and arterial flow signal. Each study was usually completed in 30 minutes.

*Results.*—Associated diagnoses were malignancy in 46 cases, parenteral nutrition in 21, hemodialysis in 6, chemotherapy in 4, and other long-term venous access in 7. The 52 women and 32 men had a mean age of 51.2 years. Correlative imaging and/or the results of attempted surgical line placement were available in 55 patients with 5 patients having both types of data. Satisfactory central venous access was achieved in 28 patients in whom MRA predicted a patent site. In all 17 cases in which correlation with contrast venography was available, there was agreement with MRA concerning the level of occluded veins (Table 2). Not all patent veins were demonstrated with contrast venography. Spin-echo MRI was used in some cases for further evaluation of an associated tumor mass.

*Conclusion.*—Two-dimensional time-of-flight MRA was an extremely accurate method of evaluating systemic chest veins and diagnosing central venous occlusion. Because of MRA's advantages over contrast venography, the latter technique is used at the study institution only as an adjunct to thrombolysis in patients who have had an MRA. The safety and reproducibility of MRA make it especially useful in patients requiring serial studies.

▶ These authors have convinced me that MRA can reliably visualize chest veins. They suggest the technique may be helpful in surgical line placement. Perhaps, but I wonder if the expense will not make such use problematic?

---

**Time-of-Flight MR Angiography of the Portal Venous System: Value Compared With Other Imaging Procedures**
Hughes LA, Hartnell GG, Finn JP, et al (Harvard Med School, Boston)
*AJR* 166:375–378, 1996                                                    3–11

---

*Objective.*—Magnetic resonance angiography can provide information about the complicated vascular anatomy of the liver that is equivalent or superior to that obtained with other imaging techniques. In this study, the results of portal MR angiography were compared with those of other available imaging techniques.

*Methods.*—During 1992, 152 patients, aged 10–81 years, underwent 165 portal MR angiography studies. Examinations were performed with an MR system operating at 1T to obtain two-dimensional (2D), flow-compensated, time-of-flight (TOF) sequences. Selective spatial presaturation, bolus tracking, and 3D reconstruction were used as indicated. The findings were compared with those found on sonography, CT, conventional digital subtraction angiography (DSA), and during surgery.

*Results.*—Magnetic resonance venograms were abnormal in 57% of the patients. Portal MR angiography showed more extensive varices than were seen by any of the alternative imaging techniques. There was 99% agreement between MR angiography and available correlative imaging studies.

*Conclusions.*—Magnetic resonance angiography reliably and accurately depicts the portal venous anatomy with more detail than any other imaging technique.

▶ I am impressed that this well-known radiology department concludes that MR angiography of the portal venous system produces images superior to, or at least as good as, images obtained by any other modality. Indeed, the accompanying portal images are most impressive. I tentatively accept their conclusion. This may indeed become the future imaging modality of choice for the portal venous system.

## Venous Imaging

### Venous Thromboembolism: Detection by Duplex Scanning
Nicholls SC, O'Brien JK, Sutton MG (Univ of Washington, Seattle)
*J Vasc Surg* 23:511–516, 1996                                    3–12

*Background.*—Transcranial Doppler ultrasound is clinically helpful in identifying intra-arterial emboli. It has been used to identify patients with symptomatic or asymptomatic carotid lesions who may have had active emboli in the distribution of the middle cerebral artery. The use of Doppler ultrasound to identify venous emboli was studied, including an evaluation of the effects of anticoagulant treatment on the embolism rate.

*Methods.*—Two hundred eighteen patients with suspected deep vein thrombosis (DVT) underwent a standard venous duplex examination. The signals were evaluated for the presence of a "Doppler embolic signal," revised criteria for which were developed. The ability to detect emboli was enhanced by the use of low-gain settings, low-frequency probes, and continuous-wave Doppler imaging.

*Results.*—Sixty patients were diagnosed as having DVT, and 43% of these showed embolism in the Doppler spectrum. Nineteen percent of patients showed emboli on B-mode images; the estimated embolus size ranged from 200 to 5,000 μm. Embolus counts of 5 to 800 per minute were observed. Two patients had DVT of the iliofemoral vein, 8 of the superficial femoral/profunda vein, 1 of the saphenofemoral junction, 1 of the popliteal vein, and 10 of the calf.

Of the 158 patients without DVT, 3% had positive scans for emboli. Heparin treatment halved the embolus count within 24 hours and eliminated all emboli within 72 hours. There were 2 deaths as the result of pulmonary embolism.

*Conclusions.*—Embolism is common among patients who are found to have DVT on duplex scanning. The microemboli appear to resolve promptly with heparin treatment. More research is needed to clarify the link between microembolism, DVT, and pulmonary embolism.

▶ These investigators from the University of Washington have widely published their observations on the use of transcranial Doppler to identify emboli in the cerebral circulation, presumably arising from the carotid arteries. They have now adopted the same technology to study veins upstream from established venous thrombosis. They believe they detected embolism upstream DVT in 26 of 60 patients, and, interestingly, in 4 of 158 patients without DVT. In patients being given heparin, the number of emboli decreased within 24 hours and vanished by 72 hours. On balance, this information confirms what we thought we already knew, namely, that most DVT do produce emboli, usually before the initiation of anticoagulant treatment. In fact, if the truth were known, 100% of DVT probably produce emboli.

---

**Limited B-Mode Venous Imaging Versus Complete Color-Flow Duplex Venous Scanning for Detection of Proximal Deep Venous Thrombosis**
Poppiti R, Papanicolaou G, Perese S, et al (Univ of Southern California, Los Angeles)
*J Vasc Surg* 22:553–557, 1995                                    3–13

---

*Introduction.*—Several studies have demonstrated the efficacy of B-mode compression technique (BMCT) for the detection of proximal deep venous thrombosis (DVT), with sensitivity and specificity approaching 100%. These findings raise concern about whether the technically demanding and time-consuming complete color-flow duplex venous evaluation (CDVE) is absolutely necessary for the diagnosis of proximal DVT. It is hypothesized that a BMCT examination is as accurate as complete CDVE for the detection of proximal DVT.

*Study Design.*—In a prospective study, 20 men and 52 women referred for venous duplex examination underwent a BMCT followed by a CDVE. Two technologists blinded to each other performed either examination independently. For BMCT, 2 sites per limb were assessed: the saphenofemoral junction including the superficial femoral and deep femoral vein confluence and the saphenopopliteal junction including tibial vein confluence. The CDVE was considered the gold standard when calculating the specificity, sensitivity, and accuracy of the studies.

*Findings.*—The BMCT failed in 3 of 144 limbs. The average time to perform BMCT was 5.5 minutes and the examination identified proximal DVT in 15 of 141 limbs. The CDVE was positive in 13 limbs. For the 2 false positive BMCT, the popliteal veins were deep to the artery leading to difficulty in compression. For the detection of proximal DVT, BMCT was 100% sensitive, 98% specific, and 99% accurate. In addition, BMCT detected a floating thrombus and chronic thrombus, and 2 small thrombi behind femoral vein valve cusps.

*Conclusions.*—The B-mode compression technique is a rapid, acceptable alternative for detecting proximal DVT. It is ideal for use in patients with abrupt onset of extremity swelling or to rule out the lower extremity as a source of pulmonary embolus. If the result of BMCT is equivocal or positive, the spectral color-flow Doppler examination should be performed to confirm the results.

▶ The problem with this study is that we do not know the diagnostic accuracy of color-coded duplex in the hands of the authors. Therefore, it is difficult to know what the new method really means in terms of detecting "true" DVT.

**D. Bergqvist, M.D., Ph.D.**

---

**Determining the Acuteness and Stability of Deep Venous Thrombosis by Ultrasonic Tissue Characterization**
Kolecki RV, Sigel B, Justin J, et al (Med College of Pennsylvania, Philadelphia; Riverside Research Inst, New York)
*J Vasc Surg* 21:976–984, 1995                                                    3–14

---

*Introduction.*—Determining the composition of the thrombus is important in indicating the acuteness and stability of deep venous thrombosis of lower extremities. A greater risk for deep venous thrombosis may be suggested by thrombi with a high red blood cell-fibrin mesh content. Ultrasonic tissue characterization tries to distinguish differences in tissue content on the basis of physical properties, such as speed of sound through tissue, attenuation, and scatterer effects. Previous studies with pigs using ultrasonic tissue characterization showed that acute red blood cell-fibrin mesh thrombi were revealed as slightly decreased slope and significantly increased intercept values, when compared with older thrombi. Ultrasonic tissue characterization was evaluated for its ability to indicate stability and acuteness of deep venous thrombosis of the lower extremities.

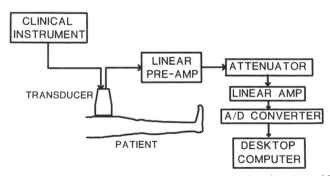

FIGURE 1.—Block diagram of UTC system for data acquisition and analysis. Unmodified signal is obtained from ultrasound transducer. Signal is amplified and converted to digital form, and digitized data are stored in computer for analysis. *Abbreviations: UTC*, ultrasonic tissue characterization. (Courtesy of Kolecki RV, Sigel B, Justin J, et al: Determining the acuteness and stability of deep venous thrombosis by ultrasonic tissue characterization. *J Vasc Surg* 21:976–984, 1995.)

TABLE 1.—Ultrasonic Tissue Characterization Basic Parameters for DVT
at Initial Examination

| Type of DVT | No. of Extremities | Slope (dB/MHz)\ | Intercept (dBr) |
|---|---|---|---|
| Acute | 19 | −3.61±0.89 | −31.0±5.3 |
| Chronic | 31 | −3.69±1.21 | −42.6±6.1 |

*P < 0.01. All values are means ± SD.
*Abbreviation: DVT*, deep vein thrombosis.
(Courtesy of Kolecki RV, Sigel B, Justin J, et al: Determining the acuteness and stability of deep venous thrombosis by ultrasonic tissue characterization. *J Vasc Surg* 21:976–984, 1995.)

*Methods.*—Forty-five patients with deep vein thrombosis who had thrombi in the common or superficial femoral or popliteal veins had ultrasonic tissue characterization analysis. The patients were divided into 2 groups: 18 patients with 19 affected extremities were classified as acute with symptoms for fewer than 4 days; 27 patients with 31 affected ex-

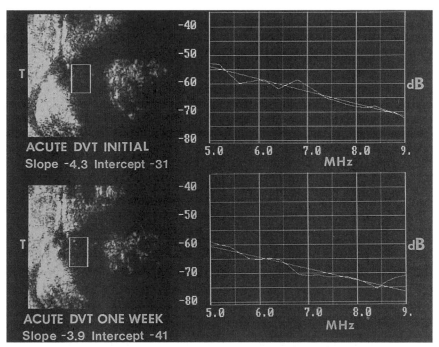

FIGURE 2.—Computer display of UTC analysis of single ROI at initial examination and at reexamination 1 week later in acute DVT extremity. Computer-reconstructed B-mode images are on left. These show femoral vein, moderately hyperechoic luminal defect, and rectangular cursor demarcating region being analyzed. Normalized power spectrum of data within ROI is on right. Power spectrum parameters are obtained from best-fit straight line applied to spectrum. These parameters are slope (dB/MHz) and intercept (dBr). Note that slope increased slightly and intercept decreased by 10 dBr after 1 week. *Abbreviations: UTC*, ultrasonic tissue characterization: *DVT*, deep vein thrombosis; *ROI*, regions of interest. (Courtesy of Kolecki RV, Sigel B, Justin J, et al: Determining the acuteness and stability of deep venous thrombosis by ultrasonic tissue characterization. *J Vasc Surg* 21:976–984, 1995.)

## INTERCEPT VALUES OF DEEP VENOUS THROMBOSIS OVER ONE WEEK

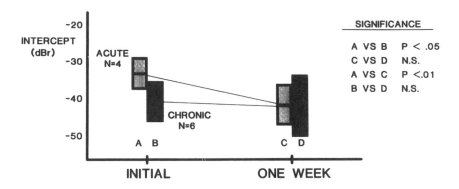

Bars indicate mean (center line segment) and standard deviation

FIGURE 6.—Graphic display of intercept values at initial and 1-week examinations and differences that occurred over time. Significance of various comparisons are on right. (Courtesy of Kolecki RV, Sigel B, Justin J, et al: Determining the acuteness and stability of deep venous thrombosis by ultrasonic tissue characterization. *J Vasc Surg* 21:976–984, 1995.)

tremities were classified as chronic with symptoms for more than 21 days. The ultrasonic tissue characterization analysis involves converting the signal from analogue to digital form and then obtaining a power spectrum by computer processing (Fig 1). At week 1, 10 of the deep vein thrombosis extremities were reexamined to assess changes in the ultrasonic tissue characterization to suggest thrombus instability.

*Results.*—Chronic deep vein thrombosis could be distinguished from acute deep vein thrombosis, which was seen in 19 of 50 extremities. In the acute group, the intercept values were 11.6 relative decibels higher than for the chronic group (Table 1). In correctly diagnosed acute deep vein thrombosis, discriminant linear analysis of the 2 parameters showed a sensitivity of 94.7% and a specificity of 90.3%. In the sample of 10 extremities that were reexamined a week later, there was a mean 9.4 relative decibel decrease in intercept values. There was no significant change in slope (Figs 2 and 6).

*Conclusion.*—This was the first study to show that a noninvasive method could discriminate between thrombus-content differences to allow for clinical staging of patients with deep vein thrombosis. Ultrasonic tissue characterization distinguished between acute and chronic deep vein thrombosis. To establish the relevance of this study, further prospective investigation is necessary.

▶ As I have stated before in the YEAR BOOK, there is a pressing need to develop a test that will allow the vascular laboratory to distinguish between a young and old venous thrombosis. These authors, in a prior YEAR BOOK,[1] suggested that electronic processing of backscatter data from the ultrasound image could be used for this purpose. They noted that an acute thrombus has a very high Y intercept, whereas a chronic thrombus has a lower intercept. Their prior study concerned experimentally induced thrombus, whereas the current study is directed toward clinical DVT. An inherent weakness in studies such as this is the inability to date the onset of thrombus with precision, although these authors appear to have done a reasonable job. The sequential observation in several patients who proceeded from acute to chronic thrombus, showing a decreasing Y intercept with time, is fascinating. I hope this information will rapidly be independently confirmed by others and, if true, will soon become available for general use. The ability of a vascular lab examination to accurately date the age of thrombi in the deep veins would be of profound clinical importance.

*Reference*

1. 1994 YEAR BOOK OF VASCULAR SURGERY, p 120.

## Contralateral Duplex Scanning for Deep Venous Thrombosis is Unnecessary in Patients With Symptoms

Strothman G, Blebea J, Fowl RJ, et al (Univ of Cincinnati, Ohio)
*J Vasc Surg* 22:543–547, 1995                                    3–15

*Background.*—Deep vein thrombosis (DVT) involves both legs in 17% to 32% of acute cases, even when the contralateral leg is asymptomatic. As a result, bilateral duplex venous scanning is the recommended evaluation. Because treatment for the symptomatic leg treats the other as well, the need for routine bilateral examinations has been questioned. This question was evaluated by review of a series of such procedures.

*Methods.*—All venous duplex scans performed at the institution during a 2-year period were reviewed retrospectively. Demographic patient data, symptoms, scan results, and incidence of bilateral DVT were recorded.

*Results.*—Of 248 patients with acute DVT, unilateral disease was significantly more common in patients with unilateral symptoms (88% of 176 patients). However, 66% (44 patients) of those with unilateral symp-

TABLE 5.—Symptoms and Duplex Scanning Results

| Duplex Scanning Results | Symptoms | | |
|---|---|---|---|
| | Unilateral | Bilateral | Total |
| Unilateral DVT | 154 | 22 | 176 |
| Bilateral DVT | 44 | 28 | 72 |
| Total | 198 | 50 | 248 |

(Courtesy of Strothman G, Blebea J, Fowl RJ, et al: Contralateral duplex scanning for deep venous thrombosis is unnecessary in patients with symptoms. *J Vasc Surg* 22:543–547, 1995.)

toms had bilateral DVT. Bilateral symptoms were accompanied significantly more often by bilateral disease (Table 5). An important finding was that every patient with contralateral DVT also had DVT in the symptomatic leg. Thus, there was no case of DVT in an asymptomatic limb that would have gone untreated.

*Conclusion.*—In patients symptomatic for DVT, duplex venous scanning of the symptomatic limb is sufficient, inasmuch as therapy will treat the contralateral limb as well when bilateral disease is present.

▶ The controversy continues. These authors conclude that contralateral venous scanning in patients with unilateral symptoms is not clinically indicated. The group from Good Samaritan Hospital in Cincinnati, however, concluded just the opposite, stating that patients suspected of having DVT should undergo bilateral lower extremity duplex ultrasound scanning regardless of the location of symptoms.[1] Whereas the authors of this paper conclude that the occasional patient will have DVT in the asymptomatic limb, they find that it never occurs there without simultaneous occurrence in the symptomatic limb. Personally, I am very concerned about missing a DVT because of its tremendous clinical importance. I will continue to obtain bilateral studies.

*Reference*

1. 1996 Year Book of Vascular Surgery, p 133.

---

**Bilateral Lower Extremity US in the Patient With Bilateral Symptoms of Deep Venous Thrombosis: Assessment of Need**
Sheiman RG, Weintraub JL, McArdle CR (Harvard Med School, Boston)
*Radiology* 196:379–381, 1995                                    3–16

---

*Objective.*—Fifty patients with bilateral lower limb symptoms suggesting deep venous thrombosis (DVT) were studied prospectively to learn how often bilateral disease is actually present in these patients.

*Method.*—The veins of the lower extremities were examined by gray-scale color Doppler flow imaging and spectral analysis, using a 5- or 7-MHz linear-array transducer. The calf veins were not studied.

*Results.*—No DVT was detected in these patients. Possible alternative causes of symptoms were present in 68% of patients. The most frequent were heart disease, superficial thrombophlebitis or cellulitis and, in 6 cases, peripheral arterial disease.

*Conclusion.*—Deep venous thrombosis is rare in patients who have bilateral symptoms suggesting this diagnosis. An initial ultrasound study is not warranted, especially if a likely alternative cause is identified.

▶ These authors have addressed a highly focused issue, namely, the likelihood of DVT in a patient with bilateral lower extremity symptoms compatible with DVT. They conclude that the likelihood approaches 0. Perhaps, but

I am not persuaded. Fear of missing a potentially fatal DVT will keep me obtaining examinations, even if they are not convincingly "cost effective." See also Abstract 3–15.

## Helical Computed Tomography

### Diagnosis of Aortic Dissection: Value of Helical CT With Multiplanar Reformation and Three-Dimensional Rendering

Zeman RK, Berman PM, Silverman PM, et al (Georgetown Univ, Washington, DC; Cleveland Clinic Found, Ohio)
*AJR* 164:1375–1380, 1995                                            3–17

*Background.*—Helical CT appears to be useful for the investigation of vascular abnormalities, perhaps including aortic dissection. The value of helical CT in the evaluation of suspected aortic dissection was studied.

*Methods.*—Twenty-three patients with suspected aortic dissection— based on chest pain or an abnormal chest radiograph—underwent helical CT. The scans used nonionic contrast material injected in a bolus at 2.0 to 2.5 mL/sec, with a mean scan delay of 47 seconds. Axial scans with 5-mm collimation, extending from the great vessels to the distal thoracic aorta just above the hiatus, were obtained. In addition, delayed helical sections through the upper abdomen were obtained. The helical data were used to create multiplanar reformations and three-dimensional (3D) models, which were compared with the findings of axial sections in 7 patients with

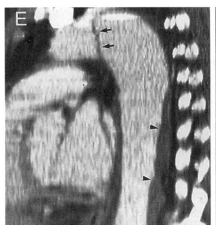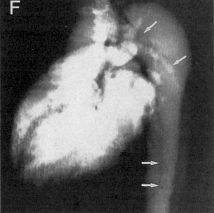

FIGURE 1.—E, multiplanar reformation in sagittal position shows intimal flap (*arrows*) extending to origin of left subclavian artery (*S*). Although intimal flap extended into lower thoracic aorta, it was not visualized on this view because it was out of plane of reformatted section. Partial thrombosis of false channel within distal aorta (*arrowheads*) is identified on this view. F, three-dimensional ray-sum projection view also depicts intimal flap (*arrows*). Flap appears to change orientation within aortic arch because it is spiraling around aorta as it extends superiorly. Both multiplanar and three-dimensional views definitively showed relationship of intimal flap to left subclavian artery. (Courtesy of Zeman RK, Berman PM, Silverman PM, et al: Diagnosis of aortic dissection: Value of helical CT with multiplanar reformation of three-dimensional rendering. *AJR* 164:1375–1380, 1995.)

proven dissection. The CT findings were compared with those of surgery, angiography, or clinical outcome.

*Results.*—The axial sections gave true negative results in 15 patients, true positive results in 7, and false positive results in 1. Axial sections had trouble delineating the extent of the intimal flaps in 3 of 7 patients with documented dissection. However, the anatomy was clarified with multiplanar reformation or 3D views (Fig 1, E and F). Ray-sum 3D projection views gave better results than surface model or maximum-intensity-projection views.

*Conclusions.*—With multiplanar reformation and 3D rendering, helical CT scanning may be a valuable adjunct to axial CT scans in detecting aortic dissection and assessing the extent of the intimal flap. More patients will have to be studied to confirm these preliminary results.

▶ The theoretical benefits of helical CT are numerous. It represents a volumetric acquisition and, therefore, misregistration artifacts are reduced. The rapid scan acquisition permits the constant use of higher intravascular levels of contrast media. Image reconstruction can be performed in such a way as to reduce volume averaging and assist in visualization of small abnormalities such as an intimal flap. The use of overlapping images results in very high quality 3D projections and multiplanar reformation can be displayed. This article describes the use of this new technology in the diagnosis of aortic dissection. Their study of a limited number of patients leads these authors to believe that extremely detailed anatomical information can be derived with optimal use of this new technology. I suspect they are correct. I do recognize that in our own institution, however, the prolonged time currently required by the radiologists to reformat 1 of these studies is a major drawback to its widespread use. I am told it takes 2–3 hours to extract complete information from such a scan.

---

**Supra- and Juxtarenal Aneurysms of the Abdominal Aorta: Preoperative Assessment With Thin-Section Spiral CT**
Van Hoe L, Baert AL, Gryspeerdt S, et al (Katholieke Universiteit Leuven, Belgium)
*Radiology* 198:443–448, 1996                                                    3–18

---

*Purpose.*—Digital subtraction angiography (DSA) and conventional incremental CT are routinely used to assess abdominal aortic aneurysms (AAAs), but because of the presence of thrombotic material in some AAAs, the real extent of aneurysmal dilatation can be underestimated with DSA. Magnetic resonance angiography and spiral CT are useful for evaluating AAAs, but most patients included in the early studies had infrarenal AAAs. The utility of thin-section spiral CT in the preoperative assessment of juxtarenal and suprarenal AAAs was examined.

*Patients.*—Digital subtraction angiography and 2-mm-collimation spiral CT were performed in 26 men and 12 women, ages 60–81 years, of

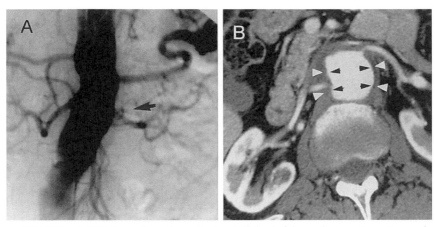

FIGURE 5.—**A**, DSA image shows the aortic size at the level of the renal arteries (*arrow*) as nearly normal; there is no evidence of suprarenal or juxtarenal extension. **B**, axial CT image shows enlargement of the aorta, involvement of both renal arteries, and attachment of thrombotic material (*arrowheads*) to the wall of the aneurysm. The suprarenal extension of this aneurysm, as shown at CT, was confirmed during surgery. (Courtesy of Van Hoe L, Baert AL, Gryspeerdt S, et al: Supra- and juxtarenal aneurysms of the abdominal aorta: Preoperative assessment with thin-section spiral CT. *Radiology* 198:443–448, 1996. Radiological Society of North America.)

whom 23 had infrarenal AAAs, 8 had juxtarenal AAAs, and 7 had suprarenal AAAs. Cine-interactive display of overlapping axial, reformatted, and maximum intensity projection images were used for CT image analysis. The DSA images and CT images were independently analyzed by 2 radiologists. The CT findings were then compared with DSA findings and surgical findings, which were used as the standard of reference.

*Results.*—All 23 infrarenal aneurysms were correctly classified with both DSA and thin-section spiral CT. The proximal extent of the AAA was correctly estimated with DSA in 7 of the 8 juxtarenal AAAs and with spiral CT in all 8 juxtarenal AAAs. Of the 7 suprarenal AAAs, 6 were correctly classified with CT and 5 with DSA (Fig 5). Digital subtraction angiography visualized 74 main and 12 accessory renal arteries. Computed tomography identified 83 of these 86 arteries (96%).

*Conclusions.*—Thin-section spiral CT can provide additional information in the preoperative assessment of AAAs involving the suprarenal or juxtarenal aorta that is not available with DSA. This imaging technique is also useful in the assessment of renal artery stenoses.

▶ We all know that conventional CT is notoriously unreliable in precisely defining the upper extent of infrarenal AAAs. These authors investigate the hypothesis that well-performed spiral CT may achieve this objective. Based on a small number of patients, they conclude that spiral CT, in their experience, was 93% accurate in determining the proximal extent of juxta- and suprarenal aneurysms. They missed a few renal arteries, however. On balance, this appears to be another extremely expensive imaging tool that will be of only incremental benefit in the clinical practice of vascular surgery. I really don't know where it will sort out in the ultimate cost/benefit analysis. I am sure the bean counters will be looking.

## Detection of Pulmonary Embolism in Patients With Unresolved Clinical and Scintigraphic Diagnosis: Helical CT Versus Angiography
Goodman LR, Curtin JJ, Mewissen MW, et al (Med College of Wisconsin, Milwaukee)
*AJR* 164:1369–1374, 1995                                                          3–19

*Background.*—The role of CT in the detection of pulmonary embolism has been the subject of much debate. Some authors suggest that CT is a reliable, noninvasive alternative to angiography, whereas others argue that the efficacy of this imaging modality has not yet been confirmed. The ability of helical CT to detect pulmonary embolism in patients with unresolved clinical and scintigraphic diagnoses was therefore prospectively investigated. Findings were compared with those obtained using pulmonary angiography.

*Patients and Methods.*—Contrast-enhanced helical CT and selective pulmonary angiography were performed in 20 patients with suspected pulmonary embolism. Studies were separated by an average of 11 hours. The CT scans were done during 24-second or two 12-second breath-holds, and evaluated without knowledge of the scintigraphic and angiographic results. The angiographic studies were performed with knowledge of the ventilation/perfusion scan findings. The sensitivity and specificity of CT and angiography were evaluated for central vessels and for all other vessels.

*Results.*—Eleven patients had angiographically proven pulmonary emboli. These were located in the central vessels in 7 and in the subsegmental vessels in 4 patients. Only 1 of the 11 patients had a high probability finding on ventilation/perfusion scans. The sensitivity, specificity, and likelihood ratio of CT were 86%, 92%, and 10.7, respectively, when analyzing central vessels. When including the more difficult-to-diagnose subsegmental vessels in the analysis, CT achieved a sensitivity of only 63%, specificity of 89%, and a likelihood ratio of 5.7 (Fig 2).

*Conclusions.*—As experience with CT increases, sensitivity may be improved. Until then, pulmonary angiography should remain the preferred study for the detection of pulmonary emboli in patients with unresolved clinical and scintigraphic diagnoses.

▶ I am sorry to learn that well-done helical CT has an unacceptably low sensitivity of only 63% in the detection of pulmonary embolus, and thus does not begin to compare with well-performed pulmonary angiography. The authors' conclusion that helical CT has a limited role in the evaluation of acute pulmonary embolism is undoubtedly correct. Too bad.

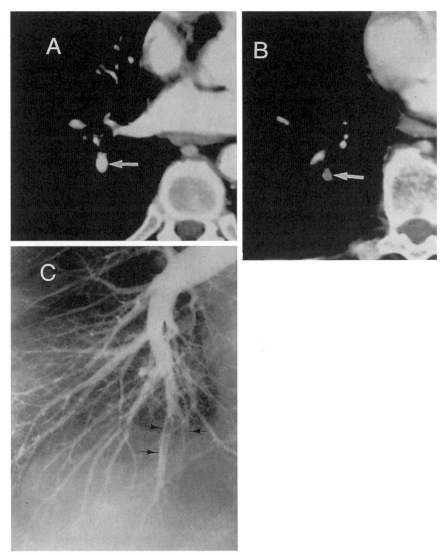

FIGURE 2.—True positive CT scan, subsegmental level. A 72-year-old man with hypoxia and increased cardiac second sound. Clinical suspicion was moderate and scintigraphic suspicion ws low. **A,** CT scan shows normal posterior part of basilar segmental artery (*arrow*). **B,** CT scan 9 mm farther caudad shows complete lack of opacification of vessel (*arrow*). **C,** selective angiogram of right pulmonary artery shows clot (*arrows*) limited to subsegmental vessels of posterior basilar segment. (Courtesy of Goodman LR, Curtin JJ, Mewissen MW, et al: Detection of pulmonary embolism in patients with unresolved clinical and scinitigraphic diagnosis: Helical CT versus angiography. *AJR* 164:1369–1374, 1995.)

## Transcranial Doppler

### The Significance of Microemboli Detection by Means of Transcranial Doppler Ultrasonography Monitoring in Carotid Endarterectomy

Ackerstaff RGA, Jansen C, Moll FL, et al (St Antonius Hosp, Nieuwegein, The Netherlands)

*J Vasc Surg* 21:963–969, 1995                                        3–20

*Objective.*—Carotid endarterectomy (CEA) can result in intraoperative and perioperative cerebral complications. Intraoperative transcranial Doppler (TCD) monitoring has been used to monitor blood flow velocities and microembolisms. The results of a prospective study to detect and describe the occurrence of embolic transients, to relate these signals to surgical technique, to evaluate the influence of the TCD signal on surgical technique, and to assess the impact of microemboli on brain function and structure are presented.

*Methods.*—Neurologic examinations were conducted in 301 patients (66 women), aged 42 to 87 years, before and after surgery and at 3 months postoperatively. Computed tomography and MR were performed before surgery, EEG and transcranial Doppler ultrasonography of the ipsilateral middle cerebral artery were used during surgery to monitor CEA, CT scans were performed 3 to 5 days postoperatively in 58 patients with TCD-detected embolic transients, and MR was performed postoperatively in 40 carotid endarterectomy patients. Pre- and postoperative scans and images were compared to assess change in brain architecture in these 2 groups of

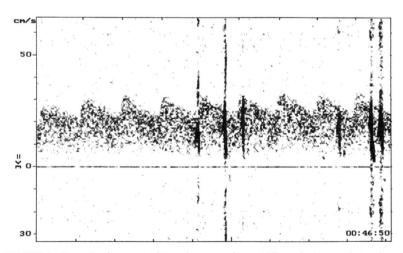

FIGURE 1.—Example of transcranial Doppler spectra from middle cerebral artery during dissection, indicating 6 embolic transients. (Courtesy of Ackerstaff RGA, Jansen C, Moll FL, et al: The significance of microemboli detection by means of transcranial Doppler ultrasonography monitoring in carotid endarterectomy. *J Vasc Surg* 21:963–969. 1995.)

TABLE 1.—Semiquantitative Analysis of Embolic Transients in 3 Different Stages of Carotid Endarterectomy ($n = 301$) and Their Impact on Intraoperative and Postoperative Ischemic Complication (*P* Values)

| Phase of Operation | Embolic Transients (%) | TIA $n = 7$ | Intraoperative Ischemic Stroke $n = 3$ | TIA $n = 1$ | Postoperative Ischemic Stroke $n = 10$ |
|---|---|---|---|---|---|
| Dissection | No ET (75) | $n = 3$ | $n = 3$ (NS) | $n = 0$ | $n = 5$ (NS) |
| | <10 ET (20) | $n = 1$ | $n = 0$ (NS) | $n = 0$ | $n = 3$ (NS) |
| | >10 ET (5) | $n = 3$ | $n = 0$ ($p < 0.002$) | $n = 1$ | $n = 2$ ($p < 0.02$) |
| After CC release | No ET (47) | $n = 1$ | $n = 3$ (NS) | $n = 1$ | $n = 3$ (NS) |
| | <10 ET (29) | $n = 3$ | $n = 0$ (NS) | $n = 0$ | $n = 2$ (NS) |
| | >10 ET (24) | $n = 3$ | $n = 0$ (NS) | $n = 0$ | $n = 5$ (NS) |
| During shunt | No ET (66) | $n = 0$ | $n = 0$ (NS) | $n = 0$ | $n = 0$ (NS) |
| manipulation | <10 ET (34) | $n = 3$ | $n = 3$ ($p < 0.007$) | $n = 1$ | $n = 3$ (NS) |

*Abbreviations: ET*, embolic transients; *TIA*, transient ischemic symptoms; *CC*, cross-clamp; *NS*, not significant.
(Courtesy of Ackerstaff RGA, Jansen C, Moll FL, et al: The significance of microemboli detection by means of transcranial Doppler ultrasonography monitoring in carotid endarterectomy. *J Vasc Surg* 21:963–969, 1995.)

patients. Pre- and intraoperative risk factors were correlated with cerebral aftermath using logistic regression analysis.

*Results.*—The combined stroke and death rate was 5.7% and included 3 intraoperative and 10 postoperative strokes and 4 deaths. Microemboli were observed in 69% of CEA, and 25% occurred during dissection (Fig 1). Patients with more than 10 microemboli had significantly more intraoperative and postoperative complications (Table 1). Postoperative MR images of these patients demonstrated a significant correlation between more than 10 microemboli and new lesions. Whereas postoperative CT scans did not show morphologic changes, transient cerebral deficits were apparent immediately after surgery.

*Conclusion.*—The presence of more than 10 microemboli during CEA is significantly related to perioperative cerebral complications and with new lesions that appear on MR images. Shunting during surgery also significantly increases the risk of intraoperative complications. Transcranial Doppler ultrasonographic monitoring during surgery can give valuable information to the operating team and may lead to a decrease in the risk of intraoperative stroke.

▶ Fifteen percent of patients could not be successfully studied by this technique because of technical problems in positioning and insonation. The effect of audible emboli on the surgeon may well lead to more caution in dissection and manipulation, even to needling the artery to measure stump pressure. Yet again, CT scanning is shown to be insensitive in the detection of small cerebral infarcts. By contrast, MR demonstrates middle cerebral infarcts small enough to be asymptomatic. The embolic transients after cross-clamp release may well be harmless air bubbles or platelet aggregates, when compared to the insoluble debris dislodged by mobilization or shunting accidents. Transcranial Doppler monitoring may be of value in heightening our awareness of risk during operation. Magnetic resonance scanning emerges as the best objective test of our success in protecting the brain.

**A.E.B. Giddings, M.D.**

▶ On balance, I do every CEA as carefully as I can. There are some things I don't want to know, including chirping noises from a TCD!

**J.M. Porter, M.D.**

---

**Interpretation of Embolic Phenomena During Carotid Endarterectomy**
Smith JL, Evans DH, Fan L, et al (Leicester Univ, England)
*Stroke* 26:2281–2284, 1995                                               3–21

---

*Introduction.*—Particulate emboli are a major source of morbidity during carotid endarterectomy (CEA), but air emboli rarely cause significant morbidity. Amplitude overload and poor time resolution have consistently limited the ability of current transcranial Doppler ultrasound (TCD) to differentiate between air and particulate emboli. These 2 limitations were overcome by rerouting embolic signals away from the audio frequency amplifier to avoid amplitude overload and substituting the Wigner distribution function for the fast Fourier transform (FFT) to improve time resolution and frequency resolution.

*Applications.*—In vitro data were obtained using a flow rig model into which controlled volumes of pure air could be introduced, ensuring that all ultrasonic properties of the blood substitute were analogous to whole blood. In vivo particulate data were acquired during routine CEA surgery in 67 patients. The effective sample volume length (SVL) was calculated as the product of embolic duration and velocity and represented the length of artery over which the embolic signal was detected. It was hypothesized that air reflected more than ultrasound and would be therefore detected over a greater SVL.

*Findings.*—The mean SVL for 75 air emboli introduced into the flow rig was 1.97 cm (range, 1.7–2.35), compared with only 0.27 cm (range, 0.16–0.43) for 185 particulate emboli detected during the initial dissection phase of CEA. Assuming an upper SVL limit of 1.28 cm for the diagnosis of particulate emboli, 97.6% of air emboli would have been correctly interpreted. For the remaining 560 emboli detected during different phases of CEA, and assuming that an embolus was particulate if the SVL was 1.28 cm or less, 32% of emboli immediately after shunt insertion were probably particulate, as well as 58% detected during shunting, 36% after restoration of flow in the external carotid artery, 9% after restoration of flow in the internal carotid artery, and 100% of those detected during the early recovery phase.

*Summary.*—This study represents an entirely new approach to analyzing embolic phenomena, providing objective physical criteria as a basis for embolus characterization, whether particulate or air. The Wigner distribution function, instead of FFT, should be used to analyze Doppler signals to improve the accuracy of measuring embolic velocity and duration. This work has major implications for patient monitoring with respect to modification of surgical technique and pharmacologic intervention.

► These authors suggest that there may be some benefit in differentiating between air and particulate cerebral emboli occurring during CEA. They present interesting and complex engineering data purporting to achieve this differentiation. Their remarkable conclusions that persistent particulate emboli may result in cognitive decline, emboli detected early during the recovery phase are frequently associated with perioperative thrombosis, and that air emboli rarely cause significant morbidity is all new information to me. I really have no idea what to make of this. I conclude that cerebral microemboli do occur during endarterectomy and that, in general, they are sometimes bad but never good. Anyone disagree?

## Carotid Imaging

**Screening for Asymptomatic Internal Carotid Artery Stenosis: Duplex Criteria for Discriminating 60% to 99% Stenosis**
Moneta GL, Edwards JM, Papanicolaou G, et al (Oregon Health Sciences Univ, Portland; Univ of Washington, Seattle)
*J Vasc Surg* 21:989–994, 1995                                            3–22

*Introduction.*—The Asymptomatic Carotid Atherosclerosis Study (ACAS) recently reported a reduced risk for ipsilateral stroke in symptom-free patients with 60% to 99% internal carotid artery (ICA) stenosis. The 5-year absolute risk reduction for ipsilateral stroke was a modest 5.8%. However, an increased number of screening duplex examinations are likely to follow this finding. The ability of duplex scanning to identify 60% to 99% ICA stenoses was evaluated. Duplex criteria that provide high accuracy and a very high positive predictive value (PPV) for asymptomatic ICA stenosis were also analyzed.

*Methods.*—A total of 352 patent ICAs were blindly compared using angiographic and duplex scanning testing. Duplex scanning criteria were determined for 95% or greater PPV for 60% or greater ICA stenosis.

*Results.*—One-hundred sixty of 352 arteries (46%) showed an angiographic ICA stenosis of 60% to 99%. In 119 ICAs, a peak systolic velocity (PSV) of more than 300 cm/sec was measured. An ICA/common carotid artery PSV ratio greater than 5.0 was measured in 105 ICAs (30%). The minimum duplex values that provided the highest combination of sensitivity and overall accuracy for determining a 60% to 99% ICA stenosis with at least 95% PPV were the combination of an ICA PSV of at least 290 cm/sec and an ICA end-diastolic velocity of at least 80 cm/sec (Table 2).

*Conclusion.*—It is reasonable, given currently available information, to require a duplex examination to have a PPV of at least 90% for a 60% or greater lesion before performing carotid angiography. The PPV should be at least 95% before expecting a patient to undergo endarterectomy on the basis of duplex scanning results alone.

TABLE 2.—Minimal PSVs, EDVs, ICA PSV/CCA PSV Ratios, and Combinations of ICA PSV and ICA EDV Associated With a 95% Positive Predictive Value for 60% to 99% ICA Stenosis

| | Sensitivity | Specificity | PPV | NPV | Accuracy |
|---|---|---|---|---|---|
| PSV (cm/sec) | | | | | |
| 360 | 58 | 98 | 96 | 74 | 80 |
| EDV (cm/sec) | | | | | |
| None | — | — | — | — | — |
| ICA/CCA PSV | | | | | |
| 6.1 | 44 | 98 | 95 | 68 | 73 |
| ICA PSV (cm/sec), EDV (cm/sec) | | | | | |
| 290, 80 | 78 | 96 | 95 | 84 | 88 |

*Abbreviations: PSV*, peak systolic velocity; *EDV*, end-diastolic velocity; *ICA*, internal carotid artery; *CCA*, common carotid artery.

(Courtesy of Moneta GL, Edwards JM, Papanicolaou G, et al: Screening for asymptomatic internal carotid artery stenosis: Duplex criteria for discriminating 60% to 99% stenosis. *J Vasc Surg* 21:989–994, 1995.)

▶ My duplex criteria friends, including Dr. Moneta, inform me that one establishes criteria retrospectively, but then they must be validated prospectively. The first half of the exercise is contained herein. The criteria for an ACAS-positive ICA are given in terms of systolic and diastolic ICA velocity for both a 92% PPV, and a 95% PPV. Without question, more and more carotid endarterectomies are being performed without preoperative arteriography. Thus, we must have rigid duplex criteria if we are to accurately define the population for surgery. This is the reason the authors have established a 95% PPV category, and I believe this reasoning to be quite logical. On balance, however, the ACAS publication has had a smaller clinical impact than I predicted. The modest clinical benefits, coupled with the indeterminate status of the procedure in women, has led some to question the significance of the ACAS results. A recent, very vocal critic has been Dr. Barnett, of North American Symptomatic Carotid Endarterectomy Trial (NASCET) fame.

## Perioperative Imaging Strategies for Carotid Endarterectomy: An Analysis of Morbidity and Cost-Effectiveness in Symptomatic Patients

Kent KC, Kuntz KM, Patel MR, et al (Beth Israel Hosp, Boston; Harvard Med School, Boston)
*JAMA* 274:888–893, 1995                                              3–23

*Introduction.*—The traditional method for evaluating carotid bifurcation before endarterectomy is contract angiography; however, some centers use noninvasive tests instead, such as duplex sonography and MR angiography. If a patient with 70% to 99% stenosis does not have carotid endarterectomy because the patient has been identified as having a low-grade stenosis by duplex sonography, the patient has a 15% greater risk of having a stroke. The appropriateness of carotid endarterectomy for the treatment of symptomatic patients with 70% to 99% stenosis has been identified by the North American Symptomatic Carotid Endarterectomy Trial. The least morbid approach for the preoperative evaluation of symptomatic candidates for carotid endarterectomy was identified. The cost-effectiveness of competing diagnostic strategies was assessed.

*Methods.*—Four diagnostic strategies for evaluating 81 potential candidates for carotid endarterectomy were assessed for their cost-effectiveness: duplex sonography, MR angiography, contrast angiography, and the combination of duplex sonography and MR angiography supplemented by contrast angiography for disparate results. The outcome measure was determined as incremental cost per quality-adjusted year of life gained.

*Results.*—Of the four options considered, the combination of tests resulted in the greatest quality-adjusted life expectancy, followed by contrast angiography, MR angiography, and duplex sonography. The MR angiography or contrast angiography were not cost-effective, after incorporating the costs of testing, surgery, and stroke. Although the combination of tests was more effective, it was more expensive than duplex sonography. The combination of tests resulted in an additional cost of $22,400 per quality-adjusted year of life gained.

*Conclusion.*—Sufficiently high accuracies must be demonstrated for the noninvasive imaging studies, which are appealing as a replacement for carotid angiography because of their lower cost. Any potential cost advantage or reduction may be offset by false negative or false positive results. Quality-adjusted life expectancy is maximized through the combination of MR angiography and duplex sonography, with carotid angiography reserved for disparate results. The next least expensive option is duplex sonography.

▶ I am not sure I either understand or agree with the conclusions presented herein. I personally find MR angiography to be almost worthless for carotid diagnosis. We have historically used carotid angiography on every patient, usually in association with duplex scanning. I have become very content with the detailed information available on carotid arteriography, and I wish we could continue to get it in all of our preoperative patients. However, I am being dragged kicking and screaming into the 21st century, and I fully realize this is no longer practical. We are currently doing more and more carotid endarterectomies based on duplex alone, and I conclude that this has been satisfactory. I am confident that, in the future, we will do a significant percentage of our carotid surgery based on duplex alone. I shed a tear for the passing of the highly detailed cut-film carotid arteriography. I suppose, however, we can no longer justify this based either on cost benefit or hazard to the patient. I am continually amazed by the remarkable morbidity reported with carotid arteriography at many centers.

## Computer-Assisted Carotid Plaque Characterisation

El-Barghouty N, Geroulakos G, Nicolaides A, et al (St Mary's Hosp, London)
*Eur J Vasc Endovasc Surg* 9:389–393, 1995                                    3–24

*Introduction.*—With the advent of high resolution B-mode ultrasound scanning, characterization of the structure and form of atheromatous plaques at the carotid bifurcation has been possible. As plaque structure has been implicated as an important factor in the development of embolic events, the importance of plaque morphology in the pathophysiology of cerebral events is accepted. In patients with symptomatic cerebrovascular disease, echolucent lipid-laden or hemorrhagic plaques are more common and are associated with a high incidence of CT brain infarctions. The relationship between incidence of CT brain infarction and computer-assisted grading of the echogenicity of carotid plaques has been determined.

*Methods.*—A prospective study was conducted of 87 consecutive patients with 148 plaques producing more than 50% internal carotid artery stenosis. In the 111 plaques studied, 25 patients had plaques associated with strokes, 19 had plaques associated with transient ischemic attacks, 35 patients had plaques associated with amaurosis fugax, and 69 had asymptomatic plaques. Computed tomographic brain scans were conducted of all patients who were found to have ipsilateral cerebral infarction. A duplex scanner was used to obtain images of the plaques, which were then transferred to a computer. An image analysis program was used to obtain a histogram of each plaque, in which the number of pixels were plotted against the gray scale (0–225). A measure of echogenicity was the median of the gray scale.

*Results.*—Ipsilateral CT brain infarction was associated with 53 of 148 plaques, or 36%. An incidence of 11% CT infarction was associated with plaques with a gray scale median of more than 32 (echogenic). There was a 55% incidence of CT infarction among plaques with a gray scale median below or equal to 32 (echolucent) (Table 2). A cut-off level of a gray scale median of 32 separates plaques with no infarction from those associated with cerebral infarction (Fig 3).

TABLE 2.—Incidence of CT Brain Infarction in Relation to the Gray Scale Median of the 11 Plaques

| Grey-Scale Median | CT Brain Infarction | | Total |
|---|---|---|---|
| | Absent | Present | |
| > 32 | 57 | 7 (11%) | 64 |
| ≤ 32 | 38 | 46 (55%) | 84 |

* $\kappa^2 = 30.35$, $P < 0.001$.
† Relative risk = 22, 95% confidence interval 4.7 to 108.
‡ Total number of plaques = 148
(Reprinted from *Eur J Vasc Endovasc Surg* 9, El-Barghouty N, Geroulakos G, Nicolaides A, et al: Computer-assisted carotid plaque characterization. pp 389–393, 1995, by permission of the publisher Academic Press Limited London.)

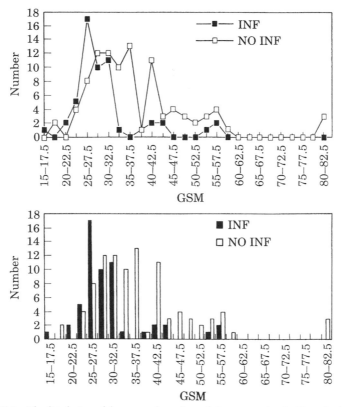

**FIGURE 3.**—The distribution of the gray scale medians of plaques associated with cerebral infarction and those with no infarction. *Abbreviations: GSM,* gray scale median. (Reprinted from *Eur J Vasc Endovasc Surg 9,* El-Barghouty N, Geroulakos G, Nicolaides A, et al: Computer-assisted carotid plaque characterization. pp 389–393, 1995, by permission of the publisher Academic Press Limited London.)

*Conclusion.*—High-risk carotid plaques can be identified by computer analysis of carotid plaque. This simple and reliable method could also identify low-risk patients. Further studies should explore the potential of such analysis in identifying asymptomatic high-risk patients.

▶ Dr. Nicolaides' group appears determined to inform us about their data on plaque echogenicity. Here is another version. Let's all accept the fact that soft mushy plaques are more likely to cause cerebral infarction than dense calcific plaques. Clearly the dividing point on the gray scale of 32 was determined by retrospective data review. To prove their point, these authors need to do a prospective study using the 32 as a cut point. I shall await the more definitive data.

### Cerebrovascular Disease Assessed by Color-Flow and Power Doppler Ultrasonography: Comparison With Digital Subtraction Angiography in Internal Carotid Artery Stenosis

Griewing B, Morgenstern C, Driesner F, et al (Ernst Moritz Arndt Univ, Greifswald, Germany)
*Stroke* 27:95–100, 1996                                      3–25

*Objective.*—Two ultrasonographic imaging techniques, color flow Doppler (CFD) imaging and the power Doppler (PD) technique, were compared with digital subtraction angiography in 54 patients who, on continuous-wave Doppler scanning, had greater than 50% stenosis of the extracranial internal carotid artery (ICA).

*Results.*—Digital subtraction angiography demonstrated 34 middle-grade (50% to 69%) stenoses; 32 high-grade (70% to 99%) stenoses and 7 complete occlusions of the ICA. Because of extensive calcification, CFD imaging failed to demonstrate 23% of stenoses, and PD, 12%. The CFD technique was less accurate in assessing both middle- and high-grade stenoses. The PD technique proved superior to both CFD imaging and angiography for characterizing the plaque surface in patients with high-grade stenoses. Power Doppler demonstrated an irregular plaque surface in 87.5% of these cases.

*Conclusion.*—The PD technique is an effective noninvasive means of diagnosing ICA stenosis and visualizing the plaque surface.

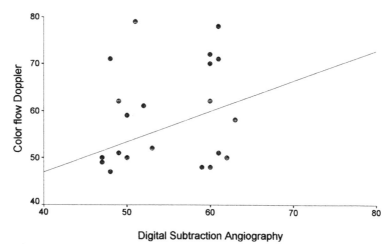

**Digital Subtraction Angiography**

FIGURE 2.—Scatterplot shows correlation of estimates of percent stenosis between digital subtration angiography (abcissa) and color-flow Doppler (ordinate) in middle-grade stenosis ($r = .23$; $P > .05$. (Griewing B, Morgenstern C, Driesner F, et al: Cerebrovascular disease assessed by color-flow and power Doppler ultrasonography: Comparison with digital subtraction angiography in internal carotid artery stenosis. *Stroke* 1996; 27:95–100. Reproduced with permission *Stroke*. Copyright 1996 American Heart Association.)

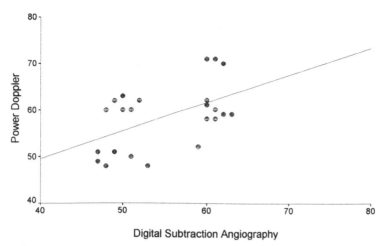

**Digital Subtraction Angiography**

FIGURE 3.—Scatterplot shows correlation of estimates of percent stenosis between power Doppler (ordinate) and digital subtraction angiography (abcissa) in middle-grade stenosis ($r = .51$; $P = .01$). (Griewing B, Morgenstern C, Driesner F, et al: Cerebrovascular disease assessed by color-flow and power Doppler ultrasonography: Comparison with digital subtraction angiography in internal carotid artery stenosis. *Stroke* 1996; 27:95–100. Reproduced with permission *Stroke*. Copyright 1996 American Heart Association.)

▶ This is one of the early clinical articles describing the use of the new PD. Perhaps PD is going to be an important new technique. The PD image indicates the density, as well as the number of red cells per unit volume of tissue. Importantly, it provides no information concerning velocity or direction of flow, but it is angle independent and free of artifacts, such as aliasing. The noise in the PD system can be assigned to homogeneous background and does not obscure the image. Preliminary information suggests that PD may be an important new imaging technique. Nobody is suggesting it is going to replace CFD, but it may provide a valuable adjunct. Time will tell.

---

**Carotid Artery Duplex Scanning: Does Plaque Echogenicity Correlate With Patient Symptoms?**
Cave EM, Pugh ND, Wilson RJ, et al (Univ Hosp of Wales, Cardiff)
*Eur J Vasc Endovasc Surg* 10:77–81, 1995                                     3–26

---

*Objective.*—Patients referred for carotid Duplex scanning because they were judged to be at risk of cerebrovascular disease were entered into a prospective study of the relationship between plaque composition and patient symptoms. Also examined was the association between plaque type and degree of vessel stenosis.

*Patients and Methods.*—Two patient groups were identified: 75 patients were symptomatic, with recent cerebrovascular symptoms referable to the ipsilateral carotid artery territory; 41 patients were asymptomatic. The 2 groups were comparable in the prevalence of a number of cardiovascular

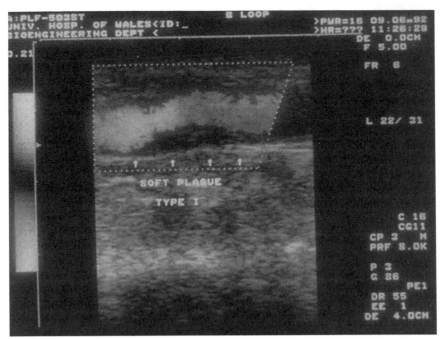

**FIGURE 1.**—Longitudinal section of the carotid bulb demonstrating a plaque type 1. The plaque is outlined by flow within the lumen demonstrated by the use of color Doppler (shown here as a black and white image). (Reprinted from *Eur J Vasc Endovasc Surg* 10. Cave EM, Pugh ND, Wilson RJ, et al: Carotid artery duplex scanning: Does plaque echogenicity correlate with patient symptoms? pp 77–81, 1995, by permission of the publisher Academic Press Limited London.)

risk factors, including angina/myocardial infarction, smoking history, and diabetes. The symptomatic group had more patients with hypertension and fewer with claudication. The ratio of echolucency to echogenicity defined 4 types of ultrasound plaque appearance: dominantly echolucent plaques (Fig 1); plaques with areas of echolucency greater than 50% (Fig 2); dominantly echogenic with areas of echolucency less than 50% (Fig 3); and uniformly echogenic plaques (Fig 4). Vessel stenosis was classified into 3 groups: less than 40%, 40% to 69%, greater than 69% and less than 100%.

*Results.*—The predominant plaque type in all 3 degrees of vessel stenosis was type 4, that described as uniformly echogenic. Compared with contralateral asymptomatic vessels in the same patients, twice as many symptomatic vessels contained plaque types 1 and 2, with echolucency predominating. The likelihood of symptoms was found to increase with the degree of plaque echolucency. Vessel stenosis was significantly associated with the presence of symptoms, especially in vessels with more than 69% stenosis. There was no significant association between vessel stenosis and plaque type, and the incidence of symptoms was more influenced by degree of stenosis than by plaque type.

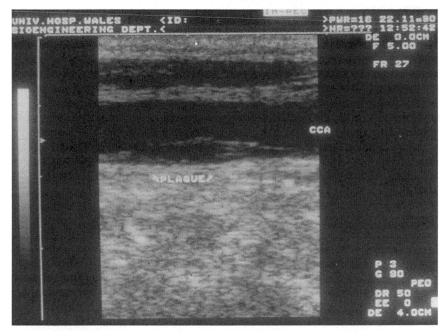

FIGURE 2.—Longitudinal section of the carotid bulb demonstrating a type 2 plaque. (Reprinted from *Eur J Vasc Endovasc Surg* 10. Cave EM, Pugh ND, Wilson RJ, et al: Carotid artery duplex scanning: Does plaque echogenicity correlate with patient symptoms? pp 77–81, 1995, by permission of the publisher Academic Press Limited London.)

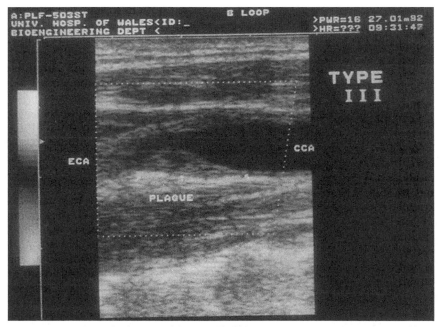

FIGURE 3.—Longitudinal section of the carotid bulb demonstrating a type 3 plaque. (Reprinted from *Eur J Vasc Endovasc Surg* 10. Cave EM, Pugh ND, Wilson RJ, et al: Carotid artery duplex scanning: Does plaque echogenicity correlate with patient symptoms? pp 77–81, 1995, by permission of the publisher Academic Press Limited London.)

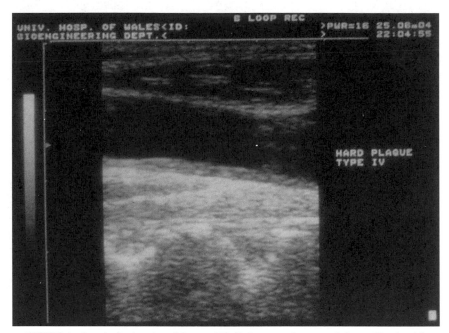

**FIGURE 4.**—Longitudinal section of the carotid bulb demonstrating a type 4 plaque. (Reprinted from *Eur J Vasc Endovasc Surg* 10. Cave EM, Pugh ND, Wilson RJ, et al: Carotid artery duplex scanning: Does plaque echogenicity correlate with patient symptoms? pp 77–81, 1995, by permission of the publisher Academic Press Limited London.)

*Conclusion.*—Both plaque echolucency and stenosis were associated with symptoms in patients at risk of cerebrovascular disease. The 2 factors act independently, and vessel stenosis had a closer association with symptoms at the time of referral.

▶ This is a study of a poorly understood phenomenon using a single vascular technologist. For very good reasons, the information from nearly half the patients studied was excluded from the analysis because of a poor history, uncertain timing, or poorly localized or nonhemispheric symptoms. Although stenosis is still the leading villain and is not associated with any particular type of plaque, echolucency warns us of the likelihood of soft debris, hemorrhage, lipid and surface ulceration, and is more frequently found in symptomatic patients. We now need to know more about the natural history of these lesions, particularly in patients who are asymptomatic and in those who have only minor degrees of stenosis. See also Abstract 3–24.

**A.E.B. Giddings, M.D.**

## Lower Extremity

### Effect of Multilevel Sequential Stenosis on Lower Extremity Arterial Duplex Scanning

Bergamini TM, Tatum CM Jr, Marshall C, et al (Univ of Louisville, Ky)
*Am J Surg* 169:564–566, 1995                                    3–27

*Introduction.*—In identifying stenoses and occlusions, lower extremity arterial duplex scanning, which noninvasively provides anatomical and physiologic data, has been highly reliable in permitting the formulation of a treatment plan before arteriography. However, the incidence of detection of second-order stenoses by duplex scanning is reduced because the reduced arterial blood flow of outflow arteries decreases the changes in peak systolic velocity that occur at distal stenotic sites. Less than 50% arterial stenosis in extremities with single-level stenosis was compared to multilevel sequential stenosis in lower extremity arterial duplex scanning.

*Methods.*—In 44 patients, lower extremity arterial duplex scanning and arteriography were performed on 80 extremities for claudication or critical limb ischemia. Duplex scanning and arteriograms of the common femoral artery, the upper and lower superficial femoral arteries, above-knee and below-knee popliteal arterial, and tibioperoneal trunk were taken with 2 months of each other and the results compared. In the 80 extremities, 404 arterial segments were analyzed. In 28 extremities, 31 arterial segments had a stenosis of less than 50%. The stenosis was categorized as: first order signified a first or only stenotic segment in the extremity, which applied to 23 patients; second order signified stenosis occurring distal to a less than 50% stenosis, which applied to 4 patients; and occlusion, which applied to 4 patients.

*Results.*—For the detection of a less than 50% arterial stenosis or occlusion in the common femoral arterial, the sensitivity of duplex scan detection was 86%, the specificity was 96%, and the positive predictive value was 67%. For the upper superficial femoral artery, the sensitivity was 95%, the specificity was 98%, and the positive predictive value was 95%. For the lower superficial femoral artery, the sensitivity was 97%, the specificity was 90%, and the positive predictive value was 88%. For the above-knee popliteal artery, the sensitivity was 84%, the specificity was 90%, and the positive predictive value was 87%. For the below-knee popliteal artery, the sensitivity was 47%, the specificity was 98%, and the positive predictive value was 90%. For the tibioperoneal trunk, the sensitivity was 25%, the specificity was 100%, and the positive predictive value was 100%. Of the 23 first-order stenoses, duplex scanning detected 18, or 78%. Of the 8 second-order stenoses in limbs with multilevel sequential disease, duplex scanning, detected only 1, or 13%. For the first-order stenoses, the peak systolic velocity at the stenotic site was higher than for the second-order stenoses.

*Conclusion.*—Significant second-order stenosis is not reliably detected by duplex scanning. More meticulous examination is necessary to identify second-order stenosis of arterial segments distal to flow-restrictive disease. In the areas of plaque formation, more attention should be given to percent changes in peak systolic velocity.

▶ I suppose this study confirms the obvious. By using velocity criteria, the first stenosis in a limb is accurately identified. However, the second stenosis is identified with diminished accuracy, having on occasion been obscured by the influence of the first stenosis on velocity. This important information has been shown by others, but it probably deserves occasional reemphasis.

## Duplex Velocity Characteristics of Aortoiliac Stenoses
de Smet AAEA, Ermers EJM, Kitslaar PJEHM (Univ Hosp Maastricht, The Netherlands)
*J Vasc Surg* 23:628–636, 1996                                              3–28

*Background.*—Doppler measurement of peak systolic velocity (PSV) change is helpful in broadly defining the degree of aortoiliac stenosis, but the potential value of other Doppler measurements is not clear. Duplex scanning was performed on 112 stenotic aortoiliac segments identified by arteriography to evaluate the usefulness of several velocity measurements.

*Methods.*—Patients with symptoms of aortoiliac disease underwent duplex ultrasonography and femoral artery pressure studies before scheduled arteriography. Doppler measurements included PSV, end-diastolic velocity (EDV), PSV ratio (ratio between stenotic and nonstenotic PSV), PSV difference (difference between stenotic and nonstenotic PSV), spectral broadening of the Doppler signal at the stenotic site, and the presence of reverse flow at the stenotic site.

*Results.*—A PSV below 200 cm/sec strongly indicated a stenosis of less than 50%, but a PSV above 200 cm/sec was less specific. The PSV ratio was able to significantly differentiate between 50% to 74% lesions and 75% to 99% lesions. The PSV difference, as with the absolute PSV, was not significantly discriminatory among lesions of 50% or larger. A significant increase in EDV was seen between 20% to 49% stenoses (0 cm/sec), 50% to 74% stenoses 5 cm/sec), and 75% to 99% stenoses (50 cm/sec). Reverse flow was present in all stenoses less than 20%, but in none from 75% to 99%. Conversely, spectral broadening was present in only 20% of stenoses less than 20%, but in all stenoses from 75% to 99%. The combination of a PSV ratio less than 1.5 and the presence of reverse flow, with absent spectral broadening, correctly predicted all cases of stenosis less than 20%. By combining PSV ratio and EDV, it was fairly possible to separate lesions into quartiles by percent of stenosis (Table 3).

*Conclusion.*—Various Doppler measurements, especially the combination of PSV and EDV, can accurately quantitate the degree of aortoiliac stenosis.

TABLE 3.—Two-way Contingency Table of Duplex Scanning Based on PSV Ratio and EDV by Arteriography

| | Arteriography | | | | |
| | 0% to 20% | 20% to 49% | 50% to 74% | 75% to 99% | n |
|---|---|---|---|---|---|
| Duplex | | | | | |
| PSV ratio <1.5 | 19 | 4 | | | 23 |
| PSV ratio ≥1.5 and <2.8 | 7 | 17 | 7 | 1 | 32 |
| PSV ratio ≥2.8 and <5.0 | | 9 | 23 | 9 | 41 |
| PSV ratio ≥5.0 and EDV ≥40 | | | 3 | 13 | 16 |
| n | 26 | 30 | 33 | 23 | 112 |

*Abbreviations: PSV*, peak systolic velocity; *EDV*, end-diastolic velocity.
(Courtesy of de Smet AAEA, Ermers EJM, Kitslaar PJEHM: Duplex velocity characteristics of aortoiliac stenoses. *J Vasc Surg* 23:628–636, 1996.)

▶ I note with interest that the Doppler does not appear to be gaining much popularity in localization of peripheral arterial stenoses. Most of us still depend on palpable pulse status, intravascular pressure, or multicuff-determined arterial pressure. Whereas most people who do use Doppler depend almost exclusively on PSV, these authors correctly note that other parameters may offer a little bit of help, including systolic velocity ratios and EDV. I suspect they are correct, but I doubt duplex is ever going to have a major role in the localization of peripheral arterial stenoses. It is too technician dependent and too time consuming.

## Postocclusive Hyperaemic Duplex Scan: A New Method of Aortoiliac Assessment

Currie IC, Wilson YG, Baird RN, et al (Bristol Royal Infirmary, England)
*Br J Surg* 82:1226–1229, 1995                                    3–29

*Objective.*—Abdominal duplex scanning is an accurate but time-consuming and technically demanding procedure for the assessment of the aortoiliac segment. Given that measurement during hyperemic blood flow improves the accuracy of hemodynamic tests, a method was sought to conduct a fast, noninvasive screening test for aortoiliac disease by observing the postocclusive hyperemic response in patients with or without significantly diseased aortoiliac segments.

*Methods.*—Using color duplex scanning, common femoral Doppler ultrasonographic waveforms were recorded after 3 minutes of arterial occlusion using a thigh cuff in 25 patients with normal aortoiliac segments and 25 patients with significant aortoiliac disease. In addition, the diagnostic value of the postocclusive hyperemic duplex (PHD) test was evaluated prospectively in 50 limbs of 39 patients, and the results were compared with clinical assessment and traditional intra-arterial pressure measurements.

*Results.*—Patients with aortoiliac disease had significantly higher end-diastolic velocity (EDV) and lower resting peak-to-peak pulsatility index and resting peak systolic velocity, compared with patients with normal aortoiliac segments. These differences were enhanced during the PHD test. By using receiver operating characteristic curve analysis, the EDV—70 seconds after cuff release—gave the best discrimination between aortoiliac disease and disease-free state, with a sensitivity of 88% and accuracy of 92%. When used prospectively in 6 limbs with critical ischemia and 44 limbs with claudication, the PHD test performed well with a sensitivity of 86% and accuracy of 84%. When compared with intra-arterial pressure measurements, the PHD test represented considerable improvement over femoral pulse palpation and compared quite favorably with arteriography for the assessment of aortoiliac disease. Most patients tolerated the PHD test, but 8% could not tolerate thigh cuff inflation.

*Conclusions.*—The PHD test is a simple and fast noninvasive assessment for aortoiliac disease. The prolonged hyperemia response in the diseased state may be measured by its effect on common femoral artery diastolic blood flow. When combined with femoral duplex scanning, the PHD test allows rapid assessment of claudicants at the initial outpatient clinical visit without the need for additional complex equipment or calculation. Duplex scanning can be reserved for patients in whom iliac disease is likely.

▶ The group in Bristol has been searching in vain for decades for a noninvasive test that accurately predicts the presence of significant aortoiliac occlusive disease. Remember the pulsatility index? At any rate, these authors now suggest that after 3 minutes of thigh cuff occlusion, detailed noninvasive studies of the femoral artery waveforms allow assessment of aortoiliac disease. Specially, they found that EDV 70 seconds after cuff release was the best discriminant of an abnormal aortoiliac segment. Perhaps so, but I am not convinced. I continue to believe that simple palpation of the femoral pulse is most important, and I continue to derive considerable help from the 4-cuff system, paying considerable attention to the proximal high-thigh cuff. If in doubt, intra-arterial pressure measurements easily obtained at angiography provide definitive information. Although I have no idea whether I can duplicate the authors' results, I do note that at their best they are only about 85% sensitive. I do not think this is good enough.

---

**Colour Duplex Ultrasonographic Imaging and Provocation of Popliteal Artery Compression**

Akkersdijk WL, de Ruyter JW, Lapham R, et al (Univ Hosp Utrecht, The Netherlands)
*Eur J Vasc Endovasc Surg* 10:342–345, 1995                                    3–30

---

*Background.*—Although compression of the artery during active plantar flexion has been considered diagnostic evidence of popliteal artery entrapment, surgery does not always confirm the entrapment. Duplex scanning is now recommended as a routine investigation for patients with suspected popliteal artery entrapment syndrome. Sixteen healthy volunteers took part in a study designed to assess the effects of several provocation maneuvers of the foot on flow patterns of the popliteal arteries.

*Methods.*—Study participants had a mean age of 25 years; the male:female ratio of the group was 3:1. Eight (all men) were semiprofessional rowers and 8 were not involved in intensive physical training. Under laboratory conditions, the popliteal arteries were studied with Duplex scanning in rest and during active and passive plantar and dorsal flexion of the foot. Flow velocity pattern measurements were obtained at 3 levels: 5 cm above the knee joint (proximal), at the level of the knee joint, and 1 cm proximal to the origin of the anterior tibial artery (distal).

*Results.*—Stenotic disease was excluded in all volunteers. All investigated arteries exhibited a normal triphasic flow pattern in neutral position. Median peak systolic velocity (PSV) decreased from 100 cm/sec in the proximal segment to 90 cm/sec in the distal segment of the artery. At neither level did passive foot movements or active dorsal flexion of the foot affect PSV. Only active plantar flexion brought about changes of PSV, with a median decrease in the proximal segment of the artery to 65 cm/sec. Overall, 27 arteries exhibited changes: complete occlusion in 19, significant lumen reduction in 4, and a low flow state in 4. Findings did not differ between rowers and the other volunteers.

*Conclusion.*—Neither passive foot movements nor active dorsal flexion of the foot affected PSV in the popliteal arteries of young healthy volunteers. There were changes at all levels of measurement, however, during active plantar flexion, and flow disappeared in this condition in up to 59% of investigated arteries. This finding in symptom-free volunteers suggests a physiologic phenomenon, and the provocation test alone does not appear to indicate popliteal entrapment syndrome.

▶ Previous studies have suggested that active plantar flexion can be used as a provocative test to diagnose popliteal entrapment syndrome if duplex-detected flow is markedly reduced in the popliteal artery. In this study, the Utrecht group demonstrated that active plantar flexion reduces popliteal blood flow in normal subjects, apparently by compressing the tibioperoneal trunk as it enters the soleal canal. Thus, they conclude that operative correction of popliteal entrapment should not be based on duplex ultrasound alone. I had not realized that anyone was using ultrasound for more than screening purposes, inasmuch as CT or MR scans are not only definitive for this diagnosis, but also allow clear definition of precise variants of entrapment. The question that remains is whether an experienced vascular technologist can differentiate popliteal entrapment (which usually occurs more proximally in the popliteal artery) from the more distal (tibioperoneal) reduction in blood flow that apparently occurs in normal patients during active plantar flexion. Because the authors did not compare patients with popliteal entrapment in this current study, this remains unanswered. I suspect that arterial deviation and proximal popliteal flow changes and turbulence can still lead to a relatively accurate diagnosis of popliteal entrapment by duplex scanning, but I would never rely on this alone to recommend surgical intervention. The present study points out the dangers of false positive studies in normal subjects and may explain the epidemic of popliteal entrapments reported by a few centers.

**J. Cronenwett, M.D.**

## Miscellaneous Topics

**Ischemia-Related Lesion Characteristics in Patients With Stable or Unstable Angina: A Study With Intracoronary Angioscopy and Ultrasound**
de Feyter PJ, Ozaki Y, Baptista J, et al (Erasmus Univ, Rotterdam, The Netherlands)
*Circulation* 92:1408–1413, 1995                                    3–31

*Background.*—It is a common belief that acute ischemic syndromes result from disruption of a lipid-rich atheromatous plaque. Ample evidence, primarily from postmortem studies, indicates that lipid-rich atheromatous plaques that have a thin, fibrous capsule are prone to plaque fissuring, and that acute ischemic syndromes are associated with plaque fissuring and superimposed thrombosis. Intracoronary imaging tools may characterize the composition of coronary lesions and provide clues on which plaques may rupture and those that have undergone rupture.

*Methods.*—Forty-four patients with unstable and 23 patients with stable angina were studied. The characteristics of ischemia-related lesions were assessed with coronary angiography and intracoronary angioscopy, and their compositions were evaluated with intracoronary ultrasound. With angiography, ischemia-related lesions were classified as noncomplex (smooth borders) or complex (irregular borders, multiple irregularities, or thrombus). In angioscopic images, the lesions were classified as thrombotic if they had irregular, ulcerated raised surface with thrombus, or stable if the raised surface was regular and smooth without thrombus. With ultrasound, the composition of the ischemia-related lesion was classified as poorly echo-reflective, highly echo-reflective with acoustic shadowing, or highly echo-reflective without shadowing (Fig 2).

*Findings.*—An angiographically complex lesion was present in 39% of patients with stable angina and in 55% of patients with unstable angina. Angioscopy demonstrated plaque rupture and thrombosis in 17% of patients with stable angina and 68% of patients with unstable angina. Angiographic findings correlated poorly with the clinical syndrome. An angiographic complex lesion was concordant with unstable angina in 55%, and a noncomplex lesion was concordant with stable angina in 61%. There was a good correlation between clinical status and angioscopic findings. An angioscopic thrombotic lesion was concordant with unstable angina in 68% and a stable lesion was concordant with stable angina in 83%. The ultrasound-defined composition of the plaque was similar in stable and unstable angina.

*Conclusions.*—Sequential imaging of the ischemia-related lesion with intracoronary angioscopy and ultrasound is feasible and relatively safe in patients undergoing coronary intervention. Intracoronary angioscopy provides information that is complementary to angiography with regard to

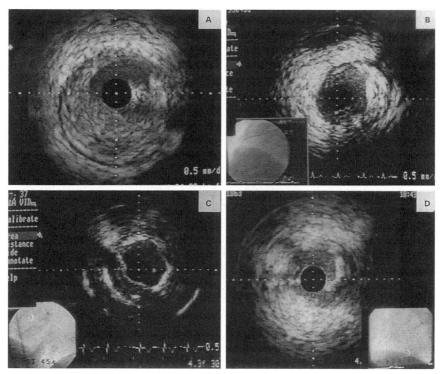

**FIGURE 2.**—Angioscopic images of the types of ultrasound-derived lesions. A, plaque with poorly echo-reflective tissue between 4 and 9 o'clock; B, plaque with highly echo-reflective tissue with eccentric location between 1 and 4 o'clock; C, with highly echo-reflective tissue with shadowing; and D, mixed plaque composed of poorly echo-reflective tissue at 6 to 11 o'clock and highly echo-reflective with shadowing at 1 to 5 o'clock. (Courtesy of de Feyter PJ, Ozaki Y, Baptista J, et al: Ischemia-related lesion characteristics in patients with stable or unstable angina: A study with intracoronary angioscopy and ultrasound. *Circulation* 1995; 92:1408–1413. Reproduced with permission *Circulation.* Copyright 1995 American Heart Association.)

distinction between stable and unstable features of the coronary lesions. Current ultrasound techniques do not discriminate between stable and unstable plaques.

▶ As noted previously, intense interest continues in characterization of the atherosclerotic fibrous cap. This study examines coronary angiography, angioscopy, and intravascular ultrasound in patients with unstable and stable angina. The authors conclude that neither angiography nor intravascular ultrasound is very good for determining plaque rupture, but that angioscopy is quite good for this purpose. Although interesting, I find this result a bit simplistic, as we are informed in abstract 1–26 that a considerable amount of coronary thrombosis occurs adjacent to plaques that have not yet ruptured. The authors of this article seem to equate plaque rupture with thrombosis. They do not seem to recognize the very real potential for thrombus associated with unruptured plaques, although they did ask the haunting question of why they did not observe thrombus in about one third of patients with unstable angina. Stay tuned. I am sure there shall be a great deal more to follow.

## Ultrasound-Guided Compression Closure of Postcatheterization Pseudoaneurysms During Concurrent Anticoagulation: A Review of Seventy-Seven Patients

Dean SM, Olin JW, Piedmonte M, et al (Cleveland Clinic Found, Ohio)
*J Vasc Surg* 23:28–35, 1996                                                                 3–32

*Purpose.*—Ultrasound-guided compression closure (UGCC) is an effective nonsurgical method for treating pseudoaneurysms that complicate therapeutic or diagnostic catheterization procedures in the vascular laboratory. A UGCC in the presence of anticoagulation is less effective, but factors responsible for anticoagulant-associated UGCC success or failure have not been identified. The results of a retrospective chart review are presented.

*Patients.*—During a recent 3-year period, 238 patients underwent attempted UGCC of pseudoaneurysms that arose after vascular procedures and had been diagnosed by duplex ultrasound with color flow imaging. Of the 238 patients, 77 were receiving uninterrupted anticoagulation. There were 44 men and 33 women, ranging in age from 35 to 88 years. Twelve patients were being treated with heparin alone, 32 with warfarin alone, and 33 with both. Multiple variables were examined in an attempt to predict UGCC success or failure.

*Results.*—Pseudoaneurysm compression was successful in 56 (73%) patients, 7 of whom (12.5%) required between 2–3 compression attempts before sustained thrombosis was achieved. Ultrasound-guided compression closure failed in the other 21 (27%) patients, 14 of whom required surgical reconstruction. Neither age, gender, sheath size, number of days after the vascular procedure, pseudoaneurysm location, nor the number of chambers in the pseudoaneurysm had any effect on UGCC outcome. Smaller pseudoaneurysm size was the only variable associated with a successful UGCC outcome.

*Conclusions.*—Ultrasound-guided compression closure to obliterate pseudoaneurysms complicating diagnostic or therapeutic vascular catheterization procedures is safe and effective, even in the presence of high levels of uninterrupted anticoagulation.

▶ Arterial pseudoaneurysms occur infrequently after diagnostic procedures and considerably more frequently after therapeutic procedures, including percutaneous angioplasty. The overall incidence seems to vary from about 0.05% to about 6.25%. Ultrasound-guided compression has generally been reported as successful in 90% to 100% of these patients.[1] These authors ask the haunting question of what is the likelihood of success in compressing patients who were fully anticoagulated. They found a success rate of

73% in this difficult group. On balance, I believe it is now well established that ultrasound compression is the treatment of choice for femoral artery, catheter-induced pseudoaneurysms, and that even anticoagulated patients have an excellent chance of a satisfactory outcome.

*Reference*

1. 1995 YEAR BOOK OF VASCULAR SURGERY, p 363.

---

**Renal Artery Stenosis: Evaluation of Doppler US After Inhibition of Angiotensin-Converting Enzyme With Captopril**
René PC, Oliva VL, Bui BT, et al (Hôpital Notre-Dame, Montreal)
*Radiology* 196:675–679, 1995                                               3–33

---

*Background.*—Several researchers have recently studied the Doppler waveform recorded distal to an arterial stenosis rather than at the stenosis itself in patients with renal artery stenosis (RAS). The presence of a pulsus tardus—a delayed or prolonged early acceleration—was described originally in the carotid arteries. By using an "acceleration index," some of these studies have shown a marked reduction in systolic acceleration distal to a severe RAS. Renal vascular resistance is reduced by angiotensin-converting enzyme (ACE) inhibitors, which interrupt the integrity of the intrarenal renin-angiotensin system.

*Methods.*—Sixty-two renal arteries in 31 patients with hypertension were studied. The patients had undergone Doppler scanning before and 1 hour after the administration of captopril before angiography was performed. Doppler waveforms were classified as having a normal or pulsus tardus configuration using pattern recognition criteria.

*Findings.*—Based on recognition of the pulsus tardus, precaptopril Doppler scanning demonstrated 68% of 19 significant renal artery stenoses subsequently detected on angiography. By contrast, all 19 stenoses were identified with postcaptopril Doppler scanning.

*Conclusions.*—Captopril administration significantly enhances the sensitivity of Doppler ultrasound in detecting RAS when waveforms are analyzed using pattern recognition criteria. In severe cases, standard renal Doppler ultrasound without captopril intake is adequate for detection. The diagnosis of more moderate cases apparently requires the addition of captopril.

▶ In recent years, there has been an increase in interest in diagnosing renal artery stenosis by insonating segmental and subsegmental vessels, rather than the main renal artery itself. Criteria for main renal artery stenosis have been well developed and accepted, but in many laboratories this is a difficult test. It appears generally easier to insonate segmental arteries. These authors conclude that the recognition of a specific pulse pattern called pulsus tardus, which they carefully define in this article, is about 68% sensitive for the recognition of renovascular hypertension before captopril, and increases to 100% sensitivity after oral captopril administration. Unfortunately, the number of patients in this study is too small to permit sweeping conclusions. On balance, however, I do believe this article appropriately emphasizes the potential importance of segmental renal artery insonation in the detection of renal artery hypertension.

---

### Routine Use of Limited Abdominal Aortography With Digital Subtraction Carotid and Cerebral Angiography

Hans SS, Zeskind HJ (Macomb Hosp Ctr, Warren, Mich)
*Stroke* 26:1221–1224, 1995                                                   3–34

---

*Objective.*—Patients with carotid artery stenosis may also have atherosclerotic involvement of the abdominal aorta and its visceral branches, and the detection of unsuspected aortic and iliac aneurysms may permit elective repair. A prospective study was conducted to evaluate the usefulness of limited abdominal aortography in conjunction with intra-arterial carotid digital subtraction arteriography (DSA) for identification of these clinically unsuspected lesions.

*Methods.*—Between 1988 and 1992, 401 consecutive patients with preliminary carotid Duplex imaging for evaluation of cerebrovascular disease underwent bilateral carotid intra-arterial DSAs in conjunction with abdominal aortograms. The studies typically included 2 arch angiograms, 1 abdominal aortogram, and 6 selective cervical, carotid, and cerebral injections.

*Results.*—Twenty-three (5.7%) abdominal aortic aneurysms were detected, ranging in size from 3.0 to 7.0 cm in transverse diameter; 6 patients underwent resection without additional conventional aortography. Two patients had iliac aneurysms that were resected. Renal artery stenosis was noted in 29 patients, including 24 (6%) with unilateral and 5 (2%) with bilateral stenosis. Medical treatment could not control hypertension in 7 patients; 5 patients underwent percutaneous renal artery balloon angioplasty and 2 underwent renal artery bypass without further conventional renal arteriography. Renal cell carcinoma was detected in 1 patient who subsequently underwent nephrectomy. Aortic ectasia was detected in 16 patients, 3 of whom showed progressive enlargement to more than 5.0 cm in transverse diameter during follow-up with subsequent aortic aneurysmectomy. Other findings on abdominal aortography included 1 renal cell carcinoma that was resected and 1 renal artery aneurysm. One patient experienced transient ischemic attack and 3 had hematomas in the groin without pseudoaneurysm of the femoral artery.

*Conclusion.*—Single-plane digital abdominal aortography performed in conjunction with carotid intraarterial DSA allows detection of significant pathologic lesions with little increase in morbidity and only a modest increase in time and cost. Diagnosis of unsuspected aortic and iliac aneurysms by digital abdominal aortography and surgical repair in carefully selected patients can reduce morbidity and mortality from ruptured aortic aneurysms. In addition, rare pathologic lesions, such as renal cell carcinoma and renal artery aneurysm, can be detected.

▶ Now this is a real fishing expedition. With a wild leap of logic, 401 patients undergoing carotid arteriography had a limited abdominal aortogram to see what could be found. Miraculously, a small number of diseases were discovered, including a few patients with renal artery stenosis, 1 with renal carcinoma, and a few with aneurysm. Exactly as one would predict, 19 of the 23 aneurysms were too small for surgery. For some reason, the authors seem very proud of the incidental disease detected. I, however, am monumentally unimpressed. If I were ever sure something would not pass cost-benefit muster, this is it.

---

**Complications of Peripheral Arteriography: A New System to Identify Patients at Increased Risk**
Eggling TKP, O'Moore PV, Feinstein AR, et al (Yale Univ, New Haven, Conn; Harvard Med School, Boston)
*J Vasc Surg* 22:787–794, 1995                                                    3–35

---

*Background.*—Although arteriography is a widely used diagnostic test, it is often regarded as expensive, dangerous, and difficult. Few studies have examined complications of arteriography—most citations of complication rates come from data collected in the 1970s. An attempt was made to see if those complication rates are still valid and to identify patient subgroups at increased risk of complications.

*Methods.*—The study included 549 consecutive patients undergoing various types of angiographic procedures. All were evaluated after angiography and twice during the 72-hour period after the procedure. Delayed complications were assessed by telephone interviews conducted 2 weeks or more after angiography. The sample was randomly divided into a training and a testing set to validate the suspected prognostic factors.

*Results.*—Major complications occurred in 2.9% of patients, but the rate varied according to the level of relative risk. The rate of major complications was 0.7% in patients in the lowest risk stratum, i.e., those with trauma or aneurysmal disease, and 2.0% for those in the intermediate category, who were studied for such problems as claudication or limb-threatening ischemia. The major complication rate rose to 9.1% for patients in the highest risk category, i.e., those with suspected aortic dissection, mesenteric ischemia, gastrointestinal bleeding, or symptomatic carotid artery stenosis. In the overall sample, the only factors independently associated with an elevated risk of complications were congestive heart failure and furosemide use.

*Conclusions.*—Old reports provide misleading information about the risks associated with arteriography. The risk may be lower than generally thought for patients with trauma or aneurysm but higher than previously reported for patients with other common indications. Complication rates must be stratified to determine the relative costs and benefits of arteriography, as well as other vascular imaging studies, in patients with specific clinical conditions.

▶ These authors ask the haunting question of just what is the complication rate after diagnostic arteriography in today's world. They seem to have appropriately defined a major complication as one requiring treatment or delay of an urgent surgical procedure, whereas minor complications were less than that. Using these criteria, they report 2.9% major complication and 6.4% minor complication rates. Predictably, they found that the indication for the diagnostic study was a significant predictor of complication, with the highest complications occurring in aortic dissection, mesenteric ischemia, gastrointestinal bleeding, or symptomatic carotid stenosis, whereas the lowest occurred in patients with trauma or aneurysmal disease. It is important to remember that both the North American Symptomatic Carotid Endarterectomy Trial and Asymptomatic Carotid Atherosclerosis Study studies reported very worrisome rates of arteriographic complications. On balance, studies such as this, although showing the relative safety of arteriography, demonstrate a major complication rate that is sufficiently worrisome to lead us all to have increasing enthusiasm for noninvasive studies. Clearly, this is 1 of the reasons why surgery without preceding arteriography is ever increasing in frequency.

## Screening for Abdominal Aortic Aneurysms During Lower Extremity Arterial Evaluation in the Vascular Laboratory

Wolf YG, Otis SM, Schwend RB, et al (Hadassah Univ, Jerusalem; Scripps Clinic and Research Found, La Jolla, Calif)
*J Vasc Surg* 22:417–423, 1995                                     3–36

*Introduction.*—The prevalence of abdominal aortic aneurysm (AAA) has been reported to be from 4.2% to 4.3% in men older than age 65. Patients with peripheral vascular disease have a high prevalence of AAA. The cost-effectiveness of screening for AAA during noninvasive lower extremity arterial examinations was evaluated.

*Methods.*—A total of 531 patients who underwent lower extremity arterial evaluations fasted overnight and also underwent B-mode ultrasonography. The same device was used for both evaluations. Measurements were taken in the anteroposterior and lateral dimensions of the aorta at the juxtarenal level and in the distal infrarenal portion. An anteroposterior or transverse diameter of the infrarenal aorta measuring 3.0 cm or larger was considered to be an AAA.

*Results.*—The mean aortic diameter of 475 patients in whom the aorta was adequately visualized was 19.6 mm at the juxtarenal level and 18.8 in the lower infrarenal aorta. The aortic diameter was significantly larger in men compared with women, and in smokers compared with nonsmokers.

An aortic diameter larger than 3.0 cm was identified in 32 patients. Of these, 15 were 4.0 cm or larger. The best predictors of AAA were male sex, age older than 65 years, and a history of smoking. The prevalence of AAA for patients in whom the aorta was visualized was 6.7%. In male smokers older than age 65, it was 15.2%. Aneurysms 4.0 cm or larger were detected in 3.2% of this cohort and in 8.8% of male smokers older than age 65. The additional time spent in the vascular laboratory for the aortic scan was an average of 5 minutes per patient. Eighty-three minutes of scanning time were required to detect 1 aneurysm and 36 minutes of scanning time were needed to detect aneurysms in male smokers older than age 65. This translates into a cost of $240 to $553 per aneurysm identified.

*Conclusion.*—Screening for AAA during lower extremity arterial examination was cost-effective for this high-risk population. It can be considered an appropriate and valuable addition to the examination protocol.

▶ It is an article of faith in vascular surgery that patients who have symptomatic arterial disease at 1 site have a much greater likelihood of disease at another site than does a normal control population. One of the earliest investigations of the association of aortic aneurysm with lower extremity occlusive disease was that of Cabellon et al.[1] It is well known that patients with lower extremity disease have more carotid disease than normal controls,[2] and certainly patients with symptomatic peripheral arterial disease have much more coronary disease than do control populations.[3] The important question, however, is just how much screening is both reasonable and cost-effective. I believe that carotid and abdominal duplex screening in patients with lower extremity ischemia is reasonable. I certainly would not add aortography as described in Abstract 3–34.

*References*

1. Cabellon S Jr, Moncrief CL, Pierre DR, et al: Incidence of abdominal aortic aneurysms in patients with atheromatous arterial disease. *Am J Surg* 146:575–576, 1983.
2. 1993 YEAR BOOK OF VASCULAR SURGERY, p 177.
3. 1995 YEAR BOOK OF VASCULAR SURGERY, p 167.

## Screening for Abdominal Aortic Aneurysms During Transthoracic Echocardiography

Eisenberg MJ, Geraci SJ, Schiller NB (Univ of California, San Francisco)
*Am Heart J* 130:109–115, 1995                                     3–37

*Introduction.*—Elective surgery for abdominal aneurysm is associated with a mortality rate of less than 5%, compared with more than 50% for emergent surgery for ruptured aneurysm. Various screening strategies have been explored to help in the early identification of abdominal aortic aneurysms. The equipment used for transthoracic echocardiography is the same as that used for abdominal ultrasound. Patients undergoing transthoracic echocardiography may be at risk for the development of abdominal aortic aneurysm as they often have atherosclerotic vascular disease. The abdominal aorta was evaluated by ultrasound in 323 consecutive patients in whom routine 2-dimensional transthoracic echocardiography was being performed.

*Methods.*—When the aorta was identified, it was examined in the longitudinal and transverse planes. Maximum dilation of the aorta was measured. Color Doppler was used to demonstrate blood flow away from the heart if there was doubt about which structure was the abdominal aorta.

*Results.*—The average age of 169 men and 154 women was 57 years. Of 7 patients in whom aortic dilatation was observed, 6 were men and 1 was a woman. Six patients were 50 years old or older. Four patients had a history of atherosclerotic vascular disease. One of 4 patients had a previous resection of a thoracic aortic aneurysm. One patient had an infrarenal aneurysm. Aortic dilatation was correlated with male gender and older age, but not with a history of ischemic heart disease.

*Conclusion.*—Only a small number of patients undergoing transthoracic echocardiography had abdominal aortic aneurysms when aortic ultrasound was performed. However, the brief time and low cost of this additional procedure may make it a worthwhile addition to routine transthoracic echocardiographic evaluations.

▶ Another variation on the theme discussed in Abstracts 3–34 and 3–36. On balance, patients undergoing transthoracic echocardiography frequently had significant atherosclerotic coronary arterial disease and abnormal left ventricular function. As far as I can tell, only 2 of 265 patients had an aorta larger than 3 cm in diameter. Despite this remarkably low pick-up rate, these authors conclude that this appears to be a reasonable thing to do in patients undergoing transthoracic echocardiography. In this cohort, I disagree.

# 4 Nonatherosclerotic Conditions

**Long-term Outcome of Raynaud's Syndrome in a Prospectively Analyzed Patient Cohort**
Landry GJ, Edwards JM, McLafferty RB, et al (Oregon Health Sciences Univ, Portland)
*J Vasc Surg* 23:76–86, 1996                                                                 4–1

*Introduction.*—Knowledge of the long-term clinical outcome in patients with Raynaud's syndrome (RS) is lacking in the medical literature. It would be helpful to be able to predict the clinical outcome of patients with RS so that monitoring of the disease process and patient education could be planned appropriately. Of 1,039 patients with RS, 118 (11.4%) were followed prospectively for more than 10 years to determine prognostic variables on initial visit.

*Methods.*—When first seen, patients were assigned to 1 of 4 groups determined by vascular laboratory and serologic testing findings: vasospastic and serologically positive (spast, sero+), vasospastic and serologically negative (spast, sero−), obstructive and serologically positive (obst, sero+), and obstructive and serologically negative (obst, sero−) (Table 2).

*Results.*—Of the patients with spast, sero+ results, 48.6% had connective tissue disease (CTD) at initial visit, as did 72.9% of the patients with

TABLE 2.—Initial Group Classification of Patients With
Raynaud's Syndrome

| Initial Classification | All (n = 1039) | >10 yrs Follow-up (n = 118) |
|---|---|---|
| Spast, sero −* | 443 (42.6%) | 32 (27.1%) |
| Spast, sero + | 142 (13.7%) | 18 (15.3%) |
| Obst, sero − | 247 (23.3%) | 28 (23.7%) |
| Obst, sero +* | 207 (23.8%) | 40 (33.9%) |

* P < 0.005 between all and more than 10 years' follow-up.
*Abbreviations: Spast*, vasospastic; *Obst*, obstructive; *sero −*, serologically negative; *sero +*, serologically positive.
(Courtesy of Landry GJ, Edwards JM, McLafferty RB, et al: Long-term outcome of Raynaud's syndrome in a prospectively analyzed patient cohort. *J Vasc Surg* 23:76–86, 1996.)

173

obst, sero+ results. The progression to CTD in the remaining patients in these groups during follow-up occurred in 16.4% of patients with spast, sero+ results and 30.4% of patients with obst, sero+ results. At follow-up of greater than 10 years, the progression to CTD occurred in 81.8% of patients in the obst, sero+ group. The progression to CTD occurred in 2.0% of patients in the spast, sero− group. In the obst, sero− group, the rate of progression to CTD was 8.5%. Percent of digital ulcers in each group were 15.5% spast, sero+; 5.2% spast, sero−; 55.6% obst, sero+; and 48.2% obst, sero−. The respective rate of amputations for these patients were 1.4%, 1.6%, 11.6%, and 19.0%.

*Conclusion.*—Patients initially seen with RS can be classified into long-term outcome groups. They can be placed into vasospastic and obstructive categories. The development of CTD can be strongly predicted in the presence of serologic positivity. Digital ulcerations are more likely to occur in patients with obstructive RS, regardless of initial serology results. Of patients with obstructive disease, 10% to 20% needed amputation. Increased duration of disease did not increase these occurrences. In patients who were seen initially with vasospastic RS, ulcerations and amputations were rare.

▶ This is a 25-year study from a tertiary center serving a population in which RS is relatively common. Patients with digital ischemia caused by drugs, thoracic outlet syndrome, and palmar occupational occlusive disease were few and were excluded. Diagnosis has been clarified, patients with obstructive disease being clearly identified by a positive Nielsen test result, blunt or peaked waveforms, and a gradient of more than 20 mm Hg between brachial and digital arteries. They are at greatest risk, as are seropositive patients, but on initial assessment, more than 40% of those with RS will have negative test results and can be reassured that they have little to fear but a recurring nuisance. Arteriography can be reserved for those with a suggestion of more proximal disease. A few patients will have negative test results initially but deteriorate because of associated atherosclerosis or Buerger's disease; follow-up in the remainder is likely to be less important and less complete because they are inconvenienced but not threatened.

**A.E.B. Giddings, M.D.**

---

**Cold Exposure Increases Cyclic Guanosine Monophosphate in Healthy Women But Not in Women With Raynaud's Phenomenon**
Leppert J, Ringqvist Å, Ahlner J, et al (Central Hosp, Västerås, Sweden; Univ of Uppsala, Sweden; Univ of Linköping, Sweden)
*J Intern Med* 237:493–498, 1995                4–2

---

*Background.*—Previous studies have shown that patients with Raynaud's phenomenon have reduced venous dilation after bradykinin stimulation, suggesting an endothelial-specific defect in muscle relaxation. One mechanism of vasodilation involves arginine-derived nitrous oxide

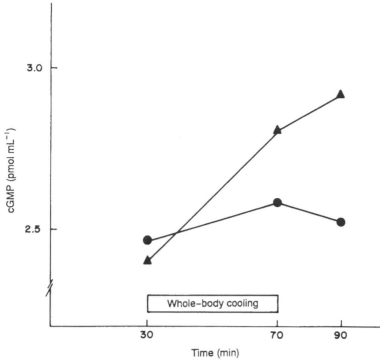

**FIGURE 1.**—Mean values of venous cGMP before, during, and after whole-body cooling in women with Raynaud's phenomenon (*circles*) and in healthy controls (*triangles*). Venous cGMP levels increased significantly compared with baseline at 70 (end of whole-body cooling) and 90 minutes (20 minutes after termination of whole-body cooling). *Abbreviation: cGMP*, cyclic guanosine monophosphate. (Courtesy of Leppert J, Ringqvist Å, Ahlner J, et al: Cold exposure increases cyclic guanosine monophosphate in healthy women but not in women with Raynaud's phenomenon. *J Intern Med* 237:493–498, 1995; Blackwell Science Ltd.)

stimulation of guanylate cyclase, which results in increased cyclic guanosine monophosphate (cGMP), causing a reduction in intracellular calcium, and thus contractile relaxation. Venous cGMP levels were measured after exposure to cold to examine the patency of this pathway in patients with Raynaud's phenomenon.

*Patients and Methods.*—Twenty-four female patients with a 17-year mean history of Raynaud's phenomenon were compared with 21 female patients with a negative history of Raynaud's or rheumatic illness. Patients were instructed to refrain from caffeine or tobacco use 12 hours before the study. Thirty minutes before the study, an IV cannula was inserted into an antecubital vein, and the patients were allowed to rest supine in a temperature controlled room. At the beginning of the study period, 10 mL of blood was drawn, and patients were covered with a 13°C water-chilled blanket. After 40 minutes of cooling, another blood sample was drawn, and cooling was terminated. A final blood sample was taken 20 minutes later. Blood pressure and pulse were measured coincident with blood samples. Levels of cGMP were measured by radioimmunoassay.

*Results.*—Diastolic blood pressure was increased significantly during and after cold exposure only among the patients with Raynaud's phenomenon. No significant changes in systolic blood pressure or pulse was found among either group of patients. In patients without Raynaud's phenomenon, cGMP levels significantly increased on and after cold exposure, with a mean elevation of 0.58 pmol/mL noted, compared with a nonsignificant increase of 0.05 pmol/mL in patients with Raynaud's phenomenon (Fig 1).

*Conclusion.*—Although further studies are needed to determine the exact deficiency, this study suggests that the underlying defect in Raynaud's phenomenon involves the arginine-NO-cGMP signal transduction pathway.

▶ These authors observed that 21 non–Raynaud's syndrome control women were different from 24 Raynaud's syndrome women in that their level of cGMP elevated after cold exposure. I wonder what the results would have been in men, a group apparently not studied. Although I am not willing to make a great deal of this isolated observation, it is important to note that cGMP is 1 of the couplers between the receptor and the effector in smooth muscle contraction. This may prove to be an important pathophysiologic observation.

---

## Blockade of Vasospastic Attacks by $\alpha_2$-Adrenergic But Not $\alpha_1$-Adrenergic Antagonists in Idiopathic Raynaud's Disease

Freedman RR, Baer RP, Mayes MD (Wayne State Univ, Detroit)
*Circulation* 92:1448–1451, 1995                                                          4–3

---

*Objective.*—Patients with idiopathic Raynaud's disease have digital vasospastic attacks, which are usually brought on by exposure to cold. Peripheral vascular $\alpha_2$-adrenergic receptors are hypersensitive to local cooling in these patients. However, the role of the $\alpha_1$-adrenergic receptors is unknown, and the role of the adrenergic receptors in producing the actual vasospastic symptoms has not been studied. The role of adrenergic receptor subtypes in producing vasospastic attacks was assessed.

*Methods.*—The randomized study included 23 patients with idiopathic Raynaud's disease, diagnosed using conservative criteria. Vasospastic attacks were provoked in the laboratory by cooling during brachial artery infusions with the $\alpha_1$-antagonist prazosin, the $\alpha_2$-antagonist yohimbine, or both. The patients' hands were photographed to document any color changes. The number of attacks in the hand receiving $\alpha_1$-antagonist infusion was compared with that in the contralateral hand (Table 1).

*Results.*—Patients receiving yohimbine infusion had a mean of 0.3 finger involved with attacks in the infused hands compared with 2.3 fingers in those receiving prazosin and 0.6 finger in those receiving both adrenergic antagonists. The number of attacks was significantly higher in patients receiving prazosin only compared with the other 2 groups.

TABLE 1.—Finger Blood Flow Responses in Raynaud's Disease Patients and Healthy Volunteers

| | | | Period | |
| | | | After 2 Minutes of | After 4 Minutes of |
| Group | Baseline | After Heat | Ischemia | Ischemia |
|---|---|---|---|---|
| Raynaud's disease | 23.0±2.0 | 28.1±2.0 | 45.4±2.9 | 48.4±2.9 |
| Healthy | 30.0±2.9 | 37.1±3.3 | 46.5±3.6 | 49.1±3.7 |

*Note:* All values are in mL/100 mL per min (mean ± standard error of the mean).
(Freedman RR, Baer RP, Mayes MD: Blockade of vasospastic attacks by $\alpha_2$-adrenergic but not $\alpha_1$-adrenergic antagonists in idiopathic Raynaud's disease. *Circulation* 1995; 92:1448–1451. Reproduced with permission of *Circulation*, Copyright 1995 American Heart Association.)

*Conclusion.*—Activation of $\alpha_2$-adrenergic receptors but not of $\alpha_1$-adrenergic receptors is necessary for the production of vasospastic attacks in patients with idiopathic Raynaud's disease. Efforts should be made to identify the causes of the $\alpha_2$-adrenergic receptor abnormality in these patients and to identify effective treatments for it.

▶ $\alpha$-Adrenergic receptors have been subdivided into many types, the most prominent being the $\alpha_1$- and the $\alpha_2$- varieties. Many of traditional sympathetic agonists and antagonists have primarily $\alpha_1$- activities. This study provides additional evidence that the $\alpha_2$- receptors may indeed be more important in the production of Raynaud's syndrome, because selective blockade of these receptors appeared to reduce the frequency of vasospastic attacks. We have found similar results in our laboratory.[1]

*Reference*

1. Edwards JM, Phinney ES, Taylor LM, et al: $\alpha_2$-Adrenoceptor levels in obstructive and spastic Raynaud's syndrome. *J Vasc Surg* 538–545, 1987.

## Asymptomatic Functional Popliteal Artery Entrapment: Demonstration at MR Imaging

Chernoff DM, Walker AT, Khorasani R, et al (Brigham and Women's Hosp, Boston)
*Radiology* 195:176–180, 1995                                            4–4

*Background.*—Functional popliteal entrapment syndrome is thought to be related to hypertrophy of the calf muscles, and surgical correction is typically performed in symptomatic patients. Functional popliteal entrapment may also be common in patients without syndrome-related symptoms, however. Functional popliteal entrapment was studied to determine whether it can occur in healthy individuals and, if so, to identify the site and source of vascular compression.

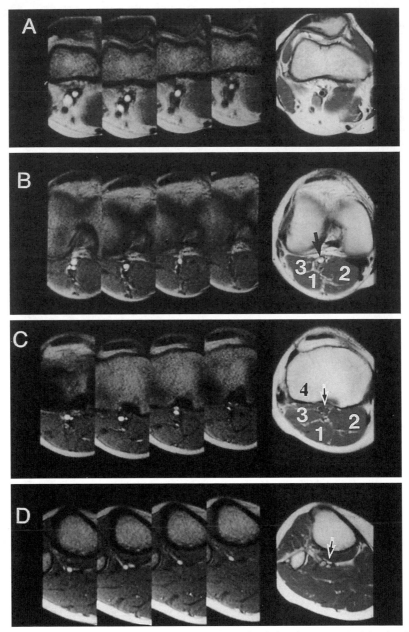

FIGURE 1.—Axial T1-weighted spin-echo images obtained with the subject at rest (*right*) and spoiled gradient recalled acquisition images obtained during graded (0%, 25%, 50%, and 75%) effort of plantar flexion at 4 anatomical levels: **(A)** just cephalic to the gastrocnemius origin; **(B)**, 1 cm above the tibial plateau; **(C)**, 1 cm below the tibial plateau; and **(D)**, at the level of the popliteal trifurcation. The popliteal artery is indicated by an *arrow* in the spin-echo images **(B–D)**. Signal intensity within the artery varies from section to section in the spin-echo images because of pulse gating during different portions of the cardiac cycle. More prominent flow artifact (ghosting) in the phase-encoding direction is shown in **(C)** during compression of the vessel, presumably because of increased flow velocity. *1,* lateral head of the gastrocnemius muscle; *2,* medial head of the gastrocnemius muscle; *3,* plantaris muscle; *4,* popliteus muscle. (Courtesy of Chernoff DM, Walker AT, Khorasani R, et al: Asymptomatic functional popliteal artery entrapment: Demonstration at MR imaging. *Radiology* 195:176–180, 1995, Radiological Society of North America.)

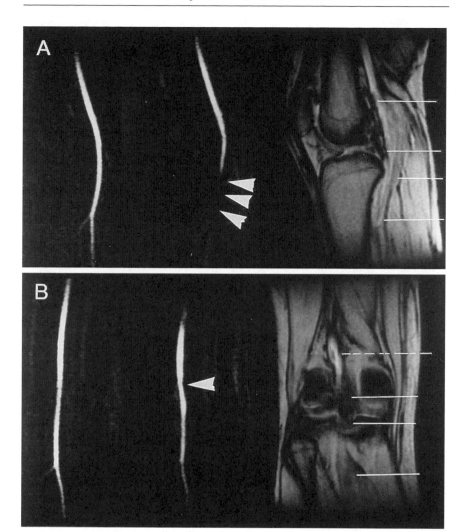

**FIGURE 2.**—Phase-contrast images in (**A**) sagittal and (**B**) coronal planes depict flow in the popliteal artery at rest (*left*) and during a submaximal contraction (*center*). Flow signal intensity is obliterated in the anteroposterior aspect over a 3-cm length below the knee during plantar flexion (**A,** *arrowheads*). The vascular lumen is narrowed from side to side and displaced to the lateral aspect of the leg above the knee during plantar flexion (**B,** *arrowhead*). The greater loss of flow signal intensity below the knee on the sagittal image is caused by a slightly greater flexing effort. Images on the right are reference (**A**) sagittal and (**B**) coronal gradient-echo images obtained at the same level as the phase-contrast images. The horizontal lines correspond to the 4 levels shown in Figure 1. (Courtesy of Chernoff DM, Walker AT, Khorasani R, et al: Asymptomatic functional popliteal artery entrapment: Demonstration at MR imaging. *Radiology* 195:176–180, 1995, Radiological Society of North America.)

*Patients and Methods.*—Thirteen individuals, including 9 men (mean age, 31 years) and 4 women (mean age, 34 years) were studied. All participants were free from symptoms related to popliteal artery entrapment. Magnetic resonance imaging was performed in the right lower extremities of all participants. Images were obtained while patients were at rest and during graded effort (0%, 25%, 50%, and 75%) of plantar flexion at 4 anatomical levels to determine whether popliteal artery blood flow can be compromised by extrinsic muscle compression and, if compressed, to define the compression location and source. Findings on MRI were correlated with those obtained during Doppler flow studies of the distal part of the leg.

*Results.*—Gradient-echo images obtained during active plantar flexion showed deformation of the popliteal artery lumen in all study participants, consistent with extrinsic compression at 1 or more levels. The observed narrowing was less than 50% of resting diameter in 1 participant and 75% to 99% of resting diameter in another 3 individuals. The lumen was entirely obliterated in the remaining 9 participants. Popliteal entrapment was attributed to compression between adjacent muscles at 2 sites— between the plantaris muscle and the medial head of the gastrocnemius muscle above the knee and between the plantaris and popliteus muscles below the knee. Figure 1 demonstrates representative MR images obtained during graded-resistance plantar flexion. The effect of a submaximal (75% effort) plantar flexion on the phase-contrast flow signal intensity in the popliteal artery lumen is shown in Figure 2. Findings obtained during Doppler flow studies were consistent with those observed on MRI. All participants had measurable Doppler pedal pulses while at rest. No change in the ankle-brachial index was noted in the individual with less than 50% narrowing. The index increased by at least 0.15 in the participants with 75% to 99% narrowing. In the remaining individuals, no detectable flow signal intensity was found in the posterior tibial or dorsalis pedis arteries during plantar flexion, and pressure measurements could not be obtained.

*Conclusion.*—Functional popliteal entrapment is common in asymptomatic individuals during normal exercise. Provocative maneuvers frequently used in the diagnosis of this condition therefore may be of limited value, given the high prevalence in patients without symptoms.

▶ It seems well established that both the popliteal artery and the popliteal vein are compressed in a significant number of completely healthy and asymptomatic individuals with either hyperextension of the leg or plantar flexion of the foot.[1] One can conclude only that the finding of pulse alteration with foot motion is a variant of normal and cannot be used to diagnose anything. See also the commentary of Abstract 3–30.

*Reference*

1. 1994 YEAR BOOK OF VASCULAR SURGERY, p 412.

## Arterial Lesions in Behçet's Disease. A Study in 25 Patients

Huong DLT, Wechsler B, Papo T, et al (Groupe Hospitalier Pitié-Salpêtrière, Paris; Hôpital Broussais, Paris)

*J Rheumatol* 22:2103–2113, 1995          4–5

*Introduction.*—Behçet's disease (BD) now is acknowledged to be a systemic disorder involving many tissues and organ systems. Vasculitis affecting arteries, veins, and capillaries is part of the process. Thrombophlebitis is more frequent than are arterial lesions such as stenosis, occlusion, and aneurysms.

*Objective.*—Prognostic factors were examined in 25 consecutive patients with BD in whom angiography demonstrated arterial lesions. The patients were followed for 78 months on average after BD was diagnosed and for 76 months after the first sign of arterial involvement.

*Observations.*—Seven of the 25 patients had occlusive lesions, 3 had aneurysms, and 15 had both. Classical features of BD were present in 16 patients when the arterial lesions was discovered. Occlusion was seen chiefly in the lower extremities. The most common clinical manifestations were intermittent claudication and gangrene of the toes or forefoot. Three patients had occlusive lesions of coronary arteries that were heralded by anterior myocardial infarction. Aneurysms involved a total of 29 arteries, mainly larger vessels. Signs were generally related to aneurysmal leakage, peripheral embolization or, rarely, rupture. Five patients had pulmonary artery aneurysms, 6 had lesions involving abdominal visceral arteries, and 7 had aneurysms of lower limb vessels.

*Treatment and Outcome.*—Five patients received 12 bypasses of occlusive or aneurysmal lesions in the lower extremity. Both autologous vein grafts and prosthetic grafts were used. In all, 15 patients underwent 27 vascular operations. Only 4 of 13 patients having aneurysmal surgery remained in remission. The use of steroids postoperatively was associated with a lesser risk of treatment failure regardless of whether immunosuppressive drugs also were used. Two of the 5 patients with bilateral pulmonary artery aneurysms died of massive hemoptysis despite steroid and immunosuppressive therapy. In all, 5 patients with aneurysms and 1 with only occlusive lesions died.

*Conclusion.*—Arterial aneurysms in patients with BD have a poorer prognosis than do occlusive lesions and should be operated on when possible. Postoperative steroid therapy may prevent a relapse and should be combined with immunosuppressive treatment. Anticoagulant therapy will help prevent graft thrombosis after bypass surgery for arterial lesions in the lower extremity.

▶ Behçet's disease consists of the clinical triad of recurrent oral and genital ulcerations, as well as iritis. The disease is endemic in certain countries, notably Turkey. A review of arterial abnormalities in a small group of patients is presented herein. It is important to remember, however, that the overwhelming majority of vascular symptoms in BD are venous, with venous thrombosis being by far the most frequent vascular condition encountered. These authors note, and I am certain correctly, that arterial repair is often unsuccessful in the occasional patient with arterial involvement. The controversial role of concomitant immunosuppressive drugs and anticoagulates is described.

## Dissection of the External Iliac Artery in Highly Trained Athletes
Cook PS, Erdoes LS, Selzer PM, et al (Saint Joseph Hosp, Denver; Univ of Arizona, Tucson; Meriter/Madison Gen Hosp, Wis; et al)
*J Vasc Surg* 22:173–177, 1995                                4–6

*Objective.*—Three highly trained athletes who experienced acute external iliac artery dissection after intense athletic events were discussed to determine whether this complication of ultraendurance events is a variant of the previously reported iliac occlusive syndromes in athletes.

*Patients.*—The patients were a 45-year-old man who competed in the Ironman Triathlon in Hawaii (Fig 1), a 50-year-old female marathoner, and a 50-year-old man who had recently increased his running mileage and

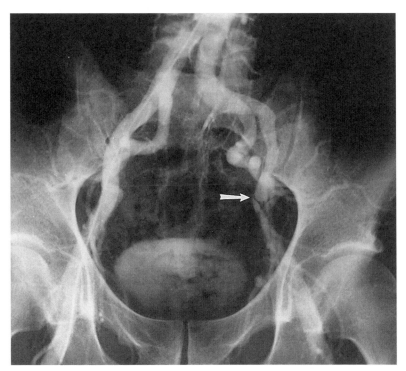

FIGURE 1.—Arterographic appearance of left external iliac artery dissection (anteroposterior projection). *Arrow* indicates area of dissection. (Courtesy of Cook PS, Erdoes LS, Selzer PM, et al: Dissection of the external iliac artery in highly trained athletes. *J Vasc Surg* 22:173–177, 1995.)

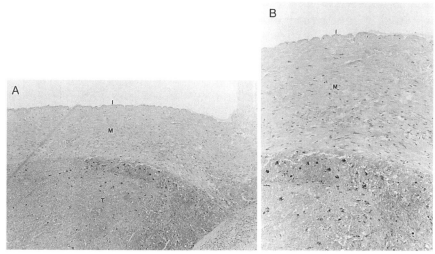

FIGURE 2.—Same patient as in Figure 1. **A,** lower-power micrograph shows arterial dissection within media. Organized thrombus is seen within media; hematoxylin and eosin, original magnification ×50. **B,** higher-power view shows normal intima with dissection in media; hematoxylin and eosin, original magnification ×120. *Abbreviations: I,* intima; *M,* media; *T,* thrombus. (Courtesy of Cook PS, Erdoes LS, Selzer PM, et al: Dissection of the external iliac artery in highly trained athletes. *J Vasc Surg* 22:173–177, 1995.)

started to practice calisthenics and use a rowing machine. Arteriography confirmed dissection of the external iliac artery in all 3 patients (Fig 2); the 50-year-old man was found to have bilateral lesions.

*Treatment and Outcome.*—The patient with bilateral involvement was treated conservatively with low-dose aspirin and close follow-up. He was then able to exercise regularly without claudication. Treatment in the other 2 patients was initiated with percutaneous transluminal angioplasty. The 45-year-old man had a successful result, was being maintained on low-dose aspirin therapy, and was training again for athletic events. The woman required operative repair and placement of a graft. She continued to run 6–9 miles per week. With a mean follow-up of 32 months, all 3 patients had normal resting hemodynamics.

*Discussion.*—All 3 patients with external iliac artery dissection were older than 40 and were involved in distance running. All complained of short-distance claudication after athletic events. This complication contrasts with the previously reported syndromes of nonatherosclerotic vascular disease in young, highly trained athletes. Local hemodynamic factors appear to be important in both acute dissection and chronic stenosis, and long-term repetitive trauma is also suspected to be a factor. Dissection of the artery may be a result of the adaptive hypertension of vigorous exercise. Conservative treatment and endovascular or surgical therapy can achieve a successful outcome.

▶ An impressive body of literature in recent years speaks to the propensity for competitive athletes, especially runners, cyclists, and perhaps rugby players, to develop external iliac lesions, typically consisting of fibrous occlusion. Herein is reported a variant, namely, the occurrence of external iliac dissection, in 2 competitive athletes. It seems inescapable that the external iliac artery is prone to the development of significant abnormalities in certain types of athletic activity. One should be familiar with this propensity. Two references are listed.[1, 2]

*References*

1. Gallegos CRR, Studley JGN, Hamer DB: External iliac artery occlusion: Another complication of long distance running? *Eur J Vasc Surg* 4:195–196, 1989.
2. Mosimann F, Walder J: Intermittent leg ischaemia during competition cycling. *Lancet* 336:746, 1993.

---

## The Effects of Elevated Compartment Pressure on Tibial Arteriovenous Flow and Relationship of Mechanical and Biochemical Characteristics of Fascia to Genesis of Chronic Anterior Compartment Syndrome

Turnipseed WD, Hurschler C, Vanderby R Jr (Univ of Wisconsin, Madison)
*J Vasc Surg* 21:810–817, 1995                                      4–7

---

*Background.*—Chronic compartment syndrome (CCS), a condition most often related to overuse in well-conditioned athletes, is characterized by recurrent muscle cramping, tightness, and intermittent paresthesia. Elevated pressure within a closed myofascial space appears to be the most significant pathologic factor associated with CCS. The effects of increased compartment pressure on anterior tibial arteriovenous flow pattern were evaluated, and the associations between compartment pressure abnormalities and the mechanical and biochemical characteristics of fascia were determined.

*Patients and Methods.*—Twenty patients with chronic anterior compartment syndrome (CACS) and 20 age-matched controls were enrolled in the study. Compartment pressure measurements were obtained, and tibial arterial and venous flow were analyzed before and after fasciectomy. The thickness, stress failure, structural stiffness, total collagen content, and prevalence of collagen cross-linkage were evaluated in harvested fascia specimens.

*Results.*—Patients with CACS had significantly increased anterior compartment pressures, 23.8 mm Hg compared with 6 mm Hg in controls. Tibial arterial flow was not significantly different between groups, with mean flows of 43 cm/sec in the CACS patients and 41.9 cm/sec in controls (Table 1). Patients with CACS but not controls had profoundly impaired venous drainage. Fascia specimens obtained from symptomatic patients were thicker and stiffer, at 0.35 mm and 109 meganewtons/mm compared with 0.22 mm and 60.3 meganewtons/mm in control specimens. Postoperative compartment pressures were normalized after fasciectomy, and venous drainage also improved. Similar collagen content per unit mass was noted for the CACS and control fascia specimens. Collagen cross-linking

TABLE 1.—Diagnostic Tests

| Test | Age-matched Controls (*n* = 20) | Patients With CACS (*n* = 20) |
|---|---|---|
| PVR (resting stress) | Normal | Normal |
| Popliteal entrapment | Negative | Negative |
| Anterior compartment pressure (mean) | 4 to 7 mm Hg (6.0) | 16 to 36 mm Hg (23.8) |
| Lateral compartment pressure (mean) | 4 to 6 mm Hg (6.0) | 2 to 11 mm Hg (6.8) |
| Color-flow duplex screening | | |
| Anterior tibial venous flow (40 limbs) | | |
| Spontaneous-phasic | 34/40 (70%) | 0/40 (0%) |
| Augmentation | 40/40 (100%) | 40/40 (100) |
| Absent | 0/40 (0%) | 0/40 (0%) |
| Anterior tibial arterial flow (40 limbs) | 23 to 62 cc/min (mean 41.9) | 36 to 69 cc/min (mean 43.0) |

*Abbreviation: CACS*, chronic anterior compartment syndrome.
(Courtesy of Turnipseed WD, Hurschler C, Vanderby R Jr: The effects of elevated compartment pressure of tibial arteriovenous flow and relationship of mechanical and biochemical characteristics of fascia to genesis of chronic anterior compartment syndrome. *J Vasc Surg* 21:810–817, 1995.)

was, however, significantly lower in the CACS fascia compared with controls.

*Conclusion.*—Arterial blood flow is not severely impaired in patients with symptomatic CACS, although tibial venous drainage is severely affected, leading to subsequent muscle edema and swelling. An association between increased pressure in CACS compartments and fascia thickness and structural stiffness was noted, although neither of these latter factors was related to collagen content and cross-linkage. Delayed venous emptying accounts for lack of recovery of symptoms in patients with CACS. Fasciotomy or fasciectomy increases capacitance of the compartment, consequently decreasing compartment pressure and improving venous drain and thereby relieving symptoms.

▶ I don't know what to make of this article. I have seen possibly 1 patient with chronic compartment syndrome in 25 years, and that was doubtful. I am amazed that this group at Wisconsin has encountered 20 patients over a short time. I am always wary of highly localized endemics.

## Fecal Impaction as a Cause of Acute Lower Limb Ischemia
Hoballah JJ, Chalmers RTA, Sharp WJ, et al (Univ of Iowa, Iowa City)
*Am J Gastroenterol* 90:2055–2056, 1995                                    4–8

*Background.*—A case of compression of the common iliac artery with subsequent leg ischemia resulting from severe fecal impaction was described.

*Case Report.*—Man, 84, was transferred from a nursing home to the emergency room after a brief history of cramping abdominal pain and a cold, mottled right leg. On examination, the abdomen

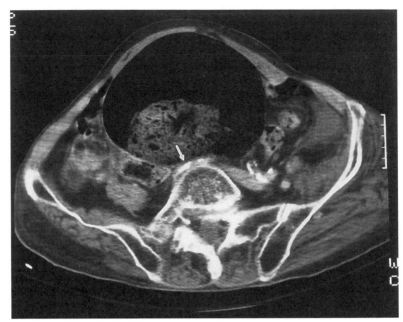

FIGURE 1.—Transverse CT scan of the pelvis. The right common iliac artery (*arrow*) is occluded between the fecaloma and the vertebral body. (Courtesy of Hoballah JJ, Chalmers RTA, Sharp WJ, et al: *Am J Gastroenterol* 90[11]:2055–2056, 1995.)

was tense and painful, but bowel sounds were present. Computed tomography scan revealed a 15 by 10 cm fecaloma that compressed the right common iliac artery against a vertebral body, occluding it (Fig 1). Bilateral hydronephrosis was also noted. All findings, including leg ischemia, resolved after disimpaction. The patient had a history of routine use of opioid analgesics and nonsteroidal anti-inflammatory medications for rheumatoid arthritis.

*Discussion.*—A rectosigmoid fecaloma can compress pelvic structures, causing obstructive uropathy and obstructed venous return through the iliac vein. In this case, sufficient pressure was exerted on the common iliac artery to cause its occlusion.

*Conclusion.*—The first documented case of compression of the common iliac artery by a fecal mass was reported. As the number of nursing home residents increases, this event may become more frequent.

▶ I include this case report because of its novelty. I'll bet you never heard of this before.

## Hydroxyurea for Patients With Essential Thrombocythemia and a High Risk of Thrombosis

Cortelazzo S, Finazzi G, Ruggeri M, et al (Ospedali Riuniti di Bergamo, Italy; Ospedale Civile S Bortolo di Vicenza, Italy)
*N Engl J Med* 332:1132–1136, 1995                                                  4–9

*Introduction.*—Patients with essential thrombocythemia who were older than 60 and those who already had a thrombolic event have been shown to have a high vascular complication rate. These patients could be candidates for platelet count reduction. Hydroxyurea reduces platelet count, but there is no evidence that it decreases thrombotic episodes in patients with essential thrombocythemia. A prospective, randomized trial was conducted to determine whether keeping the platelet count less than 600,000 cells/mm³ would reduce the incidence of thrombosis in high-risk patients.

*Methods.*—A total of 114 patients with essential thrombocythemia were 60 or older and had a median platelet count of 788,000 cells/mm³. Hemostatic and coagulation studies were done at baseline and at appropriate intervals throughout. Fifty-six patients were randomly assigned to receive hydroxyurea treatment and 58 no hydroxyurea treatment.

*Results.*—Patients were followed for a median of 27 months. All patients randomized to receive hydroxyurea had a decrease in platelet count

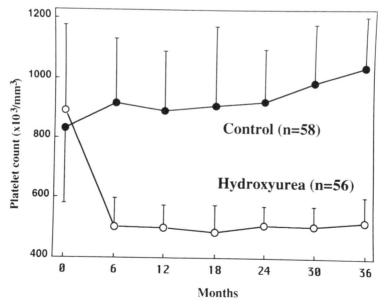

FIGURE 1.—Mean (± standard deviation) platelet counts of 114 patients with essential thrombocythemia treated with hydroxyurea or left untreated. (Reprinted by permission of *The New England Journal of Medicine* from Cortelazzo S, Finazzi G, Ruggeri M, et al: Hydroxyurea for patients with essential throbocythemia and a high risk of thrombosis. N *Engl J Med* 332:1132–1136, Copyright 1995, Massachusetts Medical Society.)

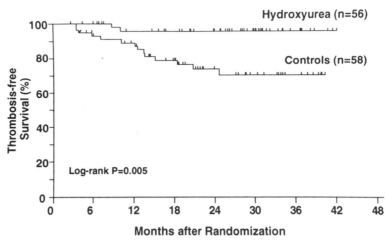

FIGURE 2.—Probability of thrombosis-free survival in 114 patients with essential thrombocythemia treated with hydroxyurea or left untreated. The *P* value is for the difference between the 2 groups (by the log-rank test). The median follow-up was 27 months. *Tick marks* indicate surviving patients who were continuously free of thrombosis. (Reprinted by permission of *The New England Journal of Medicine* from Cortelazzo S, Finazzi G, Ruggeri M, et al: Hydroxyurea for patients with essential thrombocythemia and a high risk of thrombosis. *N Engl J Med* 332:1132–1136, Copyright 1995, Massachusetts Medical Society.)

to less than 600,000 cells/mm³ (median count 459,000 cells/mm³) within 2 to 8 weeks. This level was maintained throughout long-term treatment (Fig 1). This is in agreement with an earlier finding of a reduced rate of thrombosis in patients with platelet counts less than 600,000 cells/mm³. Fourteen of 58 untreated controls and 2 of 56 patients treated with hydroxyurea had vascular occlusive events (Fig 2). Hemorrhagic complications occurred in 5 patients, all of whom were taking aspirin or ticlopidine prophylactically. Cigarette smoking was significantly associated with thrombosis, as confirmed by an earlier finding.

*Conclusion.*—Unlike busulfan, hydroxyurea is not an alkylating agent. Concerns about its leukomogenic effects, prolonged myelosupression, and pulmonary and gonadal toxicity eliminates busulfan as a first-line therapy for essential thrombocythemia. Hydroxyurea used in the treatment of essential thrombocythemia was effective in reducing platelet count and preventing thrombosis. However, it must be taken continuously. If inadvertently stopped, an excessive rebound increase in the platelet count could occur.

▶ Essential thrombocythemia with a high platelet count and symptomatic peripheral arterial occlusions, especially involving the feet and toes, is one of the more frequently encountered manifestations of nonatherosclerotic arterial occlusive disease. We have seen many such patients. In fact, a platelet count is an essential component of our hypercoagulation screen. For many years, hydroxyurea has been the primary treatment for these patients. The authors of this article attempted to determine whether maintaining the platelet count less than 600,000 cells/mm$^3$ would reduce the incidence of thrombosis in these high-risk patients. They conclude that hydroxyurea is very effective not only in reducing the platelet count but, more important, in preventing thrombosis. This is important information because heretofore we were not absolutely convinced that the number of platelets was the most important factor in thrombus production. This article suggests that it is. We, too, have had very good success with the use of hydroxyurea.

---

**Increased Incidence of Aortic Aneurysm and Dissection in Giant Cell (Temporal) Arteritis: A Population-based Study**
Evans JM, O'Fallon WM, Hunder GG (Mayo Clinic, Rochester, Minn)
*Ann Intern Med* 122:502–507, 1995                                                      4–10

---

*Purpose.*—Giant cell, or temporal, arteritis of the large and medium-sized arteries is 1 of the most common forms of vasculitis. It is occasionally complicated by aortic aneurysmal disease and even death from aortic dissection. However, data to determine the frequency and clinical relevance of this purported association are inadequate. These issues were examined in a population-based cohort study of patients with giant cell arteritis.

*Methods.*—The analysis included 96 residents of 1 Minnesota county in whom diagnosis of giant cell was made between 1950 and 1985. Each patient's records were reviewed to obtain information about the presence of aortic aneurysm, with or without dissection, along with other factors. Aneurysm was diagnosed by CT, ultrasonography, angiography, or autopsy. The incidence of aortic aneurysm was assessed, as were clinical features of giant cell arteritis that might be associated with an increased risk of aneurysm formation.

*Results.*—Aneurysms of the thoracic aorta developed in 11 of 96 patients. Two cases of aneurysm were diagnosed at the same time as giant cell arteritis. For the rest, the diagnosis of aneurysm was made a median of 6 years after that of giant cell arteritis. In 6 cases, thoracic aortic dissection led to sudden death. In 5 patients without thoracic aortic dissection, isolated abdominal aortic aneurysms developed a median of 2½ years after the diagnosis of giant cell arteritis. The incidence of aneurysms in patients with giant cell arteritis was 999/100,000 person-years for thoracic aortic aneurysms and 555/100,000 person-years for abdominal aortic aneurysms. Compared with the age- and sex-matched population of the county, patients with giant cell arteritis were 17 times more likely to have thoracic aortic aneurysm and more than twice as likely to have isolated abdominal aortic aneurysm. Survival for the cohort with giant cell arteritis was not significantly different than that of the population (Fig 3). No significant risk factors were identified beyond giant cell arteritis itself.

*Conclusion.*—Risk of aortic aneurysm is markedly increased among patients with giant cell arteritis. Abdominal and especially thoracic aortic aneurysms may occur as a late and potentially fatal complication. The

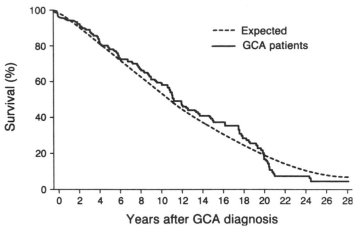

FIGURE 3.—Survival in 96 patients with giant cell arteritis compared with the expected survival rates among whites. Data obtained from the U.S. life-table of 1980. *Abbreviation: GCA,* giant cell arteritis. (Courtesy of Evans JM, O'Fallon WM, Hunder GG: Increased incidence of aortic aneurysm and dissection in giant cell (temporal) arteritis: A population-based study. *Ann Intern Med* 122:502–507, 1995.)

findings suggest that patients with giant cell arteritis should receive an annual assessment to detect aortic aneurysm, with palpation of the abdominal aorta and a radiograph of the chest, including a lateral view.

▶ We all have known for years that giant cell arteritis is prone to involve the brachiocephalic arteries, as well as the temporal arteries, and occasionally the ophthalmic arteries. It has also been known for years that the condition occasionally involves the thoracic and abdominal aorta, but we have had little information about the incidence of aortic involvement. This detailed population-based study reports a significant incidence of thoracic aortic aneurysm (11 of 96 patients) in this giant cell arteritis cohort. A number of these patients experienced symptomatic aortic valve insufficiency, and 4 had thoracic aortic dissection. Microscopic studies revealed evidence of giant cell aortitis in the 2 aortas studied at autopsy. In dealing with patients with giant cell arteritis, we must keep in mind that these patients may have a thoracic aortic aneurysm.

---

**Management of Arterial Occlusive Disease Following Radiation Therapy**
Andros G, Schneider PA, Harris RW, et al (Saint Joseph Med Ctr, Burbank, Calif)
*Cardiovasc Surg* 4:135–142, 1996                                    4–11

*Background.*—Arterial occlusive disease is a potential complication of radiation therapy. The diagnosis and management of vascular lesions associated with radiation therapy, including suggested management strategies for patients with various manifestations of radiation vasculopathy, were described.

*Methods.*—The study included 26 patients with clinically significant arterial occlusion who had previously undergone radiation therapy. The mean time since radiation therapy was 11 years, with a range of 5 months to 44 years. The lesions were located in the abdominal aorta and its branches in 10 patients, the carotid artery in 9, and the subclavian-axillary arteries in 7. Transient ischemic attack, stroke, vertebrobasilar insufficiency, carotid bruit, upper- or lower-extremity ischemia, and renovascular hypertension were the most frequent clinical manifestations.

Patients with cerebrovascular insufficiency underwent carotid endarterectomy with vein patch, interposition grafting, or subclavian to carotid bypass, and those with upper-extremity ischemia had carotid or subclavian to axillary bypass. Infrarenal reconstruction was achieved with a combination of endarterectomy and grafting with Dacron or saphenous vein. Orthotopic tunnels were placed, and musculocutaneous flaps were used as indicated to aid in wound healing. Some patients undergoing abdominal vascular reconstruction had ureteral catheters placed.

*Results.*—Operative mortality was nil, and there were no strokes or amputations. Recurrent transient ischemic attacks occurred after subclavian to carotid bypass in 1 patient. The patients were followed up for a mean of 48 months.

*Conclusion.*—A series of patients with arterial occlusive lesions occurring after radiation therapy are presented. The management of these radiation-associated lesions seems similar to that for atherosclerotic occlusive disease in other types of patients. Aggressive surgical revascularization produces good results.

▶ One must remember that radiation produces a myriad of injuries to involved arteries. Acutely, high-dose radiation may produce fibrosis and occlusion in short order. It seems, however, that low-dose radiation facilitates the development of atherosclerosis over years. That appears to be the primary lesion treated by these authors in the patients. They have encountered 26 such patients treated with a variety of standard vascular surgical procedures, with generally good results. This is a good overall review of this infrequently encountered problem.

## Sensitive Detection of Abnormal Aortic Architecture in Marfan Syndrome With High-frequency Ultrasonic Tissue Characterization

Recchia D, Sharkey AM, Bosner MS (Washington Univ, St Louis)
*Circulation* 91:1036–1043, 1995                                                4–12

*Background.*—Aneurysmal dilatation of the aorta is a major cause of morbidity and mortality in patients with Marfan syndrome, an inherited disorder of connective tissue structure and function. High-frequency ultrasonic tissue characterization was used to identify structural changes in abnormal aorta, hypothesizing that detection of such changes would help to monitor disease progression and to determine the need for medical and surgical intervention.

*Methods.*—Aortic tissue was obtained from 11 patients with Marfan syndrome who had undergone repair of an aortic aneurysm or dissection. For comparison, normal tissue obtained at autopsy from patients without evidence of aortic disease was also examined. Integrated backscatter from each specimen was measured by acoustic microscopy at 50 MHz. Specimens were mounted to ensure a direction of insonification that was orthogonal to previous 1 and parallel to the circumferential orientation of the major fiber axis of the vessel (Fig 1). Quantification of the magnitude of ultrasonic anisotropy provides a measure of the 3-dimensional organization of the tissue. A hydroxyproline assay was used to determine collagen content of the specimens.

*Results.*—Compared with normal aortas, those from patients with Marfan syndrome exhibited less backscatter. Despite considerable differences

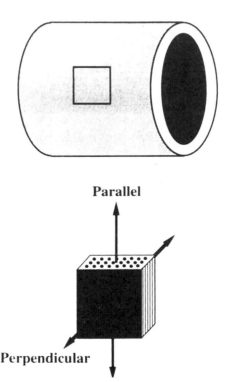

**Parallel**

**Perpendicular**

FIGURE 1.—Schematic showing orientation of the ultrasound beam in relation to the major fiber axis of the arterial wall. The area outlined by the *square* represents the sample of arterial wall removed for insonification. Elastin fibers are oriented circumferentially around the vessel wall orthogonal to the direction of blood flow. Each tissue section was insonified both perpendicular and parallel to the major fiber axis, as illustrated in the *lower panel*. (Recchia D, Sharkey AM, Bosner MS: Sensitive detection of abnormal aortic architecture in Marfan syndrome with high-frequency ultrasonic tissue characterization. *Circulation* 1995; 91:1036–1043. Reproduced with permission of *Circulation*. Copyright 1995 American Heart Association.)

## Normal Aorta        Marfan Aorta

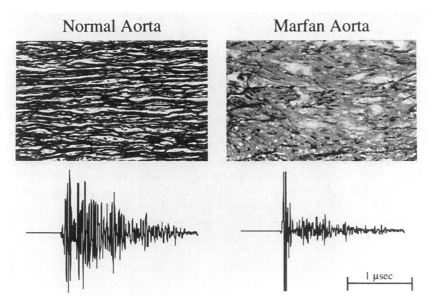

FIGURE 3.—Examples of the histologic structure and the corresponding unprocessed radiofrequency data of normal aorta from a patient without Marfan syndrome (*left*) and aneurysmal aorta from a Marfan syndrome patient (*right*). Normal tissue exhibits well-formed elastin fibers arranged in a lamellar fashion. Radiofrequency data from the normal aorta reveal a large specular echo at the water-intima interface, followed by relatively high ultrasonic scattering throughout the media. The Marfan aorta exhibits a profound decrease in the amount of elastin present and loss of the highly aligned and ordered lamellar arrangement. Radiofrequency data from the abnormal Marfan aorta also exhibit a large specular echo at the water-intima interface, but the ultrasonic scattering throughout the media is greatly reduced (van Gieson stain for elastin, original magnification ×250). (Recchia D, Sharkey AM, Bosner MS: Sensitive detection of abnormal aortic architecture in Marfan syndrome with high-frequency ultrasonic tissue characterization. *Circulation* 1995; 91:1036–1043. Reproduced with permission of *Circulation*. Copyright 1995 American Heart Association.)

in backscatter, the collagen concentrations of the normal and Marfan aortas did not differ significantly. Histologic analysis, however, showed marked contrasts between the 2 specimen types in both the amount and organization of elastin. In normal aorta, well-formed elastin fibers were arranged in a lamellar pattern. The Marfan aorta was characterized by a profound decrease in elastin content, together with loss of the highly aligned and ordered lamellar arrangement (Fig 3). Another marked difference between normal and Marfan aorta was observed in the directional dependence of scattering, or ultrasonic anisotropy, which was much smaller in Marfan aortas.

*Conclusion.*—High-frequency tissue characterization may be an important addition to MR, CT, and transthoracic and transesophageal echocardiography in detecting pathologic changes in the aortas of patients with Marfan syndrome. Findings demonstrated changes in vessel wall composition and organization, suggesting a profound extent of matrix disorganization.

▶ Marfan syndrome is a heritable disorder of connective tissue structure resulting in abnormalities in the production of the important molecule fibrillin, which forms the scaffolding on which elastin fibers appear to be assembled. In Marfan syndrome the elastin fibers are abnormal in organization and structure, leading to a marked alteration of mechanical properties of the affected tissues. These authors obtained Marfan tissue from surgery and insonated the tissue with extremely high frequency acoustic microscopy, acquiring backscattered radiofrequency signals that were then analyzed in detail. I do not begin to understand the electronics involved, but these authors concluded the backscattered radiofrequency data was distinctly different between normal and Marfan aortic tissue. The authors hypothesize that use of this type of diagnostic testing in vivo may provide a novel quantitative assessment of the altered biophysical properties of the affected tissues and permit definitive diagnosis in vivo. Perhaps. In recent years, I have noted suggestions that sophisticated electronic techniques may be used for a variety of purposes, including dating the age of venous thrombi (see Abstract 3–14). Remain tuned. There will surely be more.

# 5 Perioperative Considerations

## Hemostasis

**Protamine Use During Peripheral Vascular Surgery: A Prospective Randomized Trial**

Dorman BH, Elliott BM, Spinale FG, et al (Univ of South Carolina, Charleston)

*J Vasc Surg* 22:248–256, 1995                                                           5–1

*Background.*—Although protamine is commonly used for reversal of systemic heparin anticoagulation, the practicality of protamine-induced heparin neutralization in patients undergoing peripheral vascular operations is not clear-cut. Such patients typically receive a fairly low initial heparin dose, and heparin is cleared from the plasma with a half-life at normothermia ranging between 90 and 120 minutes. The use of protamine in this clinical setting therefore may do little to improve objective measures of blood loss. This hypothesis was tested by comparing clinical and laboratory assessments of hemostasis between patients undergoing peripheral vascular surgical procedures who had or had not received protamine for heparin neutralization.

*Patients and Methods.*—Of 120 patients included in this prospective, double-blind, randomized study, 40 were undergoing aortic reconstruction, 49 were undergoing infrainguinal bypass, and 31 were undergoing carotid endarterectomy. During surgery, all patients underwent systemic heparinization with 90 units/kg of body weight. After revascularization, 60 patients were randomly assigned to treatment with protamine and 60 to treatment with saline solution for heparin reversal. Blood loss during surgery, perioperative hematocrit, blood product requirements, objective coagulation indices, and subjective clinical assessment of coagulation status were evaluated and compared between groups.

*Results.*—Age, sex, weight, liver function test results, serum chemistry values, and preoperative coagulation status were similar between groups. No significant between-group differences in total blood loss during surgery were observed. At 20 minutes and 1 hour after administration, patients receiving saline solution had significantly higher plasma heparin concentration, partial thromboplastin time, and activated clotting time compared with patients given protamine. At 24 hours, no significant differences in blood product requirements, IV fluid administration, hematocrit, or wound hematomas were observed between groups. The surgeons' subjective intraoperative assessments of hemostasis after administration of either study agent likewise were not significantly different between groups. After drug administration, patients in the protamine group experienced a subsequent intraoperative blood loss of 318 mL compared with 195 mL in those given saline solution.

*Conclusion.*—Patients undergoing elective peripheral vascular surgical procedures do not appear to gain any clinical benefit from protamine administration. For this reason, and because protamine use is associated with a number of harmful physiologic reactions (including anaphylaxis), its routine use for neutralization of heparin is not recommended in this particular clinical setting. The elimination of this agent from peripheral vascular surgical protocols could help reduce the occurrence of hemodynamic instability and other adverse effects.

▶ Protamine has been attracting more attention in recent years than it warrants. We have learned that its use may be hazardous and that many surgeons do not use it at all. Despite this, we at Oregon have continued to use it routinely and have not recognized significant complications. This prospectively randomized study, in which patients received either protamine or no protamine, generally found no difference between the 2 groups, although paradoxically the patients receiving protamine appeared to lose more blood. I suppose the take-away message is that protamine may not be very important. Perhaps, but I will continue to use it. My mind is made up. I wish people would stop trying to confuse me with data. See also Abstract 12–16.

---

**Fibrin Sealant Reduces Suture Line Bleeding During Carotid Endarterectomy: A Randomised Trial**
Milne AA, Murphy WG, Reading SJ, et al (Univ of Edinburgh, Scotland; Scottish Natl Blood Transfusion Service, Scotland)
*Eur J Vasc Endovasc Surg* 10:91–94, 1995                                     5–2

---

*Background.*—The efficacy of fibrin sealant in cardiac surgery suggests that it may be useful in peripheral vascular surgery as well. However, there have been no studies of the clinical use of fibrin sealant in peripheral vascular surgery. Carotid endarterectomy using a polytetrafluoroethylene (PTFE) patch has been associated with prolonged anastomotic bleeding. Fibrin sealant was studied to determine whether it could significantly decrease suture line bleeding in this setting.

*Methods and Findings.*—Seventeen patients having carotid endarterectomy were randomly assigned to a group in which fibrin sealant was used as a topical hemostatic agent at the arteriotomy suture line or to a control group. Median times to hemostasis in the treatment group was 5.5 minutes

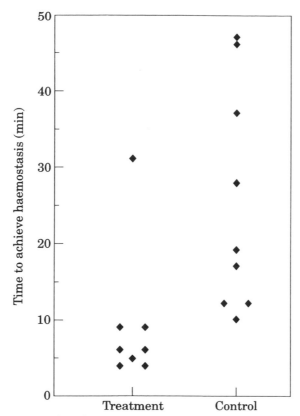

FIGURE 1.—Time to achieve hemostasis in carotid endarterectomy. (Reprinted from *Eur J Vasc Endovasc Surg*, vol 10; Milne AA, Murphy WG, Reading SJ, et al: Fibrin sealant reduces suture line bleeding during carotid endarterectomy: A randomised trial; pp 91–94; Copyright 1995 by permission of the publisher Academic Press Limited, London.)

and was 19 minutes in the control group, a significant difference (Fig 1). Total operating times were comparable in the 2 groups. The treatment group had a lower operative blood loss than the control group, but the difference was nonsignificant. One perioperative thromboembolic event occurred in a patient in the control group.

*Conclusion.*—Fibrin sealant is an effective topical hemostatic agent in vascular surgery. Concerns about the possibility of viral transmission with fibrin sealant use have resulted in production methods designed to minimize the risk of such transmission.

▶ A fibrin preparation was manufactured by a blood transfusion service from heat-treated human fibrinogen obtained from pool donor plasma cryo-supernatant. Treated human thrombin preparation was added to result in the fibrin sealant. The authors conclude, not surprisingly, that fibrin sealant is an effective topical hemostatic agent after testing the product in a group of patients undergoing carotid endarterectomy. Unfortunately, there is a possibility of viral transmission with the use of this human product. We use bovine thrombin and Gelfoam in similar situations and have recognized no problems with this combination.

---

**Essential Thrombocytosis: Underemphasized Cause of Large-vessel Thrombosis**
Johnson M, Gernsheimer T, Johansen K (Univ of Washington, Seattle)
*J Vasc Surg* 22:443–449, 1995                                                   5–3

---

*Background.*—Patients with essential thrombocytosis (ET) may have evidence of either bleeding, typically in the form of ecchymoses or mucosal bleeding, or thrombosis, usually recognized as cutaneous or digital ischemia. Few cases of large-vessel thrombosis in patients with ET have been reported. Five patients who underwent surgery for arterial or venous thrombosis associated with ET were described.

*Patients.*—The 5 patients were treated during a 2-year period. Thrombosis was found in the femoral, popliteal, and tibial arteries in 1 patient; in the aorta in 1; in the portal vein in 2; and in the inferior vena cava in 1. All required surgery. In 3 patients the diagnosis of ET was made only after surgery, when platelet counts continued to exceed 500,000/mm³. Causes of reactive thrombosis were ruled out in all patients, and the 3 new cases showed evidence of megakaryocyte hyperplasia on bone marrow biopsy. Cytoreductive therapy returned platelet levels to normal in all patients. There were no additional episodes of thrombosis over a mean follow-up of 18 months.

*Discussion.*—Essential thrombocytosis may account for more cases of large-vessel thrombosis than is generally recognized. In the authors' experience, ET is responsible for more large-vessel thromboses than all other hypercoagulable states combined.

▶ This case report reminds us of 1 hemostatic defect (ET) causing thrombosis, especially arterial. The prevalence is not clear from this study, and therefore we do not really know if it is underemphasized. At least it is important to know of its existence. See also Abstract 4–9.

**D. Bergqvist, M.D., Ph.D.**

---

**Does Desmopressin Improve Hemostasis and Reduce Blood Loss From Aortic Surgery? A Randomized, Double-blind Study**
Clagett GP, Valentine RJ, Myers SI, et al (Univ of Texas, Dallas)
*J Vasc Surg* 22:223–230, 1995                                                   5–4

---

*Introduction.*—Desmopressin acetate, 1-deamino-8-D-arginine vasopressin (DDAVP) has been used to improve hemostasis in patients with mild hemophilia and von Willebrand's disease. In the postoperative cardiopulmonary bypass setting, it has helped improve hemostasis in patients with ongoing hemorrhage and severe platelet dysfunction. It has even produced significant reductions in blood loss and transfusion as reported in a trial of patients undergoing spinal fusion. These findings have led to consideration of prophylactic DDAVP for surgeries associated with major blood loss. The effect of DDAVP on blood loss, transfusion requirements, and thromboembolic complications in patients undergoing elective aortic operations was analyzed.

*Methods.*—Patients undergoing repair of abdominal aortic aneurysm or aortofemoral bypass for occlusive disease were randomized in this double-blind investigation to receive either DDAVP or placebo. The DDAVP or placebo was administered intravenously for 15 minutes immediately after IV heparinization with 100 units/kg just before aortic cross-clamp application was accomplished. Some patients received a second supplemental dose of heparin, 50 units/kg, 45 minutes after the first dose. Protamine sulfate was used for heparin reversal at the completion of surgery. Blood loss, blood transfusion requirements, and arterial and venous thromboembolic complications were monitored. Bleeding times were performed at appropriate intervals.

*Results.*—Forty-three male patients received DDAVP, and 48 received placebo. Equivalent proportions of patients with aneurysms and occlusive disease were in each randomized group. The use of DDAVP provided a mild prolongation in postoperative bleeding times and moderate thrombocytopenia. It had no beneficial effect on blood loss or transfusion requirements. Patients receiving DDAVP required a mean of 3.1 blood transfusions compared with a mean of 2.7 required by patients in the placebo group. Of interest, the greatest amount of operative blood loss occurred between heparinization with cross-clamp application and reversal of heparin with protamine sulfate administration.

*Conclusion.*—Administration of DDAVP did not improve hemostasis or reduce transfusion requirements in patients with elective aortic operations or occlusive disease. These findings do not rule out the possibility of beneficial effects of DDAVP in patients with preexisting hemostatic aberrations undergoing aortic surgical procedures. It is not likely that DDAVP will cause major thrombotic complications in patients with diffuse vascular disease who are treated because of bleeding complications.

▶ Desmopressin acetate, a synthetic vasopressin analogue that lacks vasoconstrictor activity, acutely increases the levels of factor VIII and von Willebrand factor when administered intravenously. It has been used effectively in patients with mild hemophilia and von Willebrand's disease. These authors address the potential of this drug to reduce blood loss and transfusion requirement in patients undergoing aortic operation. Unfortunately, they found that DDAVP had no beneficial effect on blood loss or transfusion requirements in vascular surgery patients. Too bad.

### Aprotinin in Aortocoronary Bypass Surgery: Increased Risk of Vein-Graft Occlusion and Myocardial Infarction? Supportive Evidence From a Retrospective Study

van der Meer J, for the CABADAS Research Group of the Interuniversity Cardiology Institute of The Netherlands (Univ Hosp, Groningen, The Netherlands; Antonius Hosp, Nieuwegein, The Netherlands; Ignatius Hosp, Breda, The Netherlands; et al)

*Thromb Haemost* 75:1–3, 1996                                              5–5

*Introduction.*—In cardiac surgery, aprotinin has been shown to reduce blood loss and transfusion requirement, however, with improved hemostasis, this drug may increase the risk of thrombosis. A few previous studies have shown that graft occlusion and myocardial infarction were observed more frequently in patients who had received aprotinin. Data derived from a randomized clinical trial that compared 3 antithrombotic drug regimens in the prevention of vein-graft occlusion, with a focus on patients who were treated with aprotinin, were analyzed retrospectively.

*Methods.*—The study included 948 patients, of whom 42 received aprotinin. At 1 year, graft patency was assessed by angiography. Clinical end points included myocardial infarction, major bleeding, thromboembolism, and death. Results were compared with those who received aprotinin and those who did not.

*Results.*—In the aprotinin group, occlusion rates of distal anastomoses were 20.5% compared with 17.7% in the nonaprotinin group. In the aprotinin group 44.1% of patients had occluded grafts, whereas in the nonaprotinin group 26.3% of patients had occluded grafts. In the aprotinin group perioperative myocardial infarction occurred in 14.3% patients, whereas in the nonaprotinin group it occurred in 7% of patients. In the aprotinin group the mean postoperative blood loss was 451 mL, whereas in the aprotinin group it was 1,039 mL. In the aprotinin group the mean transfusion requirements were 1.1 units, whereas in the nonaprotinin group it was 2.1 units of red blood cells.

*Conclusion.*—Transfusion requirement and blood loss are decreased with aprotinin; however, this may be at the expense of reduction of graft patency and an increased risk of myocardial infarction. Although there is support for concern for the safety of aprotinin, data are not conclusive. A prospective, randomized, placebo-controlled clinical trial is strongly recommended.

▶ Patients receiving aprotinin during aortocoronary bypass experienced diminished coronary graft patency compared with patients not receiving aprotinin. This is a potentially important observation, although derived from only a few patients. The authors appropriately call for an adequately powered prospective randomized placebo-controlled clinical trial to determine the actual thrombotic risk of aprotinin therapy. Presently this substance does not have a defined role in peripheral vascular surgery.[1]

*Reference*

1. 1996 YEAR BOOK OF VASCULAR SURGERY, p 38.

## A Randomized Comparison of Antiplatelet and Anticoagulant Therapy After the Placement of Coronary-artery Stents

Schömig A, Neumann F-J, Kastrati A, et al (Technische Univ München, Germany)
N Engl J Med 334:1084–1089, 1996                    5–6

*Background.*—The risk of thrombotic stent occlusion and hemorrhagic and vascular complications of intensive anticoagulation limit the clinical efficacy of coronary-artery stenting done with coronary angioplasty. The clinical outcomes of antiplatelet therapy and conventional anticoagulation therapy 30 days after coronary-artery stenting were compared.

*Methods.*—After successful placement of Palmaz-Schatz coronary-artery stents, patients were randomly assigned to receive antiplatelet or anticoagulant treatment. Ticlopidine plus aspirin was given to 257 patients and IV heparin, phenprocoumon, and aspirin to 260 patients. The main cardiac end point was a composite measure of death from cardiac causes or myocardial infarction, aortocoronary bypass surgery, or repeated angioplasty. Death resulting from noncardiac causes, cerebrovascular accident, severe hemorrhage, and peripheral vascular events comprised the main noncardiac end point.

*Findings.*—Six percent of patients receiving anticoagulant treatment and 1.6% given antiplatelet therapy reached a primary cardiac end point. Patients given antiplatelet treatment had an 82% lower risk of myocardial infarction than patients given anticoagulant treatment. The need for repeat interventions was 78% lower in the antiplatelet group. The stented vessel became occluded in 0.8% of the patients given antiplatelet therapy and in 5.4% of those given anticoagulant therapy. One percent of the patients receiving antiplatelet therapy, and 12% receiving anticoagulant therapy reached a primary noncardiac end point. Hemorrhagic complications were documented in 6.5% of those receiving anticoagulant therapy and in none given antiplatelet therapy. Antiplatelet treatment was associated with an 87% decrease in the risk of peripheral vascular events.

*Conclusion.*—The use of combined antiplatelet therapy may markedly improve the risk-benefit ratio for stenting. This therapy reduces the incidence of cardiac events, hemorrhagic complications, and vascular complications compared with conventional anticoagulant treatment.

► Please note, dear reader, that I include a number of articles on coronary procedures, not because I believe they are necessarily transferrable to peripheral vascular surgery but because they might be, and in many circumstances they represent the only information available. Herein the authors report a comparison of antiplatelet therapy and conventional anticoagulation after coronary artery stenting, concluding that antiplatelet therapy appears superior. It is noted that the antiplatelet therapy consisted of both ticlopidine and aspirin. The authors conclude, no doubt accurately, that platelets have a crucial role in the pathogenesis of intravascular thromboses occurring after coronary stent placement.

## Coronary Disease

**The Role of Coronary Angiography and Coronary Revascularization Before Noncardiac Vascular Surgery**
Mason JJ, Owens DK, Harris RA, et al (Stanford Univ, Calif; Veterans Affairs Med Ctr, Palo Alto, Calif)
*JAMA* 273:1919–1925, 1995                                                        5–7

*Introduction.*—Perioperative cardiac complications are an important cause of morbidity and mortality after noncardiac surgery, and the risk is particularly high for patients undergoing vascular surgery. Identification of patients at increased risk presents the clinician with a number of questions. Decision analysis was used to determine whether preoperative coronary angiography and revascularization improve short-term outcome after elective vascular surgery.

*Methods.*—The decision model considered 2 basic choices: to proceed directly to vascular surgery with close monitoring of cardiac status and aggressive treatment of myocardial ischemia or to perform a coronary angiogram, then proceed to vascular surgery, perform coronary revascularization, or cancel vascular surgery. Several outcomes are possible if vascular surgery is chosen: a technically successful and uncomplicated operation, death of the patient, a technically successful operation and a nonfatal myocardial infarction, or a technically successful operation and a nonfatal stroke. The main outcome measures—mortality, nonfatal myocardial infarction, stroke, uncorrected vascular disease, and cost—were assessed within 3 months for patients who preoperatively had either no angina or mild angina and a positive dipyridamole-thallium scan result.

*Results.*—In the base case analysis, proceeding directly to vascular surgery led to both lower morbidity and reduced costs. Preoperative coronary angiography led to higher mortality if vascular surgery would proceed in patients with inoperable coronary artery disease (CAD), but this strategy led to slightly lower mortality if vascular surgery were canceled in patients with inoperable CAD. The use of coronary angiography also led to lower mortality in patients at particularly high risk for complications during vascular surgery.

*Conclusion.*—This decision model indicates that the best strategy for a patient at increased risk for perioperative cardiac complications is to proceed with the planned elective vascular surgery. The coronary angiography strategy commits the patient to 3 procedures, thus 3 encounters with the risk of death, myocardial infarction, and stroke. Overall coronary angiography before vascular surgery leads to worse outcomes, and the procedure should be reserved for patients with a substantially higher than average risk of mortality.

▶ This is a landmark article not because of its brilliant conclusions but because these conclusions were reached by a group of vascular internists. In summary, they conclude that vascular surgery without preoperative coronary arteriography leads to better outcomes than any alternate treatments. I continue to note that the only possible benefits of extensive coronary evaluation and intervention before elective vascular surgery are reduction of perioperative vascular mortality and possible prolongation of life. Not only is there no proof that this strategy leads to a reduction of perioperative mortality, there is convincing evidence to the contrary when one considers the mortality of coronary bypass in peripheral vascular disease patients averages about 6%. The issue of prolongation of life must be approached very carefully. There are absolutely no convincing data indicating that life in patients with vascular disease is prolonged by coronary intervention. Based on the previous VA study and CASS study, about 30% of young men with angina enjoy modest prolongation of life for periods of 5–7 years. On balance, I believe that patients facing elective vascular surgery who have clear indications for coronary studies should have the studies performed. This includes especially patients with unstable angina. Under no circumstances do I believe that the need for elective vascular surgery automatically indicates the need for extensive coronary evaluation. There are no supportive data, and it simply does not make sense.

## Recent Trends in Acute Coronary Heart Disease: Mortality, Morbidity, Medical Care, and Risk Factors

McGovern PG, Pankow JS, Shahar E, et al (Univ of Minnesota, Minneapolis)
*N Engl J Med* 334:884–890, 1996
5–8

*Background.*—In the United States, mortality associated with coronary heart disease (CHD) has decreased in the past 25 years. Trends in CHD mortality and morbidity, medical care, and risk factors for CHD between 1985 and 1990 were studied in a large urban population.

*Methods.*—Data were collected on all deaths from CHD among Minneapolis–St. Paul residents aged 30–74. The 1985 and 1990 patient cohorts hospitalized for myocardial infarction (MI) were followed for at least 3 years. Surveys of 25- to 74-year-olds conducted between 1985 and 1987 and between 1990 and 1992 were analyzed for trends in risk factors for CHD.

*Findings.*—Mortality from CHD declined by 25% among men and women between 1985 and 1990. Among men, in-hospital mortality declined by 41% compared with a 17% decline in out-of-hospital mortality. Hospitalization rates for acute MI decreased by 5% to 10% between 1985 and 1990. During that period, survival rates among patients hospitalized for acute MI markedly increased. The relative risk of dying within 3 years of hospitalization for MI was 0.76 for men and 0.84 for women after adjustment for age and previous MI. Survival trends were paralleled by marked increases in the use of thrombolytic treatment, heparin, aspirin, and coronary angioplasty. The CHD risk factor profile of the population studied also generally improved during the study.

*Conclusion.*—The decrease in mortality from CHD among 30- to 74-year-olds in the Minneapolis–St. Paul area between 1985 and 1990 was apparently caused by the declining incidence in acute MI and improved survival among patients with MI. In addition, there have been continued improvements in the CHD risk factor profile, especially smoking and high serum total cholesterol concentrations. The dramatic increases seen in short-term survival among patients hospitalized for MI may be explained by the increased use of treatments such as thrombolytic agents, anticoagulants, and aspirin.

▶ Although we all have been impressed with the widely reported reduction in stroke mortality in recent years, many have not been equally informed of the similarly dramatic decline in coronary mortality. The authors conclude that the reason for the declining mortality is primarily a dramatic decline in the mortality of patients having heart attacks. In fact, the in-hospital MI mortality rate declined by 41% during this period. There also appears to have been a modest decline in the incidence of MI, but the majority of decline in death could be explained by the improvement in survival after having an MI. I wonder if we will one day come to the point where MI will be an infrequent clinical diagnosis.

## Outpatient Echocardiography as a Predictor of Perioperative Cardiac Morbidity After Peripheral Vascular Surgical Procedures

Ouriel K, Green RM, DeWeese JA, et al (Univ of Rochester, New York)
*J Vasc Surg* 22:671–679, 1995                                                5–9

*Introduction.*—The use of some diagnostic tests such as dipyridamole-thallium scintigraphy, dobutamine echocardiography, and coronary angiography in the evaluation of perioperative cardiac risk are invasive, time consuming, and expensive. Outpatient echocardiography was evaluated as a method for predicting perioperative cardiac events.

*Methods.*—During a 2-year period, 250 consecutive patients undergoing elective peripheral vascular surgical procedures were evaluated by transthoracic echocardiography. Left ventricular ejection fraction (LVEF) and observation of valvular abnormalities, wall motion abnormalities, and intracardiac thrombus were evaluated during echocardiography. The American Society of Anesthesiologists Physical Status Classification grade (ASA), the Goldman multifactorial index of cardiac risk, and the Detsky clinical indices were tabulated with a thorough cardiac history to help determine the risk of cardiac complications. No coronary angiography, angioplasty, or bypass was done before patients underwent peripheral vascular surgery.

*Results.*—Seventy-one patients (28%) had a history of myocardial infarction, and 52 (21%) had undergone a previous coronary artery bypass operation. Twenty-three (9.2%) patients had a perioperative cardiac morbid event that occurred at a median of 2.2 days after surgery. Nine (3.6%) patients died as a result of these complications. The ASA, Goldman, and Detsky clinical indices were not precise in the identification of patients who had perioperative cardiac complications. Cardiac morbid events were significantly more likely to occur when LVEF was low. When the LVEF was less than 40%, the risk of death from a myocardial complication was 50%. The risk was 25% when the LVEF was between 40% and 50% and was 20% when the LVEF was 50% or more. The sensitivity was 78%, specificity was 81%, positive predictive value was 27%, and negative predictive value of LVEF of less than 50% was 97% in the identification of patients who had cardiac morbidity. The presence of valvular abnormalities, resting wall motion abnormalities, and mural thrombus were poor echocardiographic predictors of cardiac complications. Economic analysis indicated that outpatient echocardiography was considerably less expensive than dipyridamole myocardial scintigraphy or dobutamine stress echocardiography.

*Conclusion.*—Outpatient echocardiography is definitely less sensitive than dipyridamole-thallium scanning or dobutamine stress echocardiography. It provides important information about perioperative mortality rates that cannot be obtained from clinical criteria alone. This procedure can provide crucial information to the physician and patient, particularly when one is deciding whether the potential benefits of a procedure are outweighed by cardiac risks. Outpatient echocardiography may offer a cost-efficient compromise between clinical criteria alone and provocative cardiac testing.

▶ Perhaps transthoracic echocardiography with derivation of ejection fraction and detection of valvular abnormalities and wall motion abnormalities does, in fact, permit reasonably accurate identification of patients destined to experience a perioperative cardiac event after elective vascular surgery. Whereas the sensitivity was 78% overall, the positive predictive value was a dismal 27%, an observation repeatedly made by others. I partially agree with these authors. If you are determined to perform preoperative tests of cardiac function, the transthoracic echocardiogram appears to be as good as, and a lot cheaper than, a dipyridamole-thallium scan. A better choice, however, would be to do neither (see Abstract 5–7).

### Predictors of Major Vascular Events in Patients With a Transient Ischemic Attack or Minor Ischemic Stroke and With Nonrheumatic Atrial Fibrillation

van Latum JC, Koudstaal PJ, Venables GS, et al (Univ Hosp Rotterdam Dijkzigt, The Netherlands; Royal Hallamshire Hosp, Sheffield, England; Univ Hosp Utrecht, The Netherlands)
*Stroke* 16:801–806, 1995                                                    5–10

*Background.*—The reported risk for recurrent stroke and other major vascular events after an initial episode of transient ischemic attack (TIA) or minor ischemic stroke in patients with nonrheumatic atrial fibrillation (NRAF) ranges from 2% to 5% in the first year and is approximately 5% yearly thereafter, depending on the underlying cardiac abnormality. The predictive value of a number of easily obtainable patient characteristics in identifying high-risk subgroups within this patient population was examined.

*Methods.*—The study sample consisted of 375 patients with NRAF and 1 or more recent episodes of TIA or minor stroke who had been randomized to placebo as part of a multicenter clinical trial involving 1,001 patients that investigated the value of anticoagulant therapy or aspirin in the prevention of secondary cerebral ischemic events. The mean follow-up period was 1.6 years, during which 116 ischemic events occurred. The clinical predictors identified from the patients' records were used to define high-risk, moderate-risk, and low-risk subgroups.

*Results.*—Of 9 clinical variables selected for multivariate analyses, 6 were identified as independent clinical predictors of recurrent vascular events: history of previous thromboembolism, ischemic heart disease, enlarged cardiothoracic ratio on the chest radiograph, systolic blood pressure greater than 160 mm Hg at study entry, NRAF for more than 1 year, and a visible ischemic lesion on the CT scan. Incidence rates of recurrent vascular events calculated for differing risk strata within each treatment group revealed that patients older than 75 with 3 or more of the 6 independent risk factors did not greatly benefit from aspirin or anticoagulant preventive therapy (Table 4).

*Conclusion.*—Six easily obtainable patient characteristics are helpful in estimating the potential effect of adequate secondary prevention in patients with NRAF and a recent episode of TIA or minor ischemic stroke.

▶ As readers of the YEAR BOOK OF VASCULAR SURGERY know, there has been considerable interest in recent years in defining precisely which patients with NRAF have the greatest risk for cerebral ischemic events and therefore would be best treated with anticoagulation. The variables identified in this study are not surprising. The authors wisely note that the practical application of their profile of risk factors to the clinical decision-making process in the choice of antithrombotic prophylaxis is not exactly straightforward. For example, older patients with 3 or more risk factors appeared to derive little benefit from anticoagulation compared with aspirin. The thrust is that youn-

TABLE 4.—Annual Event Rates Per Treatment Group According to Age and Number of Risk Factors

| Age, y/No. of Risk Factors | Placebo (n = 375) | | | Aspirin (n = 401) | | | Oral Anticoagulants (n = 225) | | |
|---|---|---|---|---|---|---|---|---|---|
| | %* | No. of Events† | ER (95% CI) | %* | No. of Events† | ER (95% CI) | %* | No. of Events† | ER (95% CI) |
| ≤75/0 | 4 | 2 | 6.3 (0.8–23) | 6 | 4 | 6.5 (1.8–17) | 7 | 1 | 2.6 (0.1–14) |
| >75/0 | 2 | 0 | 0.0 (0.0–15) | 4 | 5 | 15 (4.9–35) | 3 | 1 | 8.9 (0.2–50) |
| ≤75/1–2 | 35 | 41 | 15 (11–20) | 36 | 40 | 13 (9.2–17) | 41 | 10 | 4.4 (2.1–8.1) |
| >75/1–2 | 27 | 30 | 16 (11–23) | 25 | 28 | 15 (10–21) | 17 | 11 | 14 (6.9–25) |
| ≤75/≥3 | 16 | 32 | 30 (21–42) | 14 | 24 | 18 (12–27) | 20 | 9 | 8.0 (3.6–15) |
| >75/≥3 | 15 | 30 | 37 (26–53) | 15 | 28 | 30 (21–43) | 12 | 11 | 30 (15–53) |

*Note:* Events include vascular death, nonfatal stroke, nonfatal myocardial infarction, and systemic embolism (whichever occurred first).
* Percentage of patients in stratum.
† Absolute number of events.
*Abbreviations:* ER, event rate (per 100 patient-years); CI, confidence interval.
(Courtesy of van Latum JC, Koudstaal PJ, Venables GS, et al: Predictors of major vascular events in patients with a transient ischemic attack or minor ischemic stroke and with nonrheumatic atrial fibrillation. *Stroke* 16:801–806, 1995. Reproduced with permission of *Stroke.* Copyright 1995 American Heart Association.)

ger patients with a few risk factors may receive aspirin, younger patients with more risk factors should receive anticoagulant therapy, but older patients with many risk factors probably do just as well using aspirin. In general, this article is supportive of previous reports on this subject.[1]

*Reference*

1. 1995 YEAR BOOK OF VASCULAR SURGERY, p 20.

## The Effect of Peripheral Vascular Disease on Long-term Mortality After Coronary Artery Bypass Surgery

Birkmeyer JD, Quinton HB, O'Connor NJ, et al (Dartmouth Med School, Hanover, NH; Veterans Affairs Hosp, White River Junction, Vt; Med Ctr Hosp of Vermont, Burlington; et al)
*Arch Surg* 131:316–321, 1996                                                   5–11

*Background.*—The effect of myocardial revascularization on long-term mortality in patients who also have peripheral vascular disease (PVD) is unclear. The effect of PVD on mortality in 2,871 consecutive patients after coronary artery bypass graft surgery was studied.

*Methods.*—Demographic data and information regarding the patients' coronary artery disease and comorbidities were collected prospectively. Medical record review identified patients with PVD. Mortality data were obtained from the National Death Index for 5 years after enrollment.

*Results.*—Of the 2,871 patients surviving bypass surgery, the records of 755 (26%) indicated the presence of PVD, with 41% of them having only cerebrovascular disease, 33% having only lower-extremity occlusive disease, and 19% having both. Patient age, female sex, cigarette smoking, and the presence of comorbidity were significantly associated with the presence of PVD. Patients with PVD experienced significantly more 5-year mortality (20%) than patients without PVD (8%). A poorer prognosis was found for patients with lower-extremity occlusive disease than for those with cerebrovascular disease. Overall patients with both did worst. After analysis of confounding factors, patients with PVD still had an adjusted hazard ratio of 2.01 for mortality.

*Conclusion.*—Long-term mortality is greater for patients with PVD who survive coronary artery bypass graft surgery than for those who do not have PVD.

▶ Are you surprised to learn that the 5-year mortality after coronary artery bypass surgery is substantially higher in patients with indicators of PVD than in patients without indicators of PVD? This information has considerable practical importance when we consider that one of the reasons for doing coronary arteriography and coronary bypass in vascular patients is to prolong life. There is not one bit of data that coronary bypass is successful in achieving this goal. The modest prolongation of life reported in studies noted in Abstract 5–7 was derived from data obtained generally from males with angina without PVD who were in the sixth decade of life. There is no evidence these data can be transferred unmodified to vasculopaths who are 10 or 20 years older, both men and women, and many of whom do not have angina pectoris. I am not at all convinced that coronary bypass in vasculopaths prolongs life, especially when one considers the mortality of the procedure.

---

### Comparative Early and Late Cardiac Morbidity Among Patients Requiring Different Vascular Surgery Procedures

L'Italien GJ, Cambria RP, Cutler BS, et al (Harvard Med School, Boston; Univ of Massachusetts, Worcester)
*J Vasc Surg* 21:935–944, 1995                                                   5–12

---

*Objective.*—Patients requiring vascular surgery are at increased risk of coronary artery disease (CAD)-related events, but the extent to which surgery itself elevates the risk remains uncertain. For this reason the risk related to specific vascular operations was estimated in 547 patients at 2 centers who underwent vascular surgery between 1984 and 1991. Aortic surgery was done in 321 patients, infrainguinal procedures in 177, and carotid surgery in 49. Myocardial perfusion was quantified by dipyridamole thallium imaging.

*Findings.*—On logistic regression analysis, perioperative infarction was predicted by a history of angina; a fixed or reversible thallum defect; and ischemic ST changes during imaging. On Cox regression analysis, diabetes and congestive heart failure were identified as predictors of long-term adverse events (Table 2, B), and previous coronary bypass graft surgery was protective. There were 45 cardiac events in all, 30 being nonfatal infractions. Events were significantly more prevalent in patients having infrainguinal procedures than in those having aortic surgery, but the difference between infrainguinal and carotid artery operations was not significant (Table 3, A). Infrainguinal surgery was associated with a significantly elevated risk in patients whose imaging studies demonstrated risk

---

**TABLE 2, B.**—Stepwise Cox Regression Results: Predictors of Long-term Outcomes

| Variable | RR | 95% Confidence interval | p Value |
|---|---|---|---|
| Diabetes mellitus | 1.8 | 1.1–3.1 | 0.030 |
| History of angina | 1.7 | 1.0–2.9 | 0.049 |
| History of CHF | 3.6 | 2.0–6.4 | 0.0001 |
| Fixed defects | 2.6 | 1.5–4.4 | 0.001 |
| Prior CABG | 0.5 | 0.2–1.0 | 0.049 |
| Perioperative nonfatal MI | 5.5 | 3.1–9.8 | 0.0001 |

Note: Long-term outcomes refer to fatal or nonfatal MI.
*Abbreviations: CHF*, congestive heart failure; *CABG* coronary artery bypass grafting; *MI*, myocardial infarction.
(Courtesy of L'Italien GJ, Cambria RP, Cutler BS, et al: Comparative early and late cardiac morbidity among patients requiring different vascular surgery procedures. *J Vasc Surg* 21:935–944, 1995.)

## TABLE 3, A.—Perioperative Outcomes According to Surgical Procedure

| | Procedure | | | | | | | | |
| | Aortic (n = 321) | | Infrainguinal (n = 177) | | Carotid (n = 49) | | Overall | Ao vs Inf | Car vs Inf |
| Variable | No. | % | No. | % | No. | % | p value | p value | p value |
|---|---|---|---|---|---|---|---|---|---|
| Fatal/nonfatal MI | 19 | 6 | 23 | 13 | 3 | 6 | 0.019 | 0.006 | 0.18 |
| All cause of death | 16 | 5 | 6 | 3 | 0 | 0 | 0.222 | | |
| Nonfatal MI | 9 | 3 | 18 | 10 | 3 | 6 | 0.003 | 0.0005 | 0.38 |

*Abbreviations: Ao,* aortic; *Inf,* infrainguinal; *Car,* carotid artery; *MI,* myocardial infarction.
(Courtesy of L'Italien GJ, Cambria RP, Cutler BS, et al: Comparative early and late cardiac morbidity among patients requiring different vascular surgery procedures. *J Vasc Surg* 21:935–944, 1995.)

factors. Cumulative 3-year survival rates were 91% for patients having aortic operations, 81% for those having infrainguinal operations, and 81% for these having carotid operations. Patients having infrainguinal surgery were at a threefold greater risk of long-term adverse events than those having aortic surgery, but the relative risk was only 1.3 after adjustment for comorbidity.

*Conclusion.*—All vascular surgery patients should have their cardiac risk status assessed, regardless of the particular procedure planned. Those with significant CAD and patients who survive a perioperative infarct are especially at risk.

▶ I believe the authors are examining the hypothesis that specific vascular procedures may in themselves contribute to perioperative and long-term cardiac risk. They conclude, not surprisingly, that the procedure itself has little independent effect, but, rather, the effects result from the risk factors of the patients having the procedures. As many of us would have predicted, infrainguinal bypass patients fare worse than patients who have aortic or carotid operations. It is clear that by the time a patient cohort develops significant symptomatic lower-extremity arterial occlusive disease, they are very late in the course of their atherosclerotic process and have severe generalized disease, especially including the cardiac and cerebrovascular circulations. I think I understand what the authors were attempting to show. I also believe it is intuitively obvious.

---

**Comparison of Surgical and Medical Group Survival in Patients With Left Main Equivalent Coronary Artery Disease: Long-term CASS Experience**

Caracciolo EA, Davis KB, Sopko G, et al (St Louis Univ; Univ of Washington, Seattle; Natl Heart, Lung, and Blood Inst, Bethesda, Md; et al)
*Circulation* 91:2335–2344, 1995                                                5–13

---

*Introduction.*—Significant combined disease of the proximal left anterior descending and proximal left circumflex coronary arteries, also known as left main equivalent (LMEQ) disease, defines an angiographic high-risk patient subset with chronic ischemic heart disease. Numerous observational and randomized trials have reported prolonged survival in patients treated surgically compared with those treated medically for left main coronary artery disease. Few comparable investigations have made these comparisons in patients with LMEQ disease. The Coronary Artery Surgery Study (CASS) Registry published a 5-year surgical and medical group survival analysis. The initial observations were extended over 16 years and provided the longest and largest follow-up for patients with LMEQ initially treated with coronary artery bypass graft (CABG) surgery.

*Methods.*—There were 912 patients in the registry with LMEQ disease, which is defined as "combined stenosis of 70% or greater in the proximal left anterior descending coronary artery before the first septal perforator and proximal circumflex coronary artery before the first obtuse margin branch." Of 912 patients, 282 were treated medically and 630 were treated surgically.

*Results.*—The 15-year cumulative survival estimates were 31% for medically treated patients and 44% for surgically treated patients. Median survival for patients in the medically treated group was 6.2 years compared with 13.1 years in the surgically treated group. When patients were stratified by age, sex, anginal class, left ventricular (LV) function, and coronary anatomy, median survival was significantly longer in the surgical than medical group. Median survival was not significantly prolonged in patients treated with CABG surgery with normal LV systolic function, even with significant right coronary artery stenosis of 70% or greater, and mildly abnormal LV systolic function of 6 to 10. The 15-year cumulative survival was 63% in medical patients with normal LV systolic function and 54% in surgical patients with normal LV systolic function. For patients in both the medical and surgical groups, the mean survival was greater than 15 years. For patients with normal LV systolic function and right coronary artery stenosis of 70% or greater (Table 3), the 15-year cumulative survival was 63% in the surgical group and 53% in the medical group. The median survival for medical and surgical patients in this subset was greater than 15 years. Median survival was 13.8 years for patients in the surgical group and 11.6 years in the medical group. Twenty-six percent of patients in the medical group eventually had CABG surgery. It was estimated that if all medical patients would have reached 15-year survival, 65% would have needed surgery. In patients with an LV ejection fraction of 50% or greater, CABG surgery did not improve the 15-year cumulative survival compared with patients treated medically.

TABLE 3.—Median Survival in Surgical and Medical Group Patients With Left Main Equivalent Disease Stratified by Angiographic Variables

| Variable | Patients, *n* Surgical | Medical | Median Survival, *y* Surgical | Medical | *P\** |
|---|---|---|---|---|---|
| LV function score | | | | | |
| 5 | 163 | 51 | >15† | >15† | ... |
| 6–10 | 260 | 55 | 13.8 | 11.6 | .59 |
| 11–14 | 123 | 79 | 11.9 | 6.9 | .0014 |
| ≥15 | 60 | 86 | 8.0 | 1.9 | <.0001 |
| Coronary anatomy‡ | | | | | |
| RCA stenosis <70% | 97 | 77 | >15† | 10.0 | ... |
| RCA stenosis ≥70% | 476 | 187 | 13.0 | 4.6 | <.0001 |
| LV function and coronary anatomy‡ | | | | | |
| LV function score = 5 and RCA stenosis ≥70% | 105 | 30 | >15† | >15† | ... |

\* For test of differences in medians equal to zero.
† Fifty percent or more of patients in this subgroup were still alive at 15 years' follow-up.
‡ Right-dominant or balanced circulation.
*Abbreviations: LV,* left ventricular; *RCA,* right coronary artery.
(Courtesy of Caracciolo EA, Davis KB, Sopko G, et al: Comparison of surgical and medical group survival in patients with left main equivalent coronary artery disease: Long-term CASS experience. *Circulation* 1995; 91:2335–2344. Reproduced with permission of *Circulation.* Copyright 1995 American Heart Association.)

*Conclusion.*—This long-term follow-up of patients with LMEQ indicated that CABG surgery prolonged life in most clinical and angiographic subgroups. Median survival was not prolonged by CABG surgery in patients with normal LV systolic function, even in the presence of significant right coronary artery stenosis of 70% or greater or in patients with an LV ejection fraction of 50% or greater who were part of the CASS randomized trial or who were randomizable. These long-term results give a better understanding of the natural history of LMEQ disease and provide a more accurate estimate of long-term medical and surgical survival.

▶ Even in patients with LMEQ disease coronary artery bypass did not convey survival benefit over medical treatment in patients who had normal or only mildly abnormal LV function, with a greater than 15-year median survival in both medical and surgical groups. The more severe the left ventricular dysfunction, the more survival benefit from coronary bypass. The benefit group, namely, those with impaired LV function, accounted for fewer than 40% of the trial patients. Detailed studies like this are very important in permitting us to put into perspective the benefits or lack thereof of coronary interventions in patients with peripheral vascular disease.

---

**Variation in the Use of Cardiac Procedures After Acute Myocardial Infarction**
Guadagnoli E, Hauptman PJ, Ayanian JZ, et al (Harvard Med School, Boston; Brigham and Women's Hosp, Boston)
*N Engl J Med* 333:573–578, 1995                                              5–14

---

*Background.*—There are considerable geographic differences in the frequency of diagnostic procedures and in the treatment of patients who have experienced an acute myocardial infarction. The reasons for these differences and their effects, if any, on patients' quality of life and survival were evaluated.

*Methods.*—The authors studied the records of Medicare patients admitted to a total of 478 hospitals in New York and Texas between February and May, 1989, for acute myocardial infarction. Patients under the care of HMOs were not included. The frequency of postinfarction coronary angiograms and the status of the patients' postinfarction quality of life and survival were compared. All patients were between 65 and 79 years of age.

*Results.*—The records analyzed included 1,852 New York patients treated at 209 hospitals and 1,837 patients treated at 269 Texas hospitals. The majority of characteristics were comparable between the 2 groups, but significant differences did exist in 9 of the 48 parameters examined (18.8%). Postinfarction coronary angiography was performed in 45% of the Texas patients compared with 30% of the New York patients. This difference was present in all subgroups of patients except those with non–Q-wave infarctions and the high-risk group who had serious postinfarction angina. The overall rate of revascularization procedures was not significantly different between the 2 geographic groups, although the incidence of postinfarction coronary angioplasty was significantly higher in the Texas group. Unadjusted mortality rates of the 2 groups were identical after 90 days (23%) and 36% for New York and 37% for Texas after 2 years. However, when adjusted for hazard ratios, the 2-year mortality rate was significantly lower for the New York patients. Adjusted quality of life ratings by the patients themselves were similar for the 2 states, but the scores for ability to perform instrumental daily tasks were significantly better for New York patients. Texas patients were more likely to report episodes of angina and inability to perform tasks requiring energy.

*Conclusions.*—Post-infarction coronary angiography was performed more often in Texas patients than in New York patients, except in patients at a high risk of reinfarction, in whom the frequency was the same. This does not appear to result in decreased mortality or improved postinfarction health-related quality of life. The study is limited by the comparison of only 2 states, its application to a limited age group, and the fact that patients under the care of HMOs were excluded.

▶ I have been impressed for years by the wide regional variation in the use of invasive coronary procedures in patients with symptomatic myocardial ischemia. This particular study examines the outcome of a group of patients with acute myocardial infarction in New York State, where the rate of use of cardiac procedures is low, to a group of such patients in Texas, where the rate of use of such procedures is quite high. Fifty percent more of the patients in Texas underwent angiography compared with those in New York. Despite this, there was no apparent advantage with respect to mortality or health-related quality-of-life issues in the 2 states. What a surprise! My conclusion is that the more rabid interventional cardiologists need to be reined in.

---

**A Clinical Trial of the Angiotensin-converting–Enzyme Inhibitor Trandolapril in Patients With Left Ventricular Dysfunction After Myocardial Infarction**
Køber L, for the Trandolapril Cardiac Evaluation (TRACE) Study Group (Gentofte Univ, Copenhagen; Esbjerg Hosp, Denmark; Slagelse Hosp, Denmark; et al)
*N Engl J Med* 333:1670–1676, 1995                                           5–15

---

*Introduction.*—Other trials examining the effects of angiotensin-converting enzyme (ACE) inhibitors on survival after acute myocardial infarction have varied so much in timing and duration of treatment that the role of ACE inhibition remains unanswered. Patients were randomly assigned to receive either trandolapril or placebo in this double-blind, placebo-controlled investigation to determine whether patients with left ventricular dysfunction soon after myocardial infarction benefit from long-term treatment.

*Methods.*—During a 2-year period, 6,676 patients with a total of 7,001 consecutive episodes of myocardial infarction were evaluated. A total of 1,749 patients were randomized to receive daily doses of either trandolapril (876 patients) or placebo (873 patients) starting 3–7 days after myocardial infarction. Follow-up ranged from 24 to 50 months.

*Results.*—During the trial, 304 patients (34.7%) in the trandolapril group died (Fig 1) compared with 369 (42.3%) in the placebo group (see Fig 1). Trandolapril significantly reduced the risk of death from cardiovascular causes and sudden death compared with placebo alone. The progression to severe heart failure was significantly less frequent in the trandolapril group than in the placebo group. The risk of fatal and non-fatal myocardial infarction recurrence was not significantly decreased in the trandolapril group compared with the placebo group.

*Conclusion.*—Long-term treatment with trandolapril begun soon after myocardial infarction in patients with decreased left ventricular function proved beneficial. The risk of overall mortality, mortality from cardiovas-

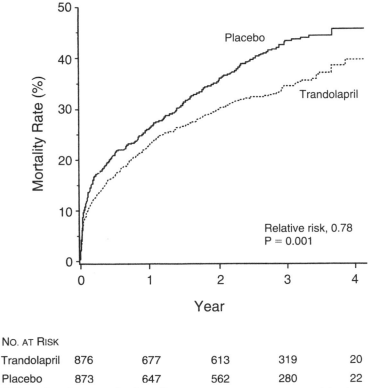

**FIGURE 1.**—Cumulative mortality from all causes among patients receiving trandolapril or placebo. (Reprinted by permission of the *The New England Journal of Medicine* from Køber L, for the Trandolapril Cardiac Evaluation (TRACE) Study Group: A clinical trail of the angiotensin-converting–enzyme inhibitor trandolapril in patients with left ventricular dysfunction after myocardial infarction; *N Engl J Med* 333:1670–1676; Copyright 1995, Massachusetts Medical Society.)

cular causes, sudden death, and the development of severe heart failure all were significantly reduced in the treatment group. The fact that mortality was reduced in a randomized trial enrolling 25% of consecutive patients screened gives this investigation a solidness that should encourage the selective use of ACE inhibition after myocardial infarction.

▶ Because a large number of our vascular surgery patients will experience cardiac-related events, I do believe it is desirable for vascular surgeons to have at least a passing familiarity with the current state of the art in the cardiologic treatment of these patients. Although I know absolutely nothing about the specific ACE inhibitor being studied, patients with ventricular dysfunction 3 days after myocardial infarction randomized to ACE inhibitor had a significant reduction in mortality compared with other patients. Interestingly, both the ISIS-IV and the GISSI-III study showed similar trends for ACE inhibitors.

## Wound Infection

**Oral Ciprofloxacin Versus Intravenous Cefuroxime as Prophylaxis Against Postoperative Infection in Vascular Surgery: A Randomised Double-blind, Prospective Multicentre Study**
Risberg B, Drott C, Dalman P, et al (Lund Univ, Sweden; County Hosps of Bors and Halmstad, Sweden; et al)
*Eur J Vasc Endovasc Surg* 10:346–351, 1995                    5–16

*Background.*—Antibiotic prophylaxis, most commonly accomplished using IV penicillins such as methicillin or cephalosporins such as cefuroxime, is performed routinely in vascular surgery. Ciprofloxacin, a 4-quinolone with a broad range of activity, may be as efficacious as cefuroxime in preventing postoperative infections. Ciprofloxacin also can be administered orally, a route that is considerably less expensive than IV delivery. The efficacy of oral ciprofloxacin in preventing postoperative wound infections was prospectively evaluated and compared with IV cefuroxime in a group of patients undergoing peripheral vascular surgery.

*Patients and Methods.*—Five hundred eighty patients scheduled for arterial surgeries requiring an inguinal incision were enrolled in this randomized double-blind study. Of these, 293 were randomly assigned to treatment with 750 mg of oral ciprofloxacin given twice and 287 to 1.5 g of IV cefuroxime given 3 times on the day of surgery. Wound and graft infections occurring within 30 postoperative days were evaluated. Wound infection was defined as pus from a surgical wound, with or without a positive bacterial culture, and graft infections as persistent wound infection communicating with the graft.

*Results.*—Analysis according to intent to treat revealed wound infection rates of 9.2% in the ciprofloxacin group and 9.1% in the cefuroxime group. Corresponding figures were 9.5% for the former group and 9.7% for the latter when analyzed for correct treatment. There were 3 (0.5%) graft infections based on intent to treat. Most infections were identified

7–10 days after surgery. Forty percent of the wound infections were noted in the groin, 20% in the thigh, 31% in the knee, and 13% in distal incisions. The most commonly isolated bacteria was *Staphylococcus aureus*, followed by *Staphylococcus epidermidis*. Wound infections were noted in 31 (7.1%) of 433 patients without and in 22 (14.9%) of 147 patients with distal ulcers. The presence of distal ulcer was identified as the only significant prognostic factor in multivariate analysis.

*Conclusion.*—Similar rates of infection were noted between patients treated with oral ciprofloxacin and those receiving IV cefuroxime. Oral ciprofloxacin thus appears to offer a safe, effective, and cost-effective alternative to IV prophylaxis in patients able to tolerate oral agents on the day of surgery.

▶ I suppose I accept the authors' conclusions that in their experience ciprofloxacin is equivalent to cefuroxime in preventing postoperative vascular surgery infections. I note with concern, however, the significant rate of infection that they did experience. In recent years more attention has been appropriately devoted to wound infection and wound healing problems in vascular surgery. I have commented on this previously. I continue to believe that vigorous surgical soap and antiseptic prepping, coupled with careful wound closure, including the use of subcuticular sutures, maximize the likelihood of uncomplicated wound healing. Even with this careful regimen, however, we (and I suspect everyone else) still experience a disappointing incidence of wound healing problems. See Abstract 5–17.

---

**Skin Closure and the Incidence of Groin Wound Infection: A Prospective Study**
Murphy PG, Tadros E, Cross S, et al (St James' Hosp, Dublin)
*Ann Vasc Surg* 9:480–482, 1995                                      5–17

---

*Objective.*—Wound infection in the groin after bypass surgery is one of the most dreaded postoperative complications because it can lead to graft infection. The relationship between skin closure with different suture materials and the incidence of wound infection was examined.

*Patients.*—Seventy men and 44 women (mean age, of 67 years) who underwent bypass surgery with a groin incision for end-stage critical ischemia were entered into the trial. Aortofemoral bypass was performed in 25% of the patients and femorodistal bypass in the other 75%. Forty-one patients were randomized to wound closure with interrupted nylon (IN), 38 to continuous nylon (CN), 45 to subcutaneous Maxon (SC), and 49 to wound closure with clips. Before the wound was closed, cultures were taken from the area around the artery and the deepest part of the wound. Repeat cultures were taken on postoperative days 3, 5, 7, 10, and 14, at which time the wound was inspected for the presence of erythema, lymph leakage, frank pus, or wound dehiscence.

TABLE 2.—Incidence of Infection

| | Infection of the scar | Infection of the graft |
|---|---|---|
| Individual cutaneous nylon stitches | 2 (4.9%) | 1 (2.5%) |
| Continuous cutaneous nylon suture | 1 (2.6%) | — |
| Intradermal Maxon suture | 1 (2.2%) | — |
| Staples | 1 (2.0%) | — |

*Abbreviations: IN,* interrupted nylon; *CN,* continuous nylon; *SC,* subcutaneous Maxon.
(Courtesy of Murphy PG, Tadros E, Cross S, et al: Skin closure and the incidence of groin wound infection: A prospective study. *Ann Vasc Surg* 9[5]:480–482, 1995.)

*Results.*—Wound infection occurred in 5 (2.9%) of the 173 patients and graft infection in 1 (2.5%) patient (Table 2). There was no difference in the incidence of wound infection with the use of the 4 different types of wound closure. The total cost of suture materials ranged from $2 for CN to $12 for clips.

*Conclusion.*—Because this study did not demonstrate a significant difference in the incidence of wound infection with the use of different suture materials, the selection of suture material for closing groin wounds after bypass surgery should be based on the vascular surgeon's preference and cost.

▶ I am not sure this study proves much because all patients had a double-layer subcutaneous closure, followed by 1 of 4 types of skin closure. Clearly skin closure had no effect in this study. I would have been more interested in a study that involved more areas than just the groin and a single-layer subcutaneous closure.

## Perioperative Normothermia to Reduce the Incidence of Surgical-wound Infection and Shorten Hospitalization

Kurz A, for the Study of Wound Infection and Temperature Group (Univ of California, San Francisco; Univ of Vienna)
*N Engl J Med* 334:1209–1215, 1996                                          5–18

*Background.*—Perioperative hypothermia of about 2.5°C less than the normal core body temperature occurs commonly in patients undergoing colonic surgery. Vasoconstriction and impaired immunity can result, increasing a patient's susceptibility to perioperative wound infections. Hypothermia was studied to determine whether it may increase both susceptibility to surgical-wound infection and length of hospital stay.

*Methods.*—Two hundred patients undergoing colorectal surgery were studied. By random assignment, half received routine intraoperative thermal care and half received additional warming. All received cefamandole and metronidazole. Their anesthetic care was standardized.

*Findings.*—More transfusions of allogeneic blood were needed in the patients assigned to hypothermia. Mean final intraoperative core temperatures were 34.75°C in the hypothermia group and 36.65°C in the normothermia group. Nineteen percent of patients assigned to hypothermia and 6% assigned to normothermia had surgical wound infections. Patients in the hypothermia group had sutures removed 1 day later than those in the normothermia group. Hospital stays were prolonged by 2.6 days (about 20%) in patients assigned to hypothermia.

*Conclusion.*—In this study, forced-air warming combined with fluid warming maintained normothermia. Unwarmed patients had core temperatures about 2.5°C less than normal. Perioperative hypothermia lasted for more than 4 hours, including the period decisive for establishing an infection.

▶ These authors remarkably conclude that patients hypothermic at the conclusion of surgery have a surgical wound infection rate 3 times higher than that of patients normothermic at the end of surgery. They apparently believe that hypothermia itself may predispose patients to wound infections and give a number of theoretic reasons why this may be true. At the least, their observations are interesting. We think we know that hypothermic patients have a considerably rougher postoperative course than normothermic patients, including more problems with postoperative bleeding. I do believe it a reasonable objective for all of us to be attentive to the temperature of our operating rooms and the patient temperature at the conclusion of the procedure. Normothermia appears better than hypothermia.

## Miscellaneous Topics

### Implications of Small Reductions in Diastolic Blood Pressure for Primary Prevention

Cook NR, Cohen J, Hebert PR, et al (Brigham and Women's Hosp, Boston; Harvard Med School, Boston; St Louis Univ)
*Arch Intern Med* 155:701–709, 1995                                              5–19

*Background.*—The pharmacologic treatment of hypertension is effective but has some disadvantages. Although changes in lifestyle such as weight loss, reduced sodium and alcohol intake, and increased physical activity result in smaller diastolic blood pressure (DBP) decreases than drug treatment does, the impact of these changes on cardiovascular disease may be great when applied to the population as a whole. Lifestyle changes may substantially reduce the incidence of cardiovascular events without the drug therapy side effects. The effect of small BP decreases on the incidence of coronary heart disease (CHD) and stroke in the general population was estimated.

*Methods and Findings.*—Data on white men and women (aged 35–64 years) were obtained for the analysis from the Framingham Heart Study and the National Health and Nutrition Examination Survey II. The findings of observational and randomized studies suggest that a 2-mm Hg decrease in DBP would be associated with a reduction of 17% in the prevalence of hypertension, 6% in the risk of CHD, and 15% in the risk of stroke and transient ischemic attacks (TIAs). When these data were applied to 35- to 64-year-old white men and women in the United States, a successful population intervention alone was estimated to decrease CHD incidence more than medical therapy for all individuals with a DBP of 95 mm Hg or greater. Such an intervention could prevent 84% of the number prevented by medical therapy for individuals with a DBP of 90 mm Hg or higher. A population-wide 2-mm Hg decrease could also prevent 93% of strokes (including TIAs) prevented by drug treatment among persons with a DBP of 95 mm Hg or greater and 69% of such events among those with a DBP of 90 mm Hg or greater. The most effective preventive strategy would be a combination of both a population decrease in DBP and targeted medical intervention. Such a strategy could double or triple the effect of medical treatment only. Adding a population-based intervention to current hypertensive therapy was estimated to prevent an additional 67,000 CHD events (6%) and 34,000 strokes and TIAs (13%) each year among 35- to 64-year-olds.

*Conclusion.*—Reducing DBP by only 2 mm Hg in the mean of the population distribution, along with drug therapy, could substantially decrease the number of CHD and stroke events that occur in the United States each year. The results of ongoing primary prevention studies and the cooperation of the food industry, government agencies, and health education professionals will be needed to determine whether such decreases in DBP can be achieved through lifestyle interventions, especially through reduced sodium intake.

▶ I have never understood trials in hypertension management. I always thought that a reduction in BP of 2- or 3-mm Hg was within the error of repeated observations and by itself meant nothing. We are informed here that a reduction in DBP of 2-mm Hg is a marvelous thing and could well result in a 6% reduction in the risk of coronary heart disease and a 15% reduction in the risk of stroke and TIAs. I had no idea that such small changes in blood pressure were so profoundly important. Of course, these are populationwide numbers and do not apply directly to the individual. I was so amazed by this information that I thought I would share it with you. You're welcome.

## Lack of Effect of Long-term Supplementation With Beta Carotene on the Incidence of Malignant Neoplasms and Cardiovascular Disease

Hennekens CH, Buring JE, Manson JE, et al (Brigham and Women's Hosp, Boston; Harvard Med School, Boston; Harvard School of Public Health, Boston)

*N Engl J Med* 334:1145–1149, 1996                    5–20

*Background.*—Risks of cancer and cardiovascular disease appear to be somewhat lower in people with a high intake of fruits and vegetables containing β-carotene. Some plausible mechanisms for this relationship have been suggested by basic science research. The ability of long-term β-carotene supplementation to prevent cardiovascular disease and malignant neoplasms was studied.

*Methods.*—The randomized, double-blind trial was conducted as part of the Physicians' Health Study. Beginning in 1982, 22,071 male physicians, aged 40–84 years, were assigned to receive either β-carotene supplementation (50 mg on alternate days) or placebo. Eleven percent of the subjects were current smokers and 39% were former smokers at baseline. The trial was scheduled to run through the end of 1995, at which time 99% of subjects were available for follow-up. Seventy-eight percent of physicians assigned to β-carotene were compliant.

*Results.*—The β-carotene and placebo groups showed few, if any, differences in the incidence of cardiovascular diseases or malignancies or in mortality. Malignant neoplasms other than nonmelanoma skin cancer developed in 1,273 subjects in the β-carotene group vs. 1,293 in the placebo group, for a relative risk of 0.98. The incidence of lung cancer, death from cancer, death from any cause, and death from cardiovascular disease was also similar in the 2 groups. Neither were there any significant differences in the number of subjects with myocardial infarction, stroke, or any of the previous 3 end points. All of the end points were also comparable among current and former smokers.

*Conclusion.*—Long-term supplementation with β-carotene does not appear to reduce the risk of malignant neoplasms, cardiovascular disease, or death in healthy men. Neither was there any evidence that β-carotene supplementation had a harmful effect. The results provide timely guidance for public health recommendations, because the general public has been spending a great deal of money on β-carotene supplements.

▶ In this remarkable 12-year study of 22,000 male physicians, β-carotene dietary supplementation did not result in any benefit. Two prior studies, the Alpha-Tocopherol, Beta Carotene (ATBC) Cancer Prevention Study, and the Beta Carotene and Retinal Efficacy Trial (CARET) found no benefits of such supplementation in terms of alteration in the incidence of cancer or cardiovascular disease. Indeed, both found somewhat higher rates of disease among patients receiving the β-carotene. This information should lay to rest for all times the hypothesis that β-carotene diminishes the risk of cardiovascular disease or cancer.

*Reference*

1. 1996 Year Book of Vascular Surgery, p 3.

---

### Age-related Differences in the Distribution of Peripheral Atherosclerosis: When Is Atherosclerosis Truly Premature?

Hansen ME, Valentine RJ, McIntire DD, et al (Univ of Texas, Dallas)
*Surgery* 118:834–839, 1995                                    5–21

---

*Introduction.*—There is no universally accepted definition of premature peripheral atherosclerosis. A definition would be useful because it appears that the natural history of peripheral atherosclerosis in young adults is unfavorable compared with that of older adults. Age-related differences in the distribution of atherosclerotic lesions were evaluated to determine an age threshold at which such differences become evident.

*Methods.*—Of 410 patients referred for arteriographic evaluation of the lower extremities within a 5-year period, 322 patients (79%) were 50 years or older and 88 (21%) were 49 years or younger. Medical records were reviewed for demographic data, medical history, risk factors for atherosclerosis, and hyperlipidemia. Arteriograms of 59 patients 49 years and younger with lower-extremity ischemia were compared with those of 150 patients 50 years and older.

*Results.*—The mean age of 29 men and 30 women in the younger age group was 43.4. Arteriograms were available for all patients, and medical records were available for 54. Patient distribution of atherosclerotic disease was 25 (42%), proximal; 21 (36%), distal; and 13, (22%) multilevel. The number of risk factors per patient in the study group were 12 (22%), 1 risk factor; 23 (42%), 2 risk factors; 15 (27%), 3 risk factors; and 5 (9%), 4 risk factors. Those with diabetes mellitus included 12 (57%) with distal disease, 5 (20%) with proximal disease, and 5 (38%) with multilevel disease. Patients with distal disease were 6.5 times as likely to be diabetic as those with proximal disease. Twelve (57%) with distal disease, 22 (88%) with proximal disease, and 11 (85%) with multilevel disease were smokers. There were no significant between-group differences in the prevalences of hypertension and hyperlipidemia. In the older age group, 92 (66%) of patients had single-level disease compared with 46 (78%) of the study group. Fifteen (16%) of patients in the older group with single-level atherosclerosis had proximal disease compared with 25 (54%) of patients in the younger group (Table 2).

*Conclusion.*—The distribution of peripheral atherosclerosis is different in older and younger adults. In younger patients who are nondiabetic, the disease most commonly involves the aortoiliac segment. There is a marked difference in lesion distribution between patients 49 years and younger compared with patients 50 years and older. The onset of symptoms at 49 years or younger is a reasonable definition of premature peripheral atherosclerosis.

**TABLE 2.**—Distribution of Atherosclerotic Lesions and Age Group

| Age (yr) | No. | Proximal Only n (%) | Distal Only n (%) | Multilevel n (%) |
|---|---|---|---|---|
| ≤39 | 15 | 8 (53) | 6 (40) | 1 (7) |
| 40–49 | 44 | 17 (39) | 15 (34) | 12 (27) |
| 50–59 | 50 | 11 (22) | 23 (46) | 16 (32) |
| ≥60 | 90 | 4 (4) | 54 (60) | 32 (36) |

*Note: Proximal only* refers to single-level disease involving aortoiliac segment; *Distal only* refers to single-level disease involving femoropopliteal-tibial segment; and *multilevel* refers to involvement of both proximal and distal vessels.
(Courtesy of Hansen ME, Valentine RJ, McIntire DD, et al: Age-related differences in the distribution of peripheral atherosclerosis: When is atherosclerosis truly premature? *Surgery* 118:834–839, 1995.)

▶ Dr. Valentine and his associates at Southwestern have made significant contributions to our understanding of atherosclerosis in young adults. In this study, they examined differences in atherosclerotic lesion distribution in an attempt to relate this to age. Their suggestion that premature atherosclerosis be defined as beginning at or before age 49 years strikes me as a bit old. We all encounter occasional patients who appear to have run-of-the-mill atherosclerosis in their thirties and early forties. These are the patients that I have considered as having truly premature atherosclerosis. I agree with the authors that in the main the disease distribution in these very young patients is aortoiliac.

# 6 Thoracic Aorta

## Aortic Dissection

### Aortic Dissection: Percutaneous Management of Ischemic Complications With Endovascular Stents and Balloon Fenestration

Slonim SM, Nyman U, Semba CP, et al (Stanford Univ, Calif)
J Vasc Surg 23:241–253, 1996
6–1

*Background.*—About 30% of patients with aortic dissection have peripheral vascular ischemic symptoms. Standard surgery for the dissection relieves most of these ischemic complications. However, some patients do not have such surgery, and some have persistent peripheral vascular ischemia after the thoracic aortic procedure. In these patients, endovascular stents and balloon fenestration may be useful.

*Methods.*—Twenty-two patients aged 35–77 years underwent percutaneous treatment for peripheral ischemic complications. Twelve patients had type A aortic dissections, and 10 had type B.

*Findings.*—Leg ischemia occurred in 10 patients, renal in 13, and visceral in 6. Sixteen patients underwent endovascular stenting. Eleven had renal stents; 6, lower extremity; 2, superior mesenteric artery; and 2, aortic stents. Balloon fenestration of the intimal flap was performed in 3 patients. Three had balloon fenestration combined with endovascular stenting. In all 22 patients, revascularization was clinically successful. One patient died 3 days after the procedure, and another died at 13.4 months. Nineteen patients had persistent relief of clinical symptoms, with a mean 13.7 months of follow-up. (One patient was lost to follow-up.) In 1 patient, perinephric hematoma resulted from the guide wire.

*Conclusion.*—Endovascular stenting and balloon fenestration are safe and effective in the percutaneous treatment of peripheral ischemic complications of aortic dissection. The long-term durability of these techniques have not been established, however, and further research is needed before these procedures can be widely adopted.

▶ I presently conclude that percutaneous management of ischemic complications of aortic dissection with endovascular stents and balloon fenestrations is the treatment of choice. For me, this is a significant concession. I note in the patients reported herein who required both surgery and percutaneous management, the surgery always came first. I question the wisdom of this temporal relationship. I have come to believe that when the acutely dissected patient has the usual angiogram confirming dissection, any visceral or extremity lesions noted at that time should undergo immediate endovascular repair. The patient can then be taken to the operating room for any requisite surgery (usually ascending aorta or aortic valve). If this temporal sequence is not elected, you may find that by the time the patient has finished the aortic surgery, the viscera or leg may be beyond salvage. At any rate, I have finally discovered at least one area in which endovascular repair appears superior to operative repair. I am delighted to be able to share this revelation with you.

---

**Peripheral Vascular Complications of Aortic Dissection**
Hughes JD, Bacha EA, Dodson TF, et al (Emory Univ, Atlanta, Ga)
*Am J Surg* 170:209–212, 1995                                          6–2

---

*Introduction.*—When untreated, spontaneous aortic dissection has a high mortality, approximately 50%, usually from cardiac or aortic complications. Tissue ischemia or infarction may also occur distal to the site of dissection. A subgroup of patients, those with peripheral vascular complications, have been found to be at highest risk for mortality. Although peripheral vascular complications may occur in up to 60% of patients, management remains unclear. Patients with both aortic dissection and peripheral vascular complications were characterized and treatment was evaluated.

*Methods.*—Medical records from 5-year period were retrospectively reviewed for cases of spontaneous aortic dissection. Demographic data and diagnostic studies used to detect aortic dissection and peripheral vascular complications were recorded. Patients were classified by extent and manifestation (acute or chronic) of dissection and by the presence or absence of peripheral vascular complications.

*Results.*—Eighty-six cases (in 84 patients) of spontaneous aortic dissection were found. Eighteen patients (21%) had peripheral vascular complications (group A). Of these patients, 13 had type I dissection, 1 had type IIIa dissection, and 4 had type IIIb. For patients without peripheral vascular complications (group B), 16 had type I dissection, 15 had type II, 22 had type IIIa, 12 had type IIIb, and 3 had type IV dissection. Transesophageal echocardiography was used in the diagnosis of dissection in 52% of all cases, CT in 27%, angiography in 22%, and MRI in 5%. Aortic dissection was classified as acute in 15 patients in group A and in 50 patients in group B. The 18 patients in group A had involvement of 38 major vessels, including the carotid artery, subclavian artery, celiac and superior mesenteric arteries, renal arteries, and the iliofemoral artery. Four of the 18 patients underwent a peripheral vascular procedure for complications; femorofemoral bypass was performed on 3 patients, and 1 patient had an aortobiiliac bypass. Three deaths occurred among patients in group A and 6 deaths occurred in group B.

*Conclusion.*—Twenty-one percent of patients with spontaneous aortic dissection were found to develop peripheral vascular complications; most complications resolved after surgical repair of the dissection. This figure for peripheral vascular complications is lower than that reported in the literature. This may be related to the use of transesophageal echocardiography, a nonangiographic method, for diagnosis in the majority of cases. Magnetic resonance imaging and CT are also less sensitive methods compared with angiography for detecting peripheral vascular lesions.

▶ This article is an interesting counterpoint to the prior article. These authors review many years of surgical treatment of vascular complications of aortic dissection. These patients were obviously carefully selected; they all underwent surgery on a chronic or subacute elective basis. I do believe for the acute problem, endovascular repair presently offers the best hope of patient salvage (see Abstract 6–1).

## Embolization

### Natural History of Severe Atheromatous Disease of the Thoracic Aorta: A Transesophageal Echocardiographic Study
Montgomery DH, Ververis JJ, McGorisk G, et al (Emory Univ, Atlanta, Ga; Veterans Affairs Med Ctr, Decatur, Ga)
*J Am Coll Cardiol* 27:95–101, 1996                                6–3

*Introduction.*—Transesophageal echocardiography is able to image the atherosclerotic process in the thoracic aorta. Recent studies suggest an association between severe atheromatous disease of the thoracic aorta and an increased risk of embolic events. A prospective study of patients with known severe atherosclerosis of the thoracic aorta sought to characterize the morphologic progression and clinical course of the disease.

*Methods.*—A total of 191 patients had the entire aorta imaged at transesophageal echocardiography. Each aorta was graded on a scale of I to V (Fig 1) for severity of atherosclerosis. Most cases fell into grades I to III; the 19 patients with grade IV and 14 with grade V atherosclerotic disease comprised the main study group. Follow-up studies performed at least 6 months later were available for 8 patients with grade IV and 10 with grade V disease. Also available were studies of 12 grade III patients who were representative of more moderate disease. Three experienced echocardiographers reviewed the images in a blinded manner.

*Results.*—The patients with severe (grades III and IV) disease had undergone transesophageal echocardiography for a variety of indications, principally a history of embolic event (33%). During a mean period of 11.7 months, 20 of the 30 patients with a follow-up study had no change in atherosclerotic severity grade, 7 progressed a grade, and 3 decreased a grade. Eleven (61%) with severe disease showed formation of new mobile lesions. All 7 patients with persistent grade V atherosclerotic disease had evidence of new mobile lesion formation on follow-up studies. Of the total of 33 patients with grade IV or V disease, 8 died and 1 had a clinical

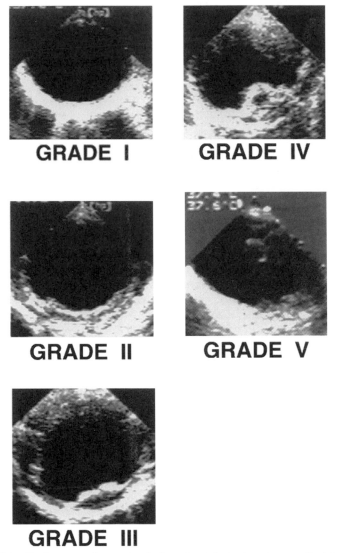

GRADE I

GRADE IV

GRADE II

GRADE V

GRADE III

FIGURE 1.—Grading system for severity of atherosclerosis in the thoracic aorta. *Grade I*, normal or minimal intimal thickening. *Grade II*, extensive intimal thickening. *Grade III*, atheroma less than 5 mm. *Grade IV*, atheroma 5 mm or more. *Grade V*, mobile lesion. (Reprinted with permission from the American College of Cardiology. *J Am Coll Cardiol* 1996; 27:95–101. Montgomery DH, Ververis JJ, McGorisk G, et al: Natural history of severe atheromatous disease of the thoracic aorta: A transesophageal echocardiographic study.)

embolic event during the study. Three morphologic categories of mobile lesions were identified; all 3 types developed and resolved during the study.

*Conclusion.*—Severe atherosclerotic disease of the thoracic aorta is associated with a high rate of mortality. Although the disease process tends to remain stable, individual lesion morphology appears dynamic and progressive. Formation of new mobile lesions occurs frequently in patients with more severe disease. A useful therapeutic strategy would encourage the healing of the lesions and the prevention of their evolution.

▶ Significant atherosclerotic lesions of the thoracic aorta appear quite dynamic over time, with many patients developing and resolving mobile lesions. Over a mean follow-up of 11 months, 24% of patients with significant thoracic aortic atherosclerosis detected by transesophageal echocardiography died, although only 3% died of a probable clinical embolic event. An unanswered question is whether the mobile lesions, which to me is the most interesting part of this particular study, have any special propensity for embolization. This is not answered by the material presented, and I am unwilling to accept that they do without convincing evidence.

---

**Atherosclerotic Disease of the Aortic Arch as a Risk Factor for Recurrent Ischemic Stroke**
Amarenco P, for the French Study of Aortic Plaques in Stroke Group (Marie Curie Univ, Paris; Universitaire de Grenoble, Paris; Universitaire de Besançon, Paris; et al)
N Engl J Med 334:1216–1221, 1996                                        6–4

---

*Background.*—Recent evidence indicates that atherosclerotic disease of the aortic arch may be a source of cerebral emboli. The risk of recurrent brain infarction and vascular events in patients with aortic arch plaques 4 mm thick or more was compared with that of patients with smaller or no plaques.

*Methods.*—A cohort of 331 patients aged 60 years or older was followed up for 2–4 years. All patients, hospitalized with brain infarction, had transesophageal echocardiography to search for atherosclerotic plaques in the aortic arch proximal to the ostium of the left subclavian artery. Three groups of patients were formed based on the thickness of the aortic arch wall: less than 1 mm (group 1), 1 to 3.9 mm (group 2), and 4 mm of greater (group 3).

*Findings.*—Group 1 consisted of 143 patients; group 2, 143; and group 3, 45. The incidence of recurrent brain infarction was 2.8 per 100 person-years in group 1, 3.5 per 100 person-years in group 2, and 11.9 per 100 person-years in group 3. The overall incidence of vascular events in the 3 groups was 5.9, 9.1, and 26 per 100 person-years. The presence of aortic plaques 4 mm thick or more independently predicted recurrent brain infarction and all vascular events after adjustment for carotid stenosis, atrial fibrillation, peripheral arterial disease, and other risk factors (Fig 2).

*Conclusion.*—In patients with brain infarction and plaques of 4 mm thick or more in the aortic arch, the recurrence rate was 11.9 per 100 person-years of follow-up, and the incidence of all vascular events was 26 per 100 person-years of follow-up. These rates are among the highest in

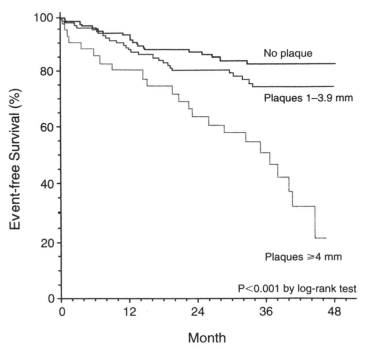

FIGURE 2.—Kaplan-Meier analysis of survival without vascular events (brain infarction, myocardial infarction, peripheral embolism, or death from vascular causes) according to plaque thickness in the aortic arch proximal to the ostium of the left subclavian artery. (Reprinted by permission of *The New England Journal of Medicine*; from Amarenco P, for the French Study of Aortic Plaques in Stroke Group: Atherosclerotic disease of the aortic arch as a risk factor for recurrent ischemic stroke. *N Engl J Med* 334:1216–1221; Copyright 1996, Massachusetts Medical Society.)

patients with ischemic stroke treated with antiplatelet drugs previously described. The high risk of vascular events in the current series may have important implications for preventive treatment in patients 60 years of age or older with plaques 4 mm thick or greater in the aortic arch. The risks and benefits of treatment in such patients should be reassessed.

▶ Here we have more testimonial to the risk of the aortic arch atherosclerotic plaque as a risk factor for cerebral infarction. The more severe the plaque, the more likely the risk of recurrent stroke. There seems little doubt that significant atheromatous involvement of the aortic arch presages a dire clinical outcome in a disturbing percentage of patients. I wonder if anticoagulant therapy would have any beneficial effect. Certainly aortic arch replacement for many of these patients is completely impractical.

## Thoracoabdominal Grafts

### The Risk of Ischemic Spinal Cord Injury in Patients Undergoing Graft Replacement for Thoracoabdominal Aortic Aneurysms

Grabitz K, Sandmann W, Stühmeier K, et al (Heinrich-Heine Univ, Düsseldorf, Germany)
*J Vasc Surg* 23:230–240, 1996                                         6–5

*Objective.*—The development of neurologic complications during graft replacement for thoracoabdominal aneurysm (TAA) remains a problem. A monitoring system that involved direct placement of epidural electrodes on the spinal cord was developed to detect spinal cord ischemia during aortic cross-clamping (AXC).

*Methods.*—Between 1981 and 1995, 260 patients underwent thoracoabdominal aortic replacement, with 80% of patients having type I, II, or III TAA. In 167 patients, 2 electrocatheters were placed before the onset of anesthesia at level L1-L2 for stimulation and at level T5-6 for recording within the epidural space. During surgery, spinal cord function was monitored by recording spinal somatosensory evoked potentials (sSSEPs).

*Results.*—With spinal cord monitoring, three groups of patients with low, moderate, and high risk for paraplegia and paraparesis were identified. Group A included 59 patients whose sSSEPs remained normal throughout surgery. The intercostal arteries (ICAs) were not reattached outside the proximal aortic anastomosis in 54 patients. In the other 5 patients, the ICAs were reimplanted separately because of possible anatomical relation to spinal cord blood supply. None of these 59 patients had postoperative neurologic deficits. Group B included 54 patients whose sSSEPs remained normal until 15 minutes after AXC but were impaired thereafter. Of these, 19 had early reimplantation of ICAs, 3 had paraparesis, and 2 had paraplegia. Neurologic deficit developed in patients without early reimplantation of ICAs. Among the 4 patients who underwent separate reimplantation of ICAs late in the procedure because of incomplete sSSEP recovery, the sSSEP subsequently returned to normal, and only 1 patient had mild paraparesis. Overall the total rate of neurologic deficits in group B was 13%, including paraplegia in 3.5% and paraparesis in 9.5%. Group C included 54 patients who exhibited rapid loss of sSSEP within 15 minutes of AXC. Twenty-eight patients underwent reimplantation of ICAs only within the proximal anastomosis; 21 showed prompt signal recovery after blood flow release into the reimplanted ICAs, and none had neurologic deficits. The other 7 patients had no or very late and incomplete sSSEP recovery; 3 had paraplegia and 4 had paraparesis. In 26 patients, ICAs were reimplanted separately to the proximal anastomosis. Among the 17 patients in whom this reimplantation was done early in the procedure, 13 had full recovery of sSSEP with normal neurologic status, and the other 4 had incomplete or no recurrence of sSSEP, followed by paraplegia in 1 and paraparesis in 3. Nineteen patients underwent reimplantation of ICAs after the aortic replacement had been completed because sSSEP recovery was not satisfactory. The sSSEP returned to normal in all patients, followed by normal neurologic status in 6 patients and mild paraparesis in 3. The neurologic complication rate in group C was 26%, including paraplegia in 7.5% and paraparesis in 18.5%. Multivariate analysis disclosed that total time of sSSEP, the time required for sSSEP regeneration, and the total AXC times predicted neurologic outcome.

*Conclusion.*—These findings indicate that the risk of ischemic spinal cord injury during replacement for TAA can be assessed continuously by monitoring the sSSEP directly from the spinal cord. Patients without sSSEP changes during aortic reconstruction do not require ICA reattachment and will eventually have normal neurologic status. Patients with impaired or loss of sSSEP longer than 15 minutes after AXC have some collateral vessels; those whose sSSEP do not return within normal recovery time after blood flow release into the proximal anastomosis should undergo reimplantation of ICAs. Loss of sSSEP within 15 minutes of AXC shows poor collateralization; early restoration of spinal cord blood supply should be done. With the return of sSSEP to normal by subsequent separate reimplantation of the ICAs, paraplegia will not occur and paraparesis will be rare and mild.

▶ These authors hypothesize that spinal cord ischemia during TAA repair can be accurately monitored by sSSEP with a stimulating catheter in the lumbar area and a monitoring catheter in the thoracic area. Abnormalities of sSSEP lead these authors to reimplant intercostal arteries. Although their results generally appear satisfactory, they appear no better than those of many others not using this technique. I remain impressed by the work of Dr. Acher et al.[1] at the University of Wisconsin in Madison, who states he does not routinely reimplant any intercostal arteries. And then we have the hypothermic spinal cord perfusers. I wonder.

*Reference*

1. Acher CW, Wynn MM, Hoch JR, et al: Combined use of cerebral spinal fluid drainage and naloxone reduces the risk of paraplegia in thoracoabdominal aneurysm repair. *J Vasc Surg* 19:236–248, 1994.

---

**Outcome and Expansion Rate of 57 Thoracoabdominal Aortic Aneurysms Managed Nonoperatively**
Cambria RA, Glovicki P, Stanson AW, et al (Mayo Clinic and Found, Rochester, Minn)
*Am J Surg* 170:213–217, 1995                                                6–6

---

*Introduction.*—Surgical repair of thoracoabdominal aortic aneurysms (TAAAs) presents a considerable challenge. Mortality rates for elective repair are reported as high as 19%, and disabling complications occur in up to 30% of patients in certain subgroups. A series of 57 nonoperatively managed patients with TAAA were reviewed for survival and the risk of aneurysm rupture.

*Methods.*—Patients with TAAAs were identified by reviewing all CT scans performed at Mayo Clinic from 1987 through 1993 that indicated a diagnosis of aortic disease. Excluded were patients with aortic dissections and ruptured aneurysms or who proceeded directly to aneurysm repair. The clinical course and CT data of eligible patients were reviewed and the aneurysms carefully measured and classified by Crawford's system. Reason for deferral of surgical repair was also noted. Mean follow-up was 37 months.

*Results.*—The mean age of the study group was 72 years; 33 patients were men and 24 were women. Common coexistent risk factors included hypertension (77%), tobacco use (75%), and history of coronary artery disease (44%). Nonoperative management of TAAAs was chosen because of aneurysm size less than 5 cm (49%), surgical risk (32%), concomitant illness (14%), or patient preference (5%). The median diameter of TAAAs at diagnosis was 5.0 cm. With the use of the Crawford classification, 35% were type I, 14% type II, 39% type III, and 12% type IV. Aneurysms of aortic segments distinct from the TAAA were present in 61% of patients. Thirty-four (60%) patients died during follow-up. Median survival time for all patients was 3.3 years, and the overall survival rate at 5 years was 39%. Excluding the 15 patients who eventually underwent aneurysm repair, the 5-year survival rate was 23%. The overall risk of aneurysm rupture for patients managed nonoperatively was 12% at 2 years; for those with aneurysms larger than 5 cm, the risk was significantly higher (18%). Twenty-nine of the 57 patients had follow-up CT scans at a mean of 2.4 years after the initial scan. Rate of expansion was related to the presence of chronic obstructive pulmonary disease but not to aneurysm size at diagnosis.

*Conclusion.*—Patients selected for nonoperative management of TAAAs had a high mortality rate. The 5-year survival rate was only 17% for those who did not eventually undergo aneurysm repair. Surgical repair should be considered for otherwise healthy patients with TAAAs larger than 5 cm in diameter.

▶ We can take a number of messages from this interesting epidemiologic paper. On balance, TAAAs expand very modestly, averaging only 0.2 cm/year. All ruptured TAAAs were greater than 5 cm in diameter, and this appeared to be the point at which rupture became distinctly more likely. Patients selected for nonoperative management of TAAA (defined as aortic diameter > 3.5 cm) had an overall survival of 39% and repair-free survival of only 17% at 5 years. All aneurysms that ruptured were greater than 5 cm in diameter. These authors conclude, and I suspect correctly, that only TAAAs less than 5 cm should be followed. Those greater than 5 cm have a distinctly increased risk of rupture and should be considered for early repair.

**Results of Contemporary Surgical Treatment of Descending Thoracic Aortic Aneurysms: Experience in 198 Patients**
Coselli JS, Plestis KA, la Francesca S, et al (Methodist Hosp, Houston)
*Ann Vasc Surg* 10:131–137, 1996                                      6–7

*Background.*—Recent years have seen important advances in the management of descending thoracic aortic aneurysms. Nevertheless, these aneurysms continue to be complex and life-threatening lesions whose management poses major challenges for the vascular surgeon. A large series of patients were treated by modern techniques for the repair of descending thoracic aortic aneurysm.

*Methods.*—The experience included 198 patients with descending thoracic aortic aneurysm. The 133 men and 65 women were treated from 1987 to 1995 by a single surgeon. Seventy-two percent of patients were symptomatic, and 62% had extensive aneurysms involving two thirds or more of the descending aorta. A simple clamp technique was used for aneurysm repair in 77% of patients; mean clamping time in this group was 25 minutes. Thirteen percent of patients considered to be at high risk underwent left atrium–to–femoral bypass, with a mean clamping time of 37 minutes. Ten percent of patients, who had extensive aneurysms involving the arch and ascending aorta, required profound hypothermia and circulatory arrest, which lasted a mean of 46 minutes.

*Results.*—There were 10 deaths, for an operative mortality of 5%; 4 patients died of pulmonary causes and 3 each of cardiac and renal causes. Three patients were left paraplegic after their operation, a rate of 1.5%. Regression analysis showed that renal failure, pulmonary complications, and paraplegia were important predictors of mortality. Clamping time was the only factor independently associated with paraplegia.

*Conclusion.*—Most patients with aneurysms of the descending thoracic aorta can be successfully managed by a simple clamp procedure. For a high-risk subgroup of patients, atriofemoral bypass is an important adjunctive technique. Ensuring that the aortic clamping time remains within safe limits is the major factor in preventing spinal cord ischemia.

▶ This is a remarkable clinical experience with generally excellent results. I am impressed that paraplegia occurred in only 3 patients. These authors continue to advocate the clamp-and-run technique. Although I admire their remarkable experience and think they are doing exactly the right thing for their environment, we have elected a slightly different approach. For both thoracoabdominal and significant thoracic aneurysms, we first perform a right axillofemoral bypass, which, if performed with a conduit 10 mm or greater, seems to preserve palpable pulsations in the distal aorta during surgery. We have observed no complications from this bypass, and in our hands this has become our shunt of choice. We generally leave the axillofemoral graft in place postoperatively and have recognized no problems resulting from this decision.

### Ruptured Thoracic Aortic Aneurysms: A Study of Incidence and Mortality Rates

Johansson G, Markström U, Swedenborg J (Karolinska Hosp, Stockholm)
*J Vasc Surg* 21:985–988, 1995                                      6–8

*Background.*—Although repair of thoracic aortic aneurysm (TAA) has become a routine surgical procedure, it still carries substantial morbidity and mortality. Relatively little is known about the natural course and surgical results of TAA. The incidence and mortality of ruptured TAA were studied in a well-defined population.

*Methods and Results.*—A review of data from various Swedish registries identified 82 cases of ruptured TAA in 1980 and 76 cases in 1989. The incidence of ruptured TAA for both years was 5 per 100,000 population. Although 41% of patients with ruptured TAA were alive when they arrived at the hospital, mortality was 100% in 1980 and 97% in 1989.

*Conclusion.*—Few patients survive a ruptured TAA. Efforts to reduce the mortality associated with TAA will require efficient screening methods for the diagnosis of unruptured TAAs. Factors associated with a high risk of rupture will have to be identified, and more operations for ruptured TAA will have to be performed.

▶ Based on the extensive record keeping in Sweden, these authors have concluded that the annual likelihood of a patient being admitted with a ruptured TAA is 5 per 100,000 patients. Unfortunately, mortality varied between 97% and 100%. These authors note that only 41% of these patients arrived at the first emergency hospital alive. Clearly the only way we are going to improve survival in patients with TAA is to resect before rupture. This is substantially true of abdominal aortic aneurysms as well, where the real rupture mortality is closer to 90% than the 50% to 60% erroneously assumed by many. The latter obviously includes only patients reaching the hospital alive (see also Abstract 6–9).

### Thoracic and Thoracoabdominal Aortic Aneurysm and Dissection: An Investigation Based on Autopsy

Svensjö S, Bengtsson H, Bergqvist D (Univ Hosps of Uppsala and Malmö, Sweden; County Hosp Kristianstad, Sweden)
*Br J Surg* 83:68–71, 1996                                      6–9

*Introduction.*—More and more patients are undergoing elective or emergency surgery for abdominal aortic aneurysm. Thoracic aortic aneurysm (TAA) is a lesion that may be decreasing in prevalence but still presents a major challenge in vascular surgery. The prevalence of TAA and the incidence of nontraumatic rupture of TAA and dissection of the thoracic aorta were studied.

*Methods.*—The investigators analyzed the autopsy records from 1958 to 1985 of the Swedish city of Malmö, which has a fairly stable population of about 230,000 and an autopsy rate of 83%. Patients with asymptomatic, ruptured, and dissected TAA were identified. The prevalence and incidence of TAA were calculated by age and sex.

*Results.*—Two hundred five subjects with asymptomatic TAA were identified: 109 men (median age, 78 years) and 96 women (median age, 85 years). Men predominated in the older age groups, and about 5% of patients of both sexes had thoracoabdominal aneurysms. Sixty-three subjects died of ruptured thoracic artery, with no age difference between men and women. Two hundred sixteen patients died of dissected thoracic artery; the men in this group died at a mean age of 69 compared with 76 for women. Rupture occurred with an incidence of 0.9 per 100,000 population for men and 1.0 per 100,000 population for women. For both men and women, the incidence of dissection was 3.2 per 100,000 population.

*Conclusion.*—At least through the mid-1980s, TAA was a lesion of low prevalence and ruptured and dissected TAA were problems of relatively low incidence. Few patients underwent operative treatment for TAA during the period studied. Because TAA is a rare lesion, centralized treatment should be considered.

▶ See also Abstract 6–8. Interestingly, in another part of the same country the calculated annual incidence of rupture of a TAA was 0.9 per 100,000, far different from the 5 per 100,000 reported in the previous paper from Stockholm. If nothing else, this points out the difficulty of attempting to derive countrywide incidence rates from specific autopsy series in various cities. I wonder if Stockholm really has 5 times the annual incidence of TAA rupture as Malmö.

# 7 Aortic Aneurysm

## Clinical Series

**Selective Management of Abdominal Aortic Aneurysms in a Prospective Measurement Program**
Brown PM, Pattenden R, Vernooy C, et al (Queen's Univ, Kingston, Ont, Canada)
*J Vasc Surg* 23:213–222, 1996                                      7–1

*Objective.*—The management of small abdominal aortic aneurysms (AAAs) remains controversial. Patients with small AAAs less than 5 cm in diameter and those believed to be unfit for operation with AAAs 5 cm diameter or greater were studied prospectively.

*Management.*—Between 1976 and 1992, 492 patients with aneurysms less than 5 cm when first seen were entered in a prospective measurement program by ultrasonography or CT (exclusively after 1988) every 6 months. The criteria for operation for patients deemed to be fit included an increase in AAA size to 5 cm, AAA expansion of more than 0.5 cm in 6 months, development of aneurysm-related symptoms or signs, and aortoiliac occlusive disease requiring treatment. Those with AAAs larger than 5 cm but deemed unfit for operation were followed-up. Another group of 91 patients with aneurysms 5 cm or greater when first seen but unfit for repair were also entered in the prospective measurement program.

*Outcome.*—Among patients with AAAs less than 5 cm at entry, surgery was undertaken as a result of an increase in AAA size to 5 cm or greater in 157, AAA expansion of more than 0.5 cm in 6 months in 24, and for other reasons in 20. The remaining 291 patients were monitored for a mean follow-up of 42 months. Expansion was significantly related to aneurysm size at entry. In particular, the rate of expansion in the group with AAAs 4.5 to 4.9 cm was 0.7 cm/yr, and this was significantly greater than that of all other groups. Patients 70 and older with AAAs less than 4 cm in diameter were far less likely to undergo operation than younger patients with AAAs equal to or greater than 4 cm in diameter. Ten ruptures occurred among the 176 patients deemed unfit for operation, including 85 patients with AAAs less than 5 cm at entry but believed to be at an unacceptable risk for operation when their AAA increased to 5 cm or more and 91 patients with AAAs 5 cm or greater. Six of these AAAs that ruptured were between 5.0 and 5.6 cm in diameter.

*Conclusion.*—Abdominal aortic aneurysms greater or equal to 5 cm are prone to rupture, whereas those smaller than 5 cm are unlikely to rupture if they are monitored closely and if operation is performed for AAA expansion greater than 0.5 cm in 6 months. In view of the risk of rupture in AAAs 5 cm or slightly greater and the progressive increase in expansion to a mean of 0.7 cm/yr in those with AAAs between 4.5 and 4.9 cm at entry, elective operation should be strongly considered for patients with AAAs between 4.5 and 5.0 cm.

▶ There is not much new information here, but it is always gratifying to have one's prejudices confirmed. In this large patient cohort, apparently no ruptures occurred in AAAs less than 5 cm, leading the authors to recommend elective surgery once the aneurysm reaches 4.5 cm, because of the unpredictable potential of rapid expansion thereafter. I do consider the matter established that the minimal size for surgery for infrarenal aortic aneurysms is 4.5 cm. I previously operated on smaller aneurysms on occasion, but no longer, based both on important publications such as this and on the refusal of managed care organizations to approve surgery of smaller aneurysms. I wonder which has been more important.

**Retroperitoneal Nonresective Staple Exclusion of Abdominal Aortic Aneurysms: Clinical Outcome and Fate of the Excluded Abdominal Aortic Aneurysms**
Blumenberg RM, Skudder PA Jr, Gelfand ML, et al (Ellis Hosp, Schenectady, NY; Albany Med College, NY)
*J Vasc Surg* 21:623–634, 1995                                            7–2

*Introduction.*—Deviations from aneurysmorrhaphy techniques to include exclusion with induced thrombosis of abdominal aortic aneurysms (AAAs) were initially developed to reduce blood loss and minimize aortic dissection in high-risk patients. Initially the exclusion technique resulted in expansion and rupture of aneurysm in a small percentage of patients. The technique has been modified to include staple exclusion of the aneurysm. The outcomes of staple exclusion of (AAAs) were prospectively evaluated.

*Methods.*—A prospective review of 100 patients undergoing elective infrarenal staple exclusion of AAA using a retroperitoneal approach was conducted. The procedure was begun with a left posterior retroperitoneal incision beginning at the lateral rectus border. After anterior mobilization of the left kidney and ligation of the lumbar tributary of the left renal vein, the infrarenal aorta was mobilized. Sufficient space is available for aortic clamping and stapling, providing an aortic segment for end-to-end anastomosis after aortic transection. Details of the procedures (clamp and operative time, transfusion requirements, complications), risk factors, and aneurysm size were recorded.

*Results.*—The average size of AAA was 5.5 cm, with 19% larger than 7 cm. Heart disease was present in 51% of patients, hypertension in 41%, and chronic obstructive pulmonary disease (COPD) in 25%. A mortality rate of 4% at 30 days was found. Patients who died were significantly older and had significantly longer anesthesia and operative times. No significant differences were noted in AAA size or transfusion requirements. Cross-clamp time was longer in those patients who died, but the difference did not reach statistical significance (80 vs. 49 minutes for survivors). Three of the patients who died had histories of myocardial infarction; the fourth patient died of lung-related causes and had advanced COPD. No patient experienced adverse postoperative coagulopathies (thrombocytopenia, hypofibrinogenemia, increased fibrin degradation products, or disseminated intravascular coagulation). Major complications included myocardial infarction (4 patients), acute renal failure (8 patients), and pulmonary complications (17 patients, 13 of whom smoked). The average length of stay was 11 days, which was extended by both pulmonary (5 days) and renal complications (9 days). Length of stay was found to correlate with patient age, aneurysm size, and risk factors (e.g., COPD or heart disease). Eighty-two of the excluded AAA thrombosed within 6 months of surgery. At 60 months of follow-up, 96.8% had thrombosis of AAA. No signs of expansion, rupture, or leakage of excluded AAA have been found. Repeat surgery has not been required.

*Conclusion.*—Staple exclusion of elective, infrarenal AAA was found to be a safe and effective procedure. Mortality associated with the procedure is low. No procedures were complicated by coagulopathies, and the aneurysm has not expanded or ruptured in any patient.

▶ When I read this, I wondered why anyone would want to do this. My reaction the second time is the same (i.e., the paper does not convince me). It's not faster, it's not safer, and the patients stay in the hospital the same length of time. The life tables as formatted don't assure us about long-term efficacy or durability. I guess the information will be of some use to those interested in "less invasive–nonresective" therapies for aneurysms. The authors state that this paper might be controversial. I agree.

**W. Abbott, M.D.**

---

**Late Survival Risk Factors for Abdominal Aortic Aneurysm Repair: Experience From Fourteen Department of Veterans Affairs Hospitals**
Feinglass J, Cowper D, Dunlop D, et al (Northwestern Univ, Chicago; Hines Veterans Affairs Hosp, Chicago; Veterans Affairs Lakeside Med Ctr, Chicago)
*Surgery* 118:16–24, 1995                                                      7–3

---

*Introduction.*—Although declining, mortality and morbidity rates associated with elective abdominal aortic aneurysm surgery are still high, estimated between 5% and 8%. Information regarding late survival probabilities after elective surgery is important in the decision for surgical treatment of abdominal aortic aneurysms. Risk factors affecting late sur-

TABLE 3.—Cox Proportional Hazards Model Results ($n = 280$)

|  | Coefficient | SE | Relative risk | 95% Confidence interval | p Value |
|---|---|---|---|---|---|
| Cerebrovascular disease | .54 | .25 | 1.72 | (1.05–2.83) | 0.04 |
| Chronic obstructive pulmonary disease | .44 | .18 | 1.55 | (1.07–2.25) | 0.02 |
| Left ventricular hypertrophy on electrocardiogram | .76 | .32 | 2.14 | (1.14–4.02) | 0.02 |
| Age >69 yr | .47 | .19 | 1.60 | (1.09–2.36) | 0.02 |

(Courtesy of Feinglass J, Cowper D, Dunlop D, et al: Late survival risk factors for abdominal aortic aneurysm repair: Experience from fourteen Department of Veterans Affairs hospitals. *Surgery* 118:16–24, 1995.)

vival after surgery for abdominal aortic aneurysms were evaluated in a cohort of male veterans.

*Methods.*—Medical records of 280 patients who had undergone surgery for abdominal aortic aneurysm between 1985 and 1987 were reviewed. Risk factors and aneurysm size at the time of surgery were recorded. A Goldman Cardiac Risk Index (CRI) score and an American Society of Anesthetists Anesthesia Physical Status Classification were also determined. The National Death Index was used to verify survival of each patient through 1991.

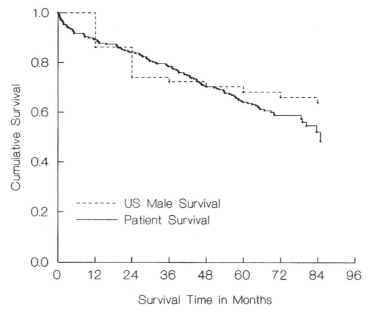

FIGURE 6.—Kaplan-Meier survival probabilities. Patient vs. age-matched U.S. 1989 male survival rates. (Courtesy of Feinglass J, Cowper D, Dunlop D, et al: Late survival risk factors for abdominal aortic aneurysm repair: Experience from fourteen Department of Veterans Affairs hospitals. *Surgery* 118:16–24, 1995.)

*Results.*—Of the 280 patients, 113 died prior to December 1991. Survival rates were 89% at 1 year and 64% at 5 years, with a cumulative survival rate of 50% at 7 years. Significantly lower survival was associated with age older than 69, a history of kidney disease, the presence of cerebrovascular disease, cardiac arrhythmias, or chronic obstructive lung disease, left ventricular hypertrophy, or a CRI score greater than 1. Multivariate analyses found age older than 69 years, chronic obstructive pulmonary disease, left ventricular hypertrophy, and history of cerebrovascular disease to be significant risk factors for increased mortality. The relative risk of mortality for cerebrovascular disease was 1.72; for chronic obstructive pulmonary disease, a 1.55 risk; for left ventricular hypertrophy, a 2.14 risk; and for age older than 69 years, a 1.60 risk (Table 3). A univariate Kaplan-Meier curve was used to compare predicted survival of study patients with that of age-matched males in the United States. Except for a higher 1-year mortality and a lower survival trend 4 years after surgery, the survival rates were comparable between the 2 groups (Fig 6).

*Conclusion.*— The late survival rate of this cohort of male patients after surgery for aortic abdominal aneurysms was found to compare favorably with the overall U.S. male life expectancy. Age, left ventricular hypertrophy, cerebrovascular disease, and chronic obstructive pulmonary disease all were found to increase the risk for mortality in this cohort of patients. Although coronary artery disease was not found to be a risk factor, this may be caused by the presence of undiagnosed coronary disease in asymptomatic patients.

▶ I am impressed that surgeons at the Department of Veterans Affairs hospitals are performing abdominal aortic aneurysm surgery with a 30-day operative mortality of 2.9%. The 1- and 5-year survival probabilities of 89% and 64%, respectively, are also impressive. It is interesting to note that a history of coronary artery disease did not predict late survival. Clearly the performance of aortic aneurysm surgery at Veterans Affairs hospitals is competitive with national standards. I congratulate the authors and their colleagues on such excellent results in a difficult population.

---

## Operative Mortality Rates After Elective Infrarenal Aortic Reconstructions

Huber TS, Harward TRS, Flynn TC, et al (Univ of Florida, Gainesville)
*J Vasc Surg* 22:287–294, 1995                                    7–4

---

*Background.*—Previous studies of abdominal aortic reconstructions have reported that the leading cause of postoperative death was complications of coronary artery disease. Since then, cardiac testing has become an important preoperative procedure before aortic reconstructions. There have also been recent reports of low cardiac mortality rates after elective vascular reconstruction and suggestions that these low rates may result from limited preoperative cardiac testing. Other reports have indicated

TABLE 3.—Cause of Death After Aortic Reconstruction

| Cause of Death | Cases | % of Total Deaths |
|---|---|---|
| MSOF | 25 | 56.8 |
| Cardiac | 11 | 25.0 |
| Hemorrhage | 3 | 6.8 |
| Respiratory | 2 | 4.5 |
| Extremity ischemia | 1 | 2.3 |
| Stroke | 1 | 2.3 |
| Refusal of therapy | 1 | 2.3 |

(Courtesy of Huber TS, Harward TRS, Flynn TC, et al: Operative mortality rates after elective infrarenal aortic reconstructions. *J Vasc Surg* 22:287–294, 1995.)

mortality rates of 3% to 6%. The leading cause of death after elective infrarenal aortic reconstruction was determined.

*Methods.*—Medical records were reviewed of all patients who had elective infrarenal aortic reconstructions between 1982 and 1994. The cause of perioperative deaths was determined. Findings were compared with findings from 266 survivors to identify risk factors for death.

*Results.*—Of 722 patients who had aortic reconstruction for aneurysmal or occlusive disease, 44 died. Mortality after aortic reconstruction alone was 4.9% but increased to 8.9% after including renal procedures and 15.8% after including lower-extremity vascular procedures. The cause of death was multisystem organ failure in 56.8% of patients (Table 3) and cardiac events in 25% of patients. The most common cause of multisystem organ failure was visceral organ dysfunction in 56% of patients and postoperative pneumonia in 36% of patients. Risk factors associated with increased operative mortality were patient age, history of myocardial infarction or congestive heart failure, ejection fraction less than 50%, length of operation, and additional surgical procedures.

*Conclusion.*—The leading cause of death in these patients was multisystem organ failure, largely from visceral organ dysfunction. More complex procedures and a higher number of comorbid conditions are associated with increased risk of multisystem organ failure and operative death.

▶ I also would have predicted that cardiac events would be the most frequent cause of death in aortic aneurysm patients undergoing elective surgery. According to these authors, I would have been wrong. According to them the most important single cause has been multisystem organ failure (the cause of 56.8% of the deaths), with visceral organ dysfunction the most frequent event leading to death. This is surprising and not in keeping with our experience at Oregon. I suspect either patients in Florida or surgeons in Florida are different.

## Routine Coronary Arteriography Before Abdominal Aortic Aneurysm Repair

Bayazit M, Göl MK, Battaloglu B, et al (Türkiye Yüksek Ihtisas Hastanesi, Ankara, Turkey)
*Am J Surg* 170:246–250, 1995                                    7–5

*Objective.*—Although mortality and morbidity after abdominal aortic aneurysm (AAA) are low, most complications are the result of cardiac events. Therefore, cardiac assessment before surgery is important. The results of a prospective evaluation of routine presurgery coronary angiography before elective AAA and effects of coronary revascularization on long-term survival were presented.

*Methods.*—Coronary arteriography was performed in 125 infrarenal or juxtarenal AAA patients (21 women and 104 men) aged 38–83 years (Table 2).

*Results.*—There were 110 patients with at least 1 operative risk factor, including coronary artery disease in 66% and hypertension in 63%. Coronary artery interventions were performed in 32 patients. There were 29 AAA patients who had concomitant operations, including 6 femoral embolectomies, 4 simultaneous coronary artery bypass grafts (CABGs), 4 cholecystectomies, and 4 splenectomies. Five patients died within 30 days postoperatively, 3 who were CABG inoperable. In 24 patients AAA surgery was performed an average of 2.3 months after CABG. Survival rates were 95% at 6 months, 95% at 1 year, 91% at 2 years, 89% at 3 years, and 85% at 6 years. Patients were followed up for an average of 3.2 years.

*Conclusion.*—Coronary angiography is a valuable tool for diagnosing coronary artery disease. In this study coronary artery revascularization appeared to improve long-term survival after AAA repair.

▶ I disagree with these authors. They followed a program of performing routine coronary arteriography in all patients before elective AAA surgery,

TABLE 2.—Results of Coronary Arteriographies in Patients With Abdominal Aortic Aneurysm

| Result | No. of Cases | PTCA | CABG |
|---|---|---|---|
| Normal coronary arteries | 59 (47%) | — | — |
| Mild to moderate coronary artery lesions | 31 (25%) | 4* | — |
| Severe operable coronary artery lesions | 28 (22%) | — | 28† |
| Inoperable coronary artery disease | 7 (6%) | — | — |

*Procedures were performed 2 or 3 days before surgery for AAA.
†In 4 cases CABG was performed a mean of 2.3 mo before AAA repair.
*Abbreviations: PTCA*, percutaneous transluminal coronary angioplasty; *CABG*, coronary artery bypass grafting; *AAA*, abdominal aortic aneurysm.

and all patients with significant lesions underwent angioplasty or bypass. Despite this, their overall aneurysm operative mortality was a very average 4%. I am surprised to learn they have apparently unlimited health care resources available in Turkey.

## Ruptured Aneurysm

**Ruptured Abdominal Aortic Aneurysms: Who Should be Offered Surgery?**
Hardman DTA, Fisher CM, Patel MI, et al (Royal North Shore Hosp, St Leonards, NSW, Australia)
*J Vasc Surg* 23:123–129, 1996                                    7–6

*Introduction.*—Mortality remains high among patients who undergo surgery for ruptured abdominal aortic aneurysm (RAAA). An increase in the elderly segment of the population and budgetary restraints on health care are factors that may influence the selection of patients for surgical intervention. Admission characteristics predictive of surgical outcome were sought in a retrospective study of patients with RAAA.

*Patients and Methods.*—Between January 1985 and December 1993, 188 patients were admitted to a university teaching hospital with RAAA; 154 underwent surgery and had records available for review. Patients were prepared for operation as soon as RAAA was diagnosed. Surgery was not undertaken in cases of serious comorbidity, patient or guardian refusal, or when the attending surgeon judged the patient unsuitable. Mortality was defined as death resulting from any cause within 30 days of operation or during hospital stay.

*Results.*—Patients who did not undergo surgery had a mean age of 81.1 years, whereas those selected for surgery had a mean age of 71.4 years. Comorbidity was the most common reason for withholding surgical intervention (Table 3). Hospital mortality was 39% for operated patients; 20 did not survive the operation, and 34 died in-hospital. Median survival was 2 hours 10 minutes for 20 of the 21 patients who did not have surgical

TABLE 3.—Reasons for Not Undertaking Operation in 21 Patients With Ruptured Abdominal Aortic Aneurysm

| Indication | No. |
|---|---|
| Patient refused | 4 |
| Comorbidity | 8 |
| Known suprarenal aneurysm* | 3 |
| Ca gallbladder | 1 |
| Cardiac arrest, refractory hypotension | 5 |

* Previously found to be unsuitable for elective reconstruction.
(Courtesy of Hardman DTA, Fisher CM, Patel MI, et al: Ruptured abdominal aneurysms: Who should be offered surgery? *J Vasc Surg* 23:123–129, 1996.)

intervention. Preoperative variables that were significant independent risk factors for mortality were ECG ischemia, loss of consciousness after arrival, age older than 76 years, creatinine level greater than 0.19 mmol/L, and hemoglobin concentration less than 9 g%. The likelihood of survival decreased as the number of risk factors in any individual patient increased. No patient with all 5 risk factors survived. Subsequent mortality for survivors of surgery was particularly high among those in whom acute renal failure developed.

*Conclusion.*—The admission risk factors identified here may help to select patients with RAAA who are likely to benefit from surgery. Patients with none of the 5 significant risk factors had a mortality rate of 16%; a single risk factor more than doubled (37%) this rate. The rate of postoperative deaths, most of which are related to major organ failure, remains high.

▶ This is another study trying to define risk factors for which surgery for RAAA is of no benefit. In this series no patient with 3 or more risk factors survived surgery. There are 2 problems, however. The number of patients in this group was only 8, making the confidence limits huge. Among the 157 patients, 21 were not operated on for various reasons (13%), and selection criteria may always play a role in this important but controversial issue—when to operate for rupture.

**D. Bergqvist, M.D., Ph.D.**

▶ In the managed care future of America, are we indeed going to define certain preoperative ruptured aneurysm patient characteristics, leading us to recommend no surgery? At the present time we do not consider surgery for ruptured aneurysm in patients with severe neurologic impairment before the rupture. This is easy. The more difficult are patients who have serious risk factors but do have at least a slim chance of survival. We do occasionally elect nonoperative treatment in patients with cardiac arrest with successful resuscitation, profound persistent shock, and so forth. I am, however, eager to develop more precise guidelines for this admittedly difficult patient group. As Professor Bergqvist notes, the numbers reported herein are too small to make this study definitive by any stretch.

**J.M. Porter, M.D.**

---

**Effect of the Duration of Symptoms, Transport Time, and Length of Emergency Room Stay on Morbidity and Mortality in Patients With Ruptured Abdominal Aortic Aneurysms**
Farooq MM, Freischlag JA, Seabrook GR, et al (Med College of Wisconsin, Milwaukee)
*Surgery* 119:9–14, 1996                                                 7–7

---

*Background.*—The morbidity and mortality associated with ruptured abdominal aortic aneurysm (AAA) continue to be high. The effect of symptom duration, length of transport time to the hospital, and length of emergency department assessment on outcomes were investigated in a retrospective study.

*Methods and Findings.*—The medical records of 122 consecutive patients treated for ruptured AAA in the past 10 years were reviewed. Twenty-six percent of the patients died intraoperatively. The 30-day mortality was 51%, and the cumulative hospital mortality was 56%. Sixty-four percent of patients with hypotension died compared with 35% of those without hypotension. Eighty-two percent of the 45 patients taken to the operating room within 2 hours of symptom onset had hypotension compared with 60% of those taken to the operating room after 2 hours. Ninety-one percent of the patients receiving CPR and 46% of those not receiving it died. Thirty percent of patients receiving more than 10 units of blood had bowel ischemia compared with 5% of those receiving 10 units or less.

*Conclusion.*—Prolonged presurgical time was correlated with better hemodynamic stability and a lower mortality in the current series of patients with ruptured AAA. A greater blood transfusion requirement indicated progressive bleeding in hemodynamically stable patients. These patients had a higher incidence of ischemic bowel complications, possibly because of splanchnic arterial ischemia augmented by preexisting atherosclerosis and extrinsic compression by mesenteric hematomas.

▶ A few things seem clear concerning ruptured AAA. In the first place, I am convinced that about 90% of patients so afflicted die, most before reaching the hospital. Thus, our perception of a 40% to 50% mortality in this condition is probably completely incorrect, because we are basing this on the number of patients reaching the emergency department alive. I do believe a majority of patients with ruptured aneurysms simply "drop dead" at home and are signed out by the coroner as having had an acute myocardial infarction. The second truism is that patients who take an extremely long time to get to the emergency department have a much better chance of survival than those who reach the emergency department extremely promptly. Dr. Johansen in Seattle showed some years ago that if you have a scoop-and-run program that brings patients into the hospital within minutes of the occurrence of rupture, you are going to have an extraodinarily high hospital mortality, because you are essentially operating on a significant number of dead people. On the other hand, if it takes your patients 24 hours to get to the hospital and they arrive still alive, they clearly represent an extraordinarily preselected cohort destined to do well. As noted in the previous commentary, we need to derive some guidelines we can use in this difficult patient group. Although I believe the history of significant neurologic impairment before rupture should lead to nonoperative treatment, I also believe the need for preoperative CPR is a relative contraindication to operative treatment. I hope we will have some clear guidelines in this difficult area in the future.

## Extracorporeal Shock Wave Lithotripsy Induced Rupture of Abdominal Aortic Aneurysm

Taylor JD, McLoughlin GA, Parsons KF (Royal Liverpool Univ, England)
*Br J Urol* 76:262–263, 1995                                            7–8

*Introduction.*—Extracorporeal shock-wave lithotripsy (ESWL) is frequently used for the treatment of renal and upper ureteric calculi. Although minor renal injury may occur as a result of this procedure, of greater concern is the fragmentation of calcific plaques in associated abdominal aortic aneurysms (AAA), resulting in embolization or rupture. Two cases of ESWL-induced rupture of AAA were described.

> *Case 1.*—Man, 77, with a history of ureteric colic underwent ESWL for fragmentation of a right renal calculi. Forty-eight hours after the procedure, the patient experienced acute, severe right loin pain. A diagnosis of right renal colic was made, and the patient was readmitted. Shortly after admission, the patient became severely hypotensive; later, a ruptured AAA was diagnosed. The patient underwent a successful aneurysmectomy and was discharged 3 weeks after the procedure.
>
> *Case 2.*—Man, 70, underwent ESWL for renal calculi in the left kidney. Twenty-four hours after the procedure, right flank pain developed and the patient was admitted with a diagnosis of right renal colic. The patient was found to have a distended abdomen and was hypotensive. The patient was transferred to the vascular service for resection of a ruptured aneurysm and was discharged 10 days later.

*Discussion.*—In both cases, AAA had been visible on prior abdominal radiographs. Aortic aneurysms have been found on ultrasonography before ESWL in 3% of men aged 65–75 years. A prevalence of 9.5% has been reported after deliberate imaging of the abdominal aorta of male urologic patients. Several factors should be considered before ESWL in patients with calcified AAA, including the distance between the stone and the aneurysm, the position and size of the aneurysm, the degree of calcification of the aneurysm, and patients' symptoms. Consideration should be given to performing resection of the aneurysm, if indicated, before ESWL, considering the mortality associated with ruptured AAA. When ESWL is performed before aneurysmectomy, the procedure should be performed in a unit prepared for aneurysm surgery.

▶ I usually do not include case reports, but I am so intrigued by these 2 that I have included them. Extracorporeal shock-wave lithotripsy continues to be a widely used procedure in this country for the treatment of renal and upper ureteric calculi. An obvious concern is the presence of a calcified AAA where the calcified wall may present an acoustic interface for the shock wave. The 2 patients presented herein, who sustained rupture of an AAA associated with ESWL are of extraordinary interest. Without question, the presence of a calcified AAA suggests great caution in selection of ESWL therapy.

# Abdominal Aortic Aneurysm and Urologic Neoplasm

**Simultaneous Abdominal Aortic Aneurysm Repair and Nephrectomy for Neoplasm**

Galt SW, McCarthy WJ, Pearce WH, et al (Northwestern Univ, Chicago; Columbus Hosp, Chicago)

*Am J Surg* 170:227–230, 1995                                                  7–9

*Background.*—More and more patients are being given concurrently diagnoses of aortic aneurysm and intra-abdominal malignancy. In this situation, the best management approach might be to perform aneurysm resection and nephrectomy at the same time. This simultaneous approach was evaluated in a review of 10 patients.

*Methods.*—Ten patients underwent simultaneous repair of an abdominal aortic aneurysm (AAA) and nephrectomy for renal neoplasm during a 10-year period. Seven patients were being evaluated for AAA when their renal neoplasm was confirmed. Another 2 patients were found to have aneurysms during investigation of hematuria, and 1 had both lesions detected at the same time. Long-term follow-up information was available for all patients.

*Results.*—Both the aneurysm repair and nephrectomy were performed successfully in all patients. The neoplasms were renal cell carcinoma in 6 patients, complex cysts in 2 patients, and hemangiopericytoma and onco-cytoma in 1 patient each. Mean follow-up was 25 months. Four patients died, 3 of causes unrelated to aneurysm or renal neoplasm and 1 of metastatic cancer. No patient experienced graft infection.

*Conclusion.*—For patients with concurrently diagnosed AAA and renal neoplasm, simultaneous aneurysm repair and nephrectomy may be a useful management strategy. This approach can avoid the difficulties and discomfort of having 2 major operations for patients who are good surgical risks and have no evidence of metastases.

▶ There is clearly an association of simultaneous AAA and renal malignancy in a number of patients. Usually the renal malignancy is identified during evaluation of the aneurysm, although occasionally the reverse is true. This report confirms our impression: With care both these lesions can be resected at the same operation. I totally agree with this management.

## Concurrent Abdominal Aortic Aneurysm and Urologic Neoplasm: An Argument for Simultaneous Intervention

Ginsberg DA, Modrall JG, Esrig D, et al (Univ of Southern California, Los Angeles)
*Ann Vasc Surg* 9:428–433, 1995                                          7–10

*Background.*—The surgical management of patients with both a urinary tract neoplasm and an abdominal aortic aneurysm (AAA) can be problematic. The management of patients with an AAA who require urologic surgery for a malignancy was described.

*Methods.*—Twenty-four patients with both an AAA and a urinary tract neoplasm were studied. The mean age of the patients was 65.5 years. The sizes of the AAA were 3.1 to 9.0 cm. The types of urinary neoplasms included transitional cell carcinoma of the bladder and renal pelvis and adenocarcinoma of the prostate. Radical prostatectomy, radical cystoprostatectomy with continent or ileal loop diversion, and radical nephroureterectomy were the surgical procedures performed. In 12 patients, the AAA was resected during the urologic procedure (group 1). In 5 patients the AAA was resected before the urologic procedure (group 2). In 7 patients the aneurysm was left in situ (group 3). The technique for replacing the AAA with a prosthetic aortoiliac graft with an orthotopic neobladder to the urethra was described in detail.

*Results.*—In group 1 all patients except 1 recovered without complications. The patient experienced a postoperative infection from fluid collection anterior to the aortic vascular graft. The fluid was drained, and the patient recovered. In group 2 all patients experienced a complicated ureteral dissection resulting from a retroperitoneal desmoplastic reaction during the urologic procedure. An ileal ureteral reconstruction for obliterative fibrosis of the ureter was later performed in 1 patient. In groups 1 and 2 there were no infectious or mechanical complications of the prothesis at a mean follow-up of 34 months. Eight patients from group 1 and 2 patients from group 2 were still alive. Of those patients who died, 3 died of metastatic disease and 2 died of myocardial infarction. Three patients in group 3 died, and 4 required AAA resection because of an increase in AAA size.

*Conclusion.*—The simultaneous correction of AAA and urologic neoplasm is recommended. This technically superior procedure minimizes perioperative complications and avoids the need for later AAA resection.

▶ See the previous commentary (Abstract 7–9). This report describes 24 patients with concurrent AAA and urinary tract neoplasm. In most of these patients, however, the urinary tract neoplasm was bladder rather than renal. Twelve of these 24 patients underwent simultaneous procedures. The remainder who underwent dyssynchronous procedures had complications with both operations. The authors conclude, and I believe appropriately, that the simultaneous correction of concomitant AAA and urologic neoplasm is both feasible and advisable, a position reached in the paper by Galt and associates as well.

## Miscellaneous Topics

### Aortic Aneurysm in Heart Transplant Recipients

Muluk SC, Steed DL, Makaroun MS, et al (Univ of Pittsburgh, Pa)
*J Vasc Surg* 22:689–696, 1995                                    7–11

*Introduction.*—Survival rates after cardiac transplantation are increasing, with a 1-year survival rate of 90% and a 5-year survival rate of 78%. Recent reports have indicated that cardiac transplant recipients are susceptible to the development of extracardiac surgical disease, in particular aortic aneurysms (AAs). Fewer than 20 cases of aortic aneurysms in cardiac transplant recipients have been reported during the past 18 years. The clinical features of AAs in cardiac transplantation patients were described.

*Methods.*—Medical records of patients who underwent orthotopic heart transplantation were retrospectively reviewed to identify cases with AA. The clinical features of each patient were recorded.

*Results.*—Twelve patients with AA were found out of 734 cardiac transplantation patients. The indication for transplantation was cardiac ischemia in 9 of the 12 patients. Nine patients had infrarenal AAs and 3 had thoracoabdominal AAs. Of the 9 patients with cardiac ischemia as an indication for transplantation, 8 had infrarenal AA, making the risk for infrarenal AA significantly higher for patients who had cardiac ischemia. All patients were asymptomatic at the time of diagnosis; 10 cases were found after transplantation (7 infrarenal AAs and all thoracoabdominal AAs), at a mean of 5 years for infrarenal AA and 2 years for thoracoabdominal AA. Surgery was performed as the initial management in 5 of 9 patients with infrarenal AAs; the mean AA size was 6.7 cm. The remaining 4 patients had been observed with serial imaging; 3 of these patients had significant AA expansion and eventually underwent surgical repair of the AA. All 3 patients with thoracoabdominal AAs died of acute aneurysm rupture. In 7 of the 12 patients, the rate of expansion of the aneurysm ranged from 0 to 2.53 cm per year over 0.9 to 11.7 years; the mean expansion rate per year was 21.5%.

*Conclusion.*—Development of AAs occurred more frequently among cardiac transplant recipients who had ischemic cardiomyopathy. Aortic aneurysms in transplant recipients were found to exhibit a rapid rate of expansion and an aggressive clinical course. When detected in cardiac transplant recipients, all AAs warrant immediate repair or close observation to reduce morbidity and mortality. Because of the higher mortality, thoracoabdominal aneurysms should be aggressively treated.

▶ This and prior studies have shown that the occurrence of AAs is far more likely in heart transplant patients in whom the indication for transplantation was ischemic cardiomyopathy. The generally good results obtained with infrarenal aortic resection in this series have also been noted by others. I am impressed with their serial radiologic data indicating that these aneurysms expanded at a mean rate of 1 cm per year for infrarenal abdominal AAAs, a rate considerably in excess of that expected. Overall the message is clear; heart transplant patients should be carefully screened for the occurrence of abdominal AAs, especially those patients transplanted because of ischemic cardiomyopathy. Similar conclusions have been reached by others.[1]

*Reference*

1. 1993 YEAR BOOK OF VASCULAR SURGERY, p 178.

---

**Subsequent Proximal Aortic Operations in 123 Patients With Previous Infrarenal Abdominal Aortic Aneurysm Surgery**
Coselli JS, LeMaire SA, Büket S, et al (Methodist Hosp, Houston)
*J Vasc Surg* 22:59–67, 1995                                                          7–12

---

*Background.*—Three percent to 8% of patients undergoing operative repair of an infrarenal abdominal aortic aneurysm (AAA) will later have a new aortic aneurysm proximal to the initial lesion. There are questions about the incidence, pathogenesis, and natural history of these subsequent aneurysms. The characteristics and outcomes of a series of patients with proximal aortic aneurysms developing after surgery on a previous infrarenal AAA were reviewed.

*Methods.*—The analysis included 123 patients undergoing surgery for a new proximal aortic aneurysm after previous operation for an infrarenal AAA. When admitted to the hospital, 59% of patients had chest or abdominal pain, 33% were asymptomatic, and 5% had ruptured aneurysms. Three fourths of the subsequent proximal aneurysms involved the thoracoabdominal aorta. Other locations included the juxtarenal abdominal aorta, the descending thoracic aorta, or the transverse aortic arch. More than 80% of the new aneurysms were in continuity with the previously placed prosthetic graft.

Emergency resection and graft placement were performed in patients with signs of impending aneurysmal rupture, whereas surgery was performed on an elective basis for those whose aneurysms measured more than 5.5 cm in diameter. An average of 8 years passed between the first and second operations. Mean aortic clamp time was 40 minutes, and mean visceral ischemic time was 34 minutes.

*Results.*—The second operations had an in-hospital mortality of 12%. Oliguric kidney failure occurred in 11% of patients, and 4% were left with paraplegia (Table 1). The results were better than those previously reported in patients undergoing subsequent proximal aortic operations.

*Conclusion.*—Subsequent proximal aortic aneurysms are common in patients with previous surgery for infrarenal AAA. Patients undergoing AAA replacement should undergo resection of the entire infrarenal aorta,

TABLE 1.—Results of Subsequent Proximal Aortic Operations in 123 Patients With Previous Infrarenal Aortic Aneurysmectomy

| Resected aneurysm | No. of patients | In-hospital deaths | Postoperative paraplegia | Postoperative ORF |
|---|---|---|---|---|
| Thoracoabdominal aorta | 98 | 14 (14.3%) | 5 (5.1%) | 12 (12.2%) |
| Type I | 9* | 2 | 0 | |
| Type II | 25 | 6 | 4 | |
| Type III | 29 | 1 | 0 | |
| Type IV | 35† | 5 | 1 | |
| Juxtarenal abdominal aorta | 17 | 1 (5.9%) | 0 | 1 (5.9%) |
| Transverse aortic arch | 1 | 0 | 0 | 0 |
| Descending thoracic aorta | 7‡ | 0 | 0 | 1 |
| Total | 123 | 15 (12.2%) | 5 (4.1%) | 14 (11.4%) |

*Includes 1 patient with concomitant transverse aortic arch replacement.
†Includes 2 patients with concomitant replacement of separate descending thoracic aortic aneurysm.
‡Includes 1 patient with concomitant distal arch replacement.
*Abbreviation: ORF*, oliguric kidney failure.
(Courtesy of Coselli JS, LeMaire SA, Büket S, Berzin E: Subsequent proximal aortic operations in 123 patients with previous infrarenal abdominal aortic aneurysm surgery. *J Vasc Surg* 22:59–67, 1995.)

followed by biannual monitoring with chest and abdominal CT or MRI scanning. Awareness of the possibility of subsequent proximal aortic aneurysm will facilitate early diagnosis and surgical repair. The subsequent aneurysms can be repaired on an elective or emergency basis with acceptable morbidity and mortality.

▶ The authors conclude that proximal aortic aneurysms that develop after initial infrarenal AAA repair are common, that screening CT scans should be performed biannually after infrarenal AAA repair, and that detected thoraco-abdominal aneurysms should be repaired electively if they are 5.5 cm or more in diameter. Although the Houston surgical results are excellent, I cannot agree with these conclusions. First, the authors' opinion that these aneurysms are "common" is clearly influenced by the referral nature of their practice, which also accounts for the large predominance of thoracoabdominal as opposed to juxtarenal aneurysm in this series. In fact, the development of a new, proximal aortic aneurysm after infrarenal AAA repair is distinctly uncommon. This is not surprising, because these aneurysms developed on average 8 years after AAA repair, and by this time most of these patients have died of other causes. Population-based reports have found that less than 5% of patients require further aortic surgery after infrarenal AAA repair. Thus, it is more accurate to conclude that new, proximal aortic aneurysms are more common only in Houston. This impacts on the authors' recommendation concerning the value of screening CT scans. Given the relatively low incidence of new proximal aneurysms after AAA repair, it is unlikely that biannual CT scans would ever be cost effective. More reasonable would be a single CT scan performed 5–8 years after AAA repair in surviving patients. Finally, the threshold for elective repair of these more complicated aneurysms must be carefully individualized. Even this series reports a 12% operative mortality, with 4% paraplegia overall and a 40% mortality for patients older than 80 years. Because most patients with infrarenal AAAs are in their seventies, and because new aneurysms do not develop for 8 years, the operative mortality for repair of subsequent aneurysms will be excessive in most of these elderly patients. The few younger patients who do require subsequent thoracoabdominal aneurysm repair seem to be reaching Houston, which is fortunate, because it is unlikely that their excellent results can be duplicated in most centers.

**J. Cronenwett, M.D.**

## Medial Neovascularization in Abdominal Aortic Aneurysms: A Histopathologic Marker of Aneurysmal Degeneration With Pathophysiologic Implications

Holmes DR, Liao S, Parks WC, et al (Washington Univ, St Louis)
*J Vasc Surg* 21:761–772, 1995                                         7–13

*Purpose.*—Abdominal aortic aneurysms (AAAs) are almost always associated with aortic atherosclerosis, but the exact relationship between AAA and atherosclerosis is not known. The distribution of aortic wall microvessels in normal aorta, atheroocclusive disease (AOD), and AAA was characterized; the patterns of neovascularity were compared with other cellular and morphologic changes in the aortic wall; and medial neovascularization (MNV) was evaluated to determine whether it is a good histopathologic marker of aneurysmal degeneration.

*Methods.*—Aortic tissue samples from 9 normal organ transplant donors, 10 patients with AOD, and 10 patients with AAAs were stained for elastin determination or processed for immunochemistry. *Ulex europaeus* type I lectin, an endothelial-specific antigen, was used to identify microvascular endothelial cells (ECs), and laminin was used to confirm the specificity of the microvessel-associated EC staining. Light microscopy was used to assess MNV. For each specimen the mean vessel count was determined and the capillary density was recorded as microvessels per high-power field (HPF).

*Results.*—Histochemical staining revealed distinct patterns for each of the 3 types of tissue specimens. Elastic media were entirely intact in 8 of the 10 AOD specimens. However, in 2 of the AOD and all 10 of the AAA specimens, there was partial elastin disruption at the interface between the diseased atherosclerotic intima and the elastic media. The 10 AAA samples were characterized by dense inflammatory infiltrates in the outer aortic wall and mural thrombus. Immunoperoxidase staining for ECs (Fig 2) was evident only along the intact intima and in the adventitial vasa vasorum in normal aorta and was occasionally seen in the diseased intima in AOD specimens, although there was no increase in the density or pattern of EC staining in 8 of 10 AOD specimens. In contrast, in all of the AAA specimens, neovascularization associated with chronic inflammation and destruction of elastin was pronounced in the media and periadventitial areas of the aortic wall. The mean density of MNV was 15-fold higher in AAA compared with normal aorta specimens and 3-fold higher in AAA com-

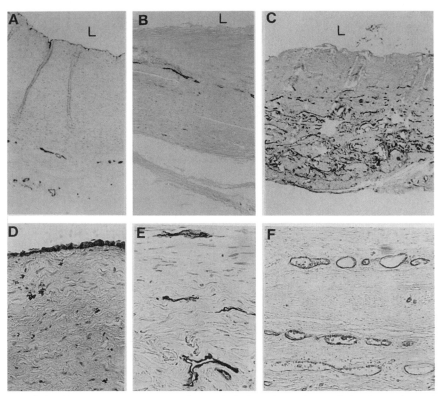

**FIGURE 2.**—Representative sections of normal (**A, D,** and **E**), athero-occlusive disease (**B**), and abdominal aortic aneurysm (**C** and **F**) stained for vascular endothelial cells. Only lumenal endothelial cells (**D**) and adventitial vasa vasorum (**E**) are identified in normal aorta. Mild neovascularization at base of atherosclerotic plaque is occasionally seen in athero-occlusive disease (**B**), whereas dense neovascularization throughout the aortic wall is typical of abdominal aortic aneurysms (**C** and **F**). Immunoperoxidase for *Ulex europaeus* lectin; original magnification ×40 (**A–C**), ×200 (**D–F**). (Courtesy of Holmes DR, Liao S, Parks WC, et al: Medial neovascularization in abdominal aortic aneurysms: A histopathologic marker of aneurysmal degeneration with pathophysiologic implications. *J Vasc Surg* 21:761–772, 1995.)

pared with AOD specimens. A close spatial correlation between neovascularization in the aortic wall and inflammatory infiltration was also noted.

*Conclusion.*—Medial neovascularization is a reliable histopathologic marker of aneurysmal degeneration that correlates with destruction of elastin and chronic inflammation.

▶ Although MNV appears to be associated with AAA formation, I wonder whether it is cause or effect. Perhaps the process of angiogenesis contributes to elastin degradation and chronic inflammation, because the newly formed vessels bring white blood cells to the site. This is an interesting area of speculation.

### Prognosis in Elderly Men With Screening-detected Abdominal Aortic Aneurysm

Ögren M, Bengtsson H, Bergqvist D, et al (Lund Univ, Malmö, Sweden; Akademiska Sjukhuset Uppsala Univ, Sweden)

*Eur J Vasc Endovasc Surg* 11:42–47, 1996                                      7–14

*Background.*—Ultrasound screening for abdominal aortic aneurysm (AAA) in asymptomatic patients is controversial. Men in a cohort study in Sweden (Men born in 1914), which has been in progress since 1969, were invited to undergo ultrasound screening to prospectively study the natural course of symptomless AAA that is so detected.

*Methods.*—Of the 423 74-year-old men enrolled in the study, 343 underwent ultrasound AAA screening. Five-year mortality from all causes was evaluated in relation to the screening and its results. A single, specially trained radiologist performed all screenings. Three men who had previ-

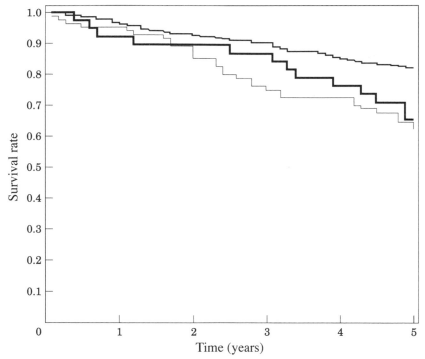

FIGURE 1.—Five-year survival rates in 74-year-old men in relation to participation in ultrasound screening for AAA and to the result of the screening procedure. *Thick bold line* indicates AAA; *thin bold line* indicates no AAA; *thin lightface line* refers to nonparticipants. *Abbreviation: AAA,* abdominal aortic aneurysm. (Reprinted from *Eur J Vasc Endovasc Surg;* vol 11; Ögren M, Bengtsson H, Bergqvist D, et al: Prognosis in elderly men with screening-detected abdominal aortic aneurysm; pp 42–47; Copyright 1996 by permission of the publisher Academic Press Limited, London.)

ously undergone abdominal aortic graft surgery were excluded from the analyses.

*Results.*—Of the 340 participating men with a native aorta, 38 (11%) showed evidence of AAA. Thirteen of these men (one third) had died by the 5-year follow-up. Myocardial infarction was the cause of death in 7 men, stroke in 3. The mortality rate (Fig 1) in men with AAA was double that of men without (80.2/1,000 person-years with AAA vs. 39.4/1,000 person-years without.) Aneurysm surgery was performed on 6 men; surgery did not alter the total mortality rate for these men, although none died of aneurysm rupture. Men not participating in the screening showed the highest mortality rate (91.9/1,000 person-years).

*Conclusion.*—From a public health perspective, screening for early detection and intervention of AAA is of questionable value. General screening does not appear to be cost effective in reducing mortality from aneurysm rupture. Patients with AAA may have widespread atherosclerosis, and survival is limited by occurrence of myocardial infarction and stroke even when aneurysms are repaired.

▶ Here is another report of a screening study for AAA. Of the 343 patients undergoing screening by invitation, aneurysm surgery was required in only 6. The authors noted that the aneurysm population had a much higher mortality than the nonaneurysm population, a finding that is not surprising. The authors' conclusion that screening for early detection and intervention is of questionable value from a public health perspective is probably correct. Other studies have shown that we can significantly increase the yield from screening if we limit ourselves to patients with certain well-defined risk factors, such as symptomatic peripheral atherosclerosis, cigarette smoking, and history of coronary disease.

---

**Role of Physical Examination in Detection of Abdominal Aortic Aneurysms**
Chervu A, Clagett GP, Valentine RJ, et al (Univ of Texas, Dallas)
*Surgery* 117:454–457, 1995                                            7–15

---

*Introduction.*—Nearly 15,000 deaths are attributed to abdominal aortic aneurysms (AAAs) each year. Many of these deaths are the result of a ruptured AAA, which may have been preventable with early detection and surgery. Elective repair of AAA has a mortality rate of less than 5%; however, mortality with surgical repair of ruptured AAA is substantially higher, 80% to 90%. Although a practical means of detecting asymptomatic AAA has not been established, accurate physical examination is an important step in the detection. The use of physical examination in the detection of AAA was evaluated and the factors that precluded detection were identified.

*Methods.*—Medical records of patients who had undergone surgical repair of an infrarenal AAA were retrospectively reviewed. The method of

TABLE 2.—Detection of Abdominal Aortic Aneurysm by Physical
Examination vs. Incidental Radiologic Findings

|  | PE | Radiologic examination |
|---|---|---|
| Number | 93 (38%) | 150 (62%) |
| AAA size (cm) | 5.8 ± 1.6 | 5.5 ± 1.9 |
| Height (cm) | 176.6 ± 8.1 | 176.2 ± 7.9 |
| Weight (kg) | 74.2 ± 13.9 | 81.1 ± 16.4* |
| BMI (kg/m²) | 23.7 ± 3.6 | 26.0 ± 4.6* |

*$P < 0.001$; PE vs. incidental detection of AAAs.
*Abbreviations: PE*, physical examination; *AAA*, abdominal aortic aneurysm; *BMI*, body mass index.
(Courtesy of Chervu A, Clagett GP, Valentine RJ, et al: Role of physical examination in detection of abdominal aortic aneurysms. *Surgery* 117:454–457, 1995.)

diagnosis (whether on physical or radiologic examination), size of aneurysm at time of diagnosis, and whether the aneurysm was palpable before surgery were recorded. Atherosclerotic risk factors, signs of atherosclerosis, and patient characteristics were also noted.

*Results.*—A total of 243 patients who had undergone elective repair of infrarenal AAAs were included in the study. A physical examination had been performed on all patients in the year preceding the detection of the AAA. Physical examination had detected the AAA in 93 of the patients. The diagnosis was confirmed by abdominal ultrasonogram or CT. In the remaining 150 patients, the AAA was an incidental finding on radiologic examination. In the 93 patients in whom the aneurysm was detected initially on physical examination, the mean diameter of the aneurysm was 5.8 cm. This was not significantly different from the mean diameter of the AAA initially detected in the 150 patients by radiologic examination (Table 2). However, the patients whose aneurysms were detected on physical examination weighed significantly less than those whose aneurysms were initially diagnosed by radiologic examination. When examined before surgery, 188 of the 243 patients were reported to have the AAA palpable by physical examination. Of the 150 patients whose AAA was initially detected by radiologic examination, 64 had a palpable AAA on examination before surgery. At the time of surgery, the mean diameter of the palpable AAA was 6.2 cm, significantly larger than the nonpalpable AAA. Patients with palpable AAA also weighed significantly less and had a lower body mass index than patients with nonpalpable AAA. The percentage of AAA detected by residents at the different institutions involved in the study ranged from 23% to 48%; 71% to 88% of these aneurysms were palpable at time of surgery.

*Conclusion.*—Physical examination alone appears to underdiagnose AAAs, especially in obese patients. Proper performance of abdominal physical examinations should improve the detection of AAAs.

▶ In this group of 243 patients with aneurysms, only 38% had been detected by physical examination, whereas the remaining 62% had been found incidentally on radiologic examinations performed for other indications.

Overall at least 23% of these aneurysms were not palpable on physical examnation, even when the diagnosis was known. The authors' conclusion that AAAs are underdiagnosed by physical examination, especially in obese patients, should provoke little controversy. Presently I believe all patients older than 65 years of age, especially men, who have the associated risk factors in the commentary following (Abstract 7–14) should have either a definitive abdominal examination or an ultrasound.

---

**Spinal Cord Injury Increases the Risk of Abdominal Aortic Aneurysm**
Gordon IL, Kohl CA, Arefi M, et al (Univ of California, Irvine; VA Med Ctr, Long Beach, Calif)
*Am Surg* 62:249–252, 1996                                          7–16

---

*Introduction.*—A recent experience suggested an increased prevalence of abdominal aortic aneurysm (AAA) in patients with spinal cord injury (SCI). Patients with SCI were studied to determine whether they had increased rates of aortic enlargement.

*Methods.*—Maximum infrarenal aortic diameters ($AoD_{max}$s) were measured by B-mode ultrasound in 89 patients with SCI (average age, 60.3 years) and 223 age- and sex-matched controls. Race, height, and weight distributions were similar in the 2 groups. Aortic dilation greater than 3 cm was considered as a marker of aneurysmal degeneration.

*Results.*—The average $AoD_{max}$ in patients with SCI was 2.27 compared with 2.07 in controls; the difference was significant. In addition, 20.2% of the patients with SCI had an $AoD_{max}$ 3 cm or more compared with 8.97% of controls; this difference was highly significant. There was a positive correlation between aortic enlargement and smoking history in both SCI and control groups; cigarette consumption was significantly lower among those with $AoD_{max}$s less than 3 cm than those with $AoD_{max}$s 3 cm or more. History of hypertension did not differ between the group with $AoD_{max}$s less than 3 cm and the group with $AoD_{max}$s 3 cm or larger. Average level of spinal injury was more caudad in the SCI patients with AAAs cm or more than those with AAAs less than 3 cm (T6 vs. T8), but this was not significant.

*Discussion.*—Patients with SCI have a twofold risk of aortic enlargement. It appears that the increased risk of aneurysm in the SCI group is a direct effect of the SCI itself rather than a hidden association with an already appreciated risk factor.

▶ I had never before considered the possibility that SCI may have a causative effect on subsequent aortic enlargement. These authors conclude that it does, and I must say their numbers are relatively convincing, although a bit confounded by associated risk factors. At the least, we all should be aware when encountering older SCI patients there is a distinct possibility of an AAA.

## Variability in Measurement of Abdominal Aortic Aneurysms

Lederle FA, Wilson SE, Johnson GR, et al (Veterans Affairs Med Ctr, Minneapolis; Univ of California, Irvine; Veterans Affairs Med Ctr, West Haven, Conn; et al)
*J Vasc Surg* 21:945–952, 1995                                           7–17

*Background.*—The maximum diameter of an asymptomatic abdominal aortic aneurysm (AAA) is usually the main factor considered in deciding whether to perform elective repair. The measurements are performed mainly with ultrasound and CT. The interobserver and intraobserver variability of CT measurements of AAA diameter were evaluated, along with the level of agreement between CT and ultrasound.

*Methods.*—The analysis was performed as part of a multicenter, randomized study of the treatment of small AAAs. Each center's CT measurements were compared with measurements performed on the same scan at a central laboratory. Intraobserver variability was assessed by blinded measurement of a random subset of these scans. Computed tomography and ultrasound measurements made within 1 month of each other were compared for agreement as well.

*Results.*—A total of 806 interobserver pairs of local and central CT measurements were compared. Although 65% of paired measurements showed a difference of no more than 0.2 cm, 17% diverged by 0.5 cm or more. On comparison of 70 intraobserver pairs of CT measurements and remeasurements made at the central laboratory, only 1 pair disagreed by 0.5 cm. Comparison of 258 ultrasound and central CT measurements found a difference of 2 cm or less in 44% of cases and a difference of 0.5 cm or more in 33% of cases. Ultrasound measurements averaged 0.27 cm smaller than the CT measurements made at the central laboratory (Table 1). Measurements made at the participating study centers were likely to be recorded in half-centimeter values.

TABLE 1.—Intraobserver and Interobserver Variability in CT Measurement of Abdominal Aortic Aneurysm and Agreement Between CT and Ultrasound Measurements

| | No. of pairs | Mean difference (cm) | p Value* | Limits of agreement (cm)† |
|---|---|---|---|---|
| Central CT reading 1 vs central CT reading 2 | 70 | 0.003 | NS | 0.31, −0.30 |
| Local CT reading vs central CT reading | 806 | −0.123 | <0.0001 | 0.57, −0.81 |
| Ultrasound vs central CT reading | 258 | −0.267 | <0.0001 | 0.70, −1.24 |
| Ultrasound vs local CT reading‡ | 258 | −0.119 | <0.0001 | 0.70, −0.94 |

*Tests the hypothesis that the mean difference is not different from zero.

†The range within which 95% of the differences would be expected to occur, calculated as the mean difference ± 1.96 times the standard deviation of the differences.

‡These readings were not made blinded to each other.

(Courtesy of Lederle FA, Wilson SE, Johnson GR, et al: Variability in measurement of abdominal aortic aneurysms. *J Vasc Surg* 21:945–952, 1995.)

*Conclusion.*—Computed tomography measurements of AAA diameter can be very precise, but this level of precision may not be achieved in everyday practice. Variability is affected by differences in measurement technique and between imaging modalities. Measurement variations of more than 0.5 cm are a frequent occurrence. Steps that might be taken to address the issue of variation in measurement of AAA diameter include reaching a consensus on the precise definition of AAA diameter, restricting the number of radiologists who perform AAA measurements, and using calipers and magnifying glass to make measurements on CT scans.

▶ Because we routinely make important patient care decisions based on serial measurements of AAAs, it is important to know the agreement between imaging studies. These authors point out quite correctly that differences in aneurysm measurement in excess of 0.5 cm are frequent, and the likelihood of differences based on measurement techniques and machinery must be carefully considered before clinical decisions are made. I applaud this spin-off information from the VA AAA Detection and Management Study.

# 8 Aortoiliac Disease

---

**Exercise Training Improves Functional Status in Patients With Peripheral Arterial Disease**
Regensteiner JG, Steiner JF, Hiatt WR (Univ of Colorado, Denver)
*J Vasc Surg* 23:104–115, 1996                                    8–1

---

*Purpose.*—The benefits of a supervised treadmill training program in patients with moderate to severe intermittent claudication (IC) have previously been demonstrated, but the effects of such programs on functional status during daily activities have not previously been examined. The effects of a treadmill training program, a strength training program, or a combination of both on functional status during activities of daily living in patients with disabling IC were compared in a randomized, controlled trial. The potential benefit of extending the program by another 12 weeks was also examined.

*Patients.*—The study sample was composed of 29 men with disabling IC, of whom 10 were randomized to a 12-week exercise program of supervised treadmill walking, 9 to 12 weeks of strength training of the lower leg muscles, and 10 to a nonexercising control group. The Walking Impairment Questionnaire (WIQ) was used to assess changes in walking ability, the Physical Activity Recall (PAR) was used to measure habitual physical activity levels, and the Medical Outcomes Study questionnaire (MOS SF-20) was used to evaluate functional status. In each group a subset of patients used a Vitalog activity monitor to objectively measure changes in activity attributable to the exercise routine. At the end of the 12-week program, all patients were asked to continue training for another 12 weeks, and 21 of the 29 men agreed to do so.

*Results.*—At the end of the 12-week study, the mean peak walking time had increased by 74% for patients in the treadmill training group and by 30% for patients in the strength training group. Extending the treadmill training program by 12 weeks increased the peak treadmill walking time by an additional 49% for patients originally randomized to treadmill walking and by 54% for patients originally randomized to strength training. The peak treadmill walking time in the control patients had not increased after 12 weeks of observation, but it did increase by 99% when these patients subsequently participated in a 12-week combined walking and strength training program.

*Conclusion.*—A 12-week supervised walking exercise program improves walking ability in patients with disabling IC. Extending the program to 24 weeks increases its effectiveness. Treadmill training alone is more beneficial than strength training or a combination of both in improving functional status in these patients.

▶ Here we have a politically correct paper evaluating patients' functional assessment of improvements associated with exercise training for IC. Using a group of questionnaires, some of which they invented themselves, these authors conclude that walking improves the functional status of claudicants. Furthermore, treadmill training was more effective in improving functional status than was strength training or any combination of training modalities. I have to confess, I still have significant reservations about functional, touchy-feely, politically correct outcome assessment. I like to cite the example of the patient with severe heart disease, lung disease, and arthritis who suddenly experiences acute leg ischemia. You can fix the leg ischemia perfectly and then give a functional assessment test to the patient, and he will accurately note that he still has severe heart disease, lung disease, and arthritis and, in all likelihood will consider himself substantially unimproved by the experience. Clearly, such testing has limits.

---

**Results of Vascular Reconstructions for Atherosclerotic Arterial Occlusive Disease of the Lower Limbs in Young Adults**
van Goor H, Boontje AH (Univ Hosp Groningen, The Netherlands)
*Eur J Vasc Endovasc Surg* 10:323–326, 1995                                      8–2

---

*Introduction.*—Arterial occlusive disease is uncommon in young patients and may be more progressive than in older patients. An aggressive surgical approach has been suggested for younger patients both to limit disability and provide long-term benefits. The early and long-term results of vascular reconstructive surgery in young patients with arterial occlusive disease (AOD) were described.

*Methods.*—Medical records of 1,432 patients who underwent vascular reconstructive surgery for AOD of the aortoiliac or femoropopliteal segments (or both) during a 15-year period were retrospectively reviewed. Twenty-nine of these patients were younger than 40 years of age and fulfilled criteria for admission to the study. Records of these patients were reviewed for morbidity and mortality, additional procedures for failures, other manifestations of atherosclerotic disease, and recurrence of symptoms.

*Results.*—Nine patients died an average of 10 years after the initial surgery, with 77% of deaths related to atherosclerotic disease. Causes of death included myocardial infarction, ruptured aneurysm, and sepsis. Types of reconstructive surgery performed included aortoiliac-femoral (AIF) endarterectomy, AIF bypass (bilateral or unilateral), femoropopliteal bypass (above or below the knee), and femorofemoral bypass, for a total

**TABLE 1.**—Initial Vascular Reconstructions and Failures During Follow-up in 29 Patients

| Type of Reconstruction | (*n*) | Failures <3 Months (*n*) | 3–12 Months (*n*) | 1–3 Years (*n*) | 3–5 Years (*n*) | 5–10 Years (*n*) | Total (*n*) |
|---|---|---|---|---|---|---|---|
| AIF endarterectomy | 13 | | 1 | 3 | 2 | 3 | 9 |
| AIF bypass | | | | | | | |
| Bilateral | 3 | 1 | | 1 | | | 2 |
| Unilateral | 6 | | 1 | | 1 | 1 | 3 |
| FP bypass | | | | | | | |
| Above knee | 6 | 1 | | 1 | | 2 | 4 |
| Below knee | 5 | 1 | 4 | | | | 5 |
| Fem-Fem bypass | 1 | 1 | | | | | 1 |
| Total | 34 | 4 | 6 | 5 | 3 | 6 | 24 |

*Abbreviations:* AIF, aortoiliac-femoral; FP, femoropopliteal; Fem-Fem, femorofemoral.

(Reprinted from *Eur J Vasc Endovasc Surg*; vol 10; van Goor H, Boontje AH: Results of vascular reconstructions for atherosclerotic arterial occlusive disease of the lower limbs in young adults; pp 323–326; Copyright 1995 by permission of the publisher Academic Press Limited, London.)

of 34 procedures (Table 1). Early failures (within 3 months of surgery) occurred after 4 of the procedures in 4 patients. Twenty failures occurred 3 months or longer after the procedure in 17 patients, including all 5 of below-knee femoropopliteal bypasses. Within 10 years of the 34 initial procedures, failures occurred in 24 (71%). During this same period, 22 patients underwent a total of 54 operations for failures or for atherosclerotic disease in different segments of the lower limbs. Amputations were performed in 5 patients. Atherosclerotic disease, manifested most commonly as coronary artery disease or hypertension, developed in 15 of the 29 patients. Of the 20 patients who were still alive at follow-up (mean 12.3 years), only 5 were asymptomatic; 12 had claudication, 1 patient had pain at rest, and 2 had undergone amputations.

*Conclusion.*—A mortality rate of 31% within an average of 10 years of initial surgery was found in this series of patients, substantially higher than that found in the general population. Patients who died had more extensive and progressive atherosclerotic disease, had more cardiovascular disease develop, and had more additional surgeries than patients who survived. Initial surgery failed in 72% of patients, with only 25% of surviving patients asymptomatic at follow-up. These results question the benefits of reconstructive surgery for AOD in younger patients.

▶ These authors define young patients as those younger than 40 years of age, as opposed to the article by the group from Southwestern, who defined young patients as those younger than 49 years (see Abstract 5–21). I believe the age 40 years more accurately defines the clinical group. The authors' conclusion that patients younger than 40 years requiring surgery for occlusive arterial disease have a measurably poorer outcome than patients older than 40 years of age merely confirms the obvious. Their conclusion that vascular surgery for claudication should be undertaken infrequently in patients younger than 40 years of age also appears a restatement of the obvious. Surgery for occlusive disease in young patients should be undertaken only in the most desperate limb salvage situation because of the poor anticipated success of the surgical repair. Clearly symptomatic occlusive atherosclerotic arterial disease manifesting itself in the fourth decade of life is in every way a more virulent beast than that which afflicts patients later in life.

## Comparison of Axillofemoral and Aortofemoral Bypass for Aortoiliac Occlusive Disease

Passman MA, Taylor LM Jr, Moneta GL, et al (Oregon Health Sciences Univ, Portland)
*J Vasc Surg* 23:263–271, 1996                                              8–3

*Background.*—Aortofemoral bypass grafting has a reported 5-year patency rate of 80% or more and is standard treatment for aortoiliac occlusive disease. Axillofemoral bypass grafting is less commonly used because of lower reported patency rates. These rates have recently improved, and 5-year patency rates of more than 70% have been reported. There have been no prospective comparisons of these 2 procedures. Results of aortofemoral bypass grafting and axillofemoral bypass grafting in patients with occlusive disease were compared.

*Methods.*—Choice of procedure was based on surgical risk and surgeon's preference. There were 139 aortofemoral bypass graftings and 108 axillofemoral bypass graftings performed for lower-extremity ischemia resulting from aortoiliac occlusive disease. Results of morbidity, mortality, patency, and limb salvage were analyzed.

*Results.*—Patients who had axillofemoral bypass grafting were older and had a higher incidence of heart disease and surgery for limb salvage. There was no significant difference in operative mortality between the 2 procedures. After aortofemoral bypass grafting, there was a higher rate of major postoperative complications. For aortofemoral bypass grafting, primary patency was 80%, limb salvage was 79%, and survival was 72% at 5 years. For axillofemoral bypass grafting, primary patency was 74%, limb salvage was 89%, and survival was 45% at 5 years. Follow-up was 1 to 83 months. Although patient survival was lower for the axillofemoral procedure, primary patency and limb salvage rates for both procedures were similar.

*Conclusion.*—Patency and limb salvage rates are similar for these 2 procedures when performed in high-risk patients with aortoiliac occlusive disease and limited life expectancy. Axillofemoral bypass grafting should not be avoided because of concerns about patency or limb salvage.

▶ The authors are careful not to claim any superior attributes for axillofemoral bypass grafting, because this was not a randomized trial. But they do fairly claim good results (better than most reported) for this operation, in the range of equivalence to aortofemoral grafts, in carefully selected patients. The important factor is the surgical technique that is restated here; proximal anastomosis very far proximal on the axillary artery, gentle arcing path with no counterincision, very distal-distal anastomosis avoiding zones of "low" flow, and the use of ringed grafts. If one does these things, the results will be duplicated. See also Abstract 10–29.

**W. Abbott, M.D.**

▶ Contrary to widespread belief, kindly old Professor Abbott has actually demonstrated the ability to change his mind.[1]

**J.M. Porter, M.D.**

*Reference*

1. 1996 YEAR BOOK OF VASCULAR SURGERY, p 244.

## Sequential Aortofemoropopliteal/Distal Bypass for Treatment of Critical Lower-limb Ischaemia

Zukauskas G, Ulevicius H, Triponis V (Vilnius Univ, Lithuania; Mubarak Al-Kabeer Hosp, Kuwait)
*Cardiovasc Surg* 3:671–678, 1995                                    8–4

*Objective.*—Multilevel arterial occlusive disease of the lower limbs often results in severe ischemia with ischemic rest pain and tissue loss (Fontaine classification grades III and IV). In a retrospective fashion, a 6-year experience of the treatment of critical lower limb ischemia resulting from multisegmental occlusive arterial disease was reviewed to determine the diagnostic criteria that could help select patients for sequential aortofemoropopliteal/distal reconstruction and to compare the results after simultaneous and 2-stage surgery.

*Management.*—Between 1987 and 1992, 245 sequential aortofemorodistal (popliteal or tibial) procedures were performed for limb salvage in 239 patients with critical limb ischemia Fontaine classification grades III and IV. Two-segment reconstructions were performed in 1 stage in 161 cases (group A): Inflow procedures consisted of 70 aortofemoral, 82 iliofemoral, and 9 extra-anatomical bypasses, and distal procedures included 129 femoropopliteal and 32 femorotibial grafts. In 84 cases (group B), 2 separate operations were performed: 32 aortofemoral, 41 iliofemoral, and 11 extra-anatomical bypasses were performed as the initial inflow procedures, followed within 12 months by 68 femoropopliteal and 16 femorotibial bypass grafts when the inflow procedure failed to relieve critical leg ischemia.

*Outcome.*—The perioperative mortality rates were 3.2% in group A and 5.9% in group B. Limb salvage rates were 95.6% at 1 year and 90.4% at 5 years in group A, and 88.8% at 1 year and 80% at 5 years in group B. The primary inflow graft patency rates were 97.7% at 1 year and 91.3%

at 5 years in group A and were 93.4% at 1 year and 76.3% at 5 years in group B. Cumulative secondary inflow graft patency rates were 98.8% at both 1 and 5 years in group A and 95.3% at 1 year and 88.3% at 5 years in group B. Primary outflow bypass patency rates were 91.% at 1 year and 65.5% at 5 years for group A and 84.9% at 1 year and 59.4% at 5 years for group B. Secondary outflow patency rates were 92.2% at 1 year and 81.8% at 5 years for group A and 86.1% at 1 year and 65.9% at 5 years for group B.

*Conclusion.*—For critical ischemia of the lower limb resulting from multisegmental occlusive arterial disease, perioperative mortality, limb salvage, and primary and secondary inflow and outflow graft patency rates are better after simultaneous aortofemorodistal bypass than after separate 2-stage reconstruction. These findings indicate that a single-stage multi-segment reconstruction is a safe and effective treatment for critical limb ischemia.

▶ The occasional patient with limb ischemia needs simultaneous inflow and outflow procedures. A frequently asked question is just how do we detect such patients? By using the 4-cuff system, we assume that postoperatively the femoral brachial ratio will be 1.0. We then set up the following equation: Femoral artery brachial index (ABI) preoperatively divided by 1 equals ABI preoperatively divided by x (postoperative ABI). This allows a reasonably accurate calculation of the anticipated ABI if one does inflow only. If the calculated ABI is too low, we add a distal bypass to the inflow procedure. This situation occurs almost exclusively in patients who have the combination of severe outflow disease and only moderate inflow disease. Using a 2-team approach, we can accomplish the simultaneous repair in almost the same time it would take to do the inflow repair alone. We continue to find combined inflow/outflow surgery a useful procedure in selected patients (probably about 5% of our limb ischemia population). See also Abstract 10–16.

---

**Evaluation of Dopexamine Hydrochloride as a Renoprotective Agent During Aortic Surgery**
Welch M, Newstead CG, Smyth JV, et al (Manchester Royal Infirmary, England)
*Ann Vasc Surg* 9:488–492, 1995                                            8–5

---

*Introduction.*—Aortic surgery is frequently complicated by the development of renal impairment, caused in part by reduced renal artery blood flow. Dopamine and mannitol have been shown to provide some protection to renal function. A new synthetic catecholamine, dopexamine, has properties similar to dopamine and may provide renal protection during major surgery. The use of dopexamine in preventing renal function impairment after infrarenal aortic surgery was evaluated in a prospective, double-blind trial.

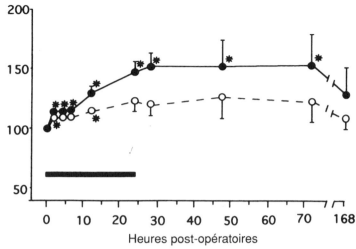

FIGURE 1.—Serum creatinine values as a percentage of the preoperative value (mean and standard error of the mean). The *line with the solid circles* is the placebo group, the *line with the open circles* is the dopexamine-treated group, * the *asterisk* refers to P < 0.001 (paired 2-tailed Student's *t* test comparing each data point with preoperative value), and the bar refers to the duration of dopexamine/placebo infusions. (Courtesy of Welch M, Newstead CG, Smyth JV, et al: Evaluation of dopexamine hydrochloride as a renoprotective agent during aortic surgery. *Ann Vasc Surg* 9[5]:488–492, 1995.)

*Methods.*—Thirty-two patients undergoing elective infrarenal aortic surgery were randomly assigned to treatment with either dopexamine at a rate of 2 M/kg per minute or a placebo (0.9% saline solution). Serum creatinine and 24-hour urinary creatinine values were determined preoperatively; serum and urinary creatinine levels were measured at 2, 4, 6, 12, and 24 hours after cross-clamping of the abdominal aorta, and at 28, 48, and 72 hours and 1 week postoperatively. At 1, 2, 3, and 7 days postoperatively, 24-hour urinary creatinine clearance was also determined. A 30% or greater increase in serum creatinine or decrease in creatinine clearance from preoperative value was considered renal impairment.

*Results.*—The baseline characteristics and surgical course of patients did not differ significantly. Two patients who received dopexamine and 8 patients who received placebo had renal impairment develop. As a group, placebo recipients had significant increases in serum creatinine (given as a percentage increase in serum creatinine) levels over baseline compared with patients given dopexamine therapy. These increases were significant at all time points measured for 3 days postoperatively for placebo; for dopexamine, percentage increases in serum creatinine values were significant only at 2 and 12 hours postoperatively (Fig 1).

*Conclusion.*—Administration of dopexamine during infrarenal aortic surgery was found to provide a significant degree of renal protection. With dopexamine, 13% of patients experienced renal impairment, whereas renal impairment occurred in 47% of patients who received a saline solution placebo. Comparisons of dopexamine with dopamine and mannitol are needed to determine which of these agents would provide optimal renal protection.

▶ An obvious concern with this paper is the volume of fluid received by the 2 groups. Although the article does not make the point clearly, it is my assessment that the saline solution (placebo) group received a very low volume of saline solution, because the authors state they received the same volume as the patients who received the dopexamine. If my suspicions are correct, what the authors are really comparing is pharmacologic diuresis to hypovolemia. Thus, what they have established is the superiority of dopexamine to dehydration. Before I ascribe any importance to this paper, I want to know that the saline-treated patients received adequate volume.

# 9 Visceral Renal Artery Disease

## Mesenteric Arteries

### Mesenteric Artery Bypass: Objective Patency Determination

McMillan WD, McCarthy WJ, Bresticker MR, et al (Northwestern Univ, Chicago)
*J Vasc Surg* 21:729–741, 1995                                    9–1

*Objective.*—Studies on the long-term patency rates after mesenteric revascularization have identified the potential benefits of the procedures in terms of relief of symptoms. The primary patency rates of mesenteric bypass grafting for acute and chronic intestinal ischemia were determined with the use of objective follow-up with mesenteric duplex ultrasound scanning or arteriography.

*Patients.*—Between 1984 and 1994, 25 patients, aged 41–78 years, underwent 38 splanchnic bypass grafts for acute (n = 9) or chronic (n = 16) intestinal ischemia. Twenty-nine grafts used saphenous vein (SVG) as conduit and 9 used polytetrafluoroethylene (PTFE). Twenty-two grafts were restored in a retrograde fashion and 16 in an antegrade fashion. Objective evidence of graft patency was obtained by mesenteric duplex scanning or visceral angiography, and life-table and log rank analysis were used to determine and compare graft patency.

*Outcome.*—The early mortality rate was 12%. Nearly 30% of patients had significant morbidity, particularly among patients undergoing surgery for acute ischemia. Twenty-two survivors with 34 bypass grafts were followed for 1 to 136 months (mean 35 months). Three graft occlusions were revealed by objective testing. None of the patients died of mesenteric infarction, and none required revision of mesenteric revascularization for recurrent symptoms. Compared with objective measures, symptomatic evaluation of patency had a sensitivity for graft occlusion of only 33%. Life-table analysis revealed a primary patency rate of 89% at 72 months (Fig 3), and life-table survival was 75% at 36 months. Patency rates were similar for antegrade and retrograde bypasses (93% vs. 95% at 36 months), for SVG and PTFE bypasses (95% vs. 89% at 36 months), and

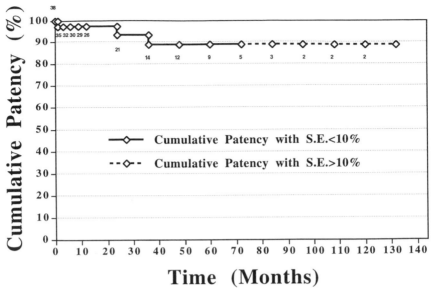

FIGURE 3.—Life-table patency rates for mesenteric bypass grafts. *Solid line,* cumulative patency rates with standard error less than 10%. *Numbers,* grafts at risk at beginning of each interval. (Courtesy of McMillan WD, McCarthy WJ, Bresticker MR, et al: Mesenteric artery bypass: Objective patency determination. *J Vasc Surg* 21:729–741, 1995.)

for patients with acute ischemia and chronic ischemia (92% vs. 88% at 36 months).

*Conclusion.*—Splanchnic bypass for mesenteric ischemia is an extremely durable form of revascularization, with a primary patency rate of 89% at 72 months. Mesenteric duplex scanning provides a safe, noninvasive objective measure of mesenteric bypass patency and represents a significant improvement over symptomatic follow-up of splanchnic reconstruction.

▶ I am surprised these authors state in the introduction that no prior authors objectively measured patency of mesenteric grafts. This is incorrect. Others have assessed the patency of all splanchnic grafts, and this information has been published.[1] I am sorry these authors comingled acute and chronic ischemia, because these are 2 distinctly different patient populations with different anticipated outcomes. As best I can calculate, their objective testing during follow-up revealed 3 patients who had graft occlusion among 22 surviving patients, for a graft failure rate of 14%. On balance, I find little of interest in this paper.

*Reference*

1. Taylor LM, Moneta GM: Intestinal ischemia. *Ann Vasc Surg* 5:403–406, 1991.

## Noninvasive Diagnosis of Mesenteric Ischemia Using a SQUID Magnetometer

Richards WO, Garrard CL, Allos SH, et al (Vanderbilt Univ, Nashville, Tenn; Living State Physics Group, Nashville, Tenn)
*Ann Surg* 221:696–705, 1995                              9–2

*Background.*—In small-bowel ischemia, the best outcome can be achieved if prompt intervention is started before widespread necrosis occurs. At present no noninvasive, sensitive, diagnostic test can detect acute ischemia before smooth muscle necrosis ensues. Previous studies indicate a reduction in frequency and amplitude of small-bowel basic electrical rhythm (BER) within 5–10 minutes of ischemia. In contrast, histopathologic changes in the muscle could not be detected until 60 minutes after the onset of ischemia. Superconducting Quantum Interference Device (SQUID) magnetometers can detect the magnetic fields generated by the electrical current of the smooth muscle of the small intestine. Decreases in BER frequency have been detected in the exteriorized small

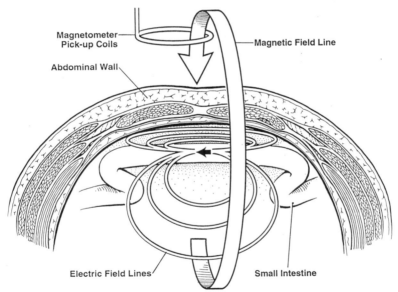

FIGURE 1.—Cross-section of an abdomen illustrating why magnetic fields of the small intestine can be recorded noninvasively in animal and human subjects. The SQUID magnetometers detect the magnetic field generated by the electrical current of the smooth muscle of the small intestine. The magnetic field is relatively insensitive to the alternating layers of insulators present within the abdominal wall (i.e., the peritoneum, preperitoneal fat, fascia, muscles, subcutaneous fat, and skin). The electric field generated by this current flow are, however, greatly attenuated by the alternating layers of insulators present in the abdominal wall. Thus, the electric fields measured by cutaneous electrodes have an extremely low signal/noise ratio. Because the magnetic fields are not attenuated as much by the insulators of the abdominal wall, the signal/noise ratio is much higher than it is for cutaneous electrode recordings. *Abbreviation: SQUID*, Superconducting Quantum Interference Device. (Courtesy of Richards WO, Garrard CL, Allos SH, et al: Noninvasive diagnosis of mesenteric ischemia using a SQUID magnetometer. *Ann Surg* 221:696–705, 1995.)

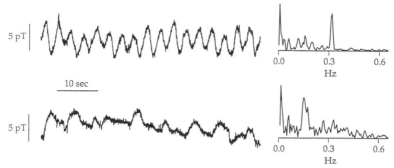

FIGURE 6.—The SQUID magnetometer recordings of intestinal magnetic fields during baseline and then after 20 minutes of superior mesenteric artery occlusion. There is a dramatic shift to lower frequencies in the dominant frequency of the BER as determined by the fast-Fourier transformation. *Abbreviations*: *SQUID*, Superconducting Quantum Interference Device; *BER*, basic electrical rhythm. (Courtesy of Richards WO, Garrard CL, Allos SH, et al: Noninvasive diagnosis of mesenteric ischemia using a SQUID magnetometer. *Ann Surg* 221:696–705, 1995.)

intestine of anesthetized rabbits during mesenteric ischemia. Given the relative insensitivity of magnetic fields to the electrically insulating layers of the fat in the abdominal wall, BER frequency of the small bowel was measured through the intact abdominal wall in a rabbit model using SQUID magnetometers (Fig 1).

*Methods.*—By using the SQUID magnetometer, BER of rabbit ileum was noninvasively measured transabdominally in normal and ischemic conditions. The SQUID recordings were compared with simultaneous recordings of electrical activity obtained with surgically implanted serosal electrodes before, during, and after snare occlusion of the superior mesenteric artery.

*Results.*—The transabdominal SQUID recordings of BER frequency correlated highly with the measurements obtained by the serosal electrodes. The BER decreased significantly from a mean baseline value of 16.4 to 8.3 cpm after 29 minutes of ischemia (Fig 6). With reperfusion of ischemic bowel, BER frequency recovered to a mean value of 14.3 cpm 10 minutes after blood flow was restored. In 10 animals studied, BER decreased by 40% to 50% within 30 minutes of ischemia and returned to normal range within 15 minutes of reperfusion. The ability of the SQUID magnetometer to detect ischemic bowel had a sensitivity of 100%, specificity of 100%, and positive predictive value of 100%.

*Conclusion.*—A SQUID magnetometer can noninvasively and reliably detect mesenteric ischemia in an animal model. Mesenteric ischemia can be detected at an early stage as evidenced by a significant drop in BER frequency. Thus, the SQUID magnetometer can be an extremely useful test for acute mesenteric ischemia. Furthermore, because the study can be performed continuously, intraoperative and postoperative recordings may assist in determining the efficacy of the therapeutic interventions. These positive findings have encouraged the development of clinically useful, noninvasive detection of intestinal magnetic fields using SQUID magnetometers.

▶ Dear ladies and gentlemen, we have a real Rube Goldberg gadget. I'll bet you've never before heard of a "Superconducting Quantum Interference Device magnetometer." For your information, the SQUID detects BER of the bowel. The authors conclude that in rabbits the SQUID device affixed to the abdominal wall is capable of reliably and noninvasively detecting mesenteric ischemia by measuring a significant drop in BER frequency. I am impressed. The next time I encounter a rabbit whom I suspect of having visceral ischemia, I will surely request the use of this device to confirm my suspicions. If the authors can convince us that this device is accurate in humans, it will, of course, represent a significant advance. Although we may hear more about this in the future, that's not the way to bet.

## Renal Arteries

**Safety and Efficacy of Transaortic Renal Endarterectomy as an Adjunct to Aortic Surgery**
Clair DG, Belkin M, Whittemore AD, et al (Malcolm Grow Med Ctr, Andrews AFB, Md; Brigham and Women's Hosp, Boston)
*J Vasc Surg* 21:926–934, 1995                                                            9–3

*Introduction.*—Atherosclerotic renovascular disease (ASRD) is frequently present in patients with atherosclerotic disease of the aortoiliac and infrainguinal arteries. It has been shown to contribute to both hypertension and kidney failure and often progresses to occlusion. For these reasons, an aggressive approach to renal revascularization has been suggested under appropriate circumstances, such as performing renal artery surgery during aortic reconstruction. Transaortic orificial renal endarterectomy (REA) was evaluated as an adjunct to aortic surgery in patients with ASRD.

*Methods.*—Medical records of patients with ASRD who underwent transaortic REA during a 10-year period were retrospectively reviewed. Indications for surgery, operative morbidity and mortality, and technical features of the surgery were recorded and efficacy of the procedures determined.

*Results.*—Forty-three patients with ASRD underwent transaortic REA. Indications for surgical evaluation included ASRD (12 patients), aortic aneurysm (17 patients), aortoiliac occlusive disease (9 patients), or combined aortorenal disease (5 patients). At the time of surgery, infrarenal aortic aneurysms were repaired in 30 patients and symptomatic aortoiliac occlusive disease in 9. Renal revascularization had been performed for hypertension or kidney failure in 41 patients; the remaining 2 patients had asymptomatic disease that was angiographically significant. A transab-

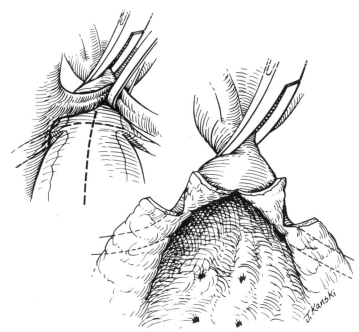

FIGURE 1.—Anterior incision through infrarenal aneurysm between renal arteries to level just distal to clamp below superior mesenteric artery to afford adequate exposure of renal artery orifices for eversion endarterectomy. Left renal vein, renal arteries, and perimesenteric aorta are widely mobilized. (Courtesy of Clair DG, Belkin M, Whittemore AD, et al: Safety and efficacy of transaortic renal endarterectomy as an adjunct to aortic surgery. *J Vasc Surg* 21:926–935, 1995.)

dominal approach was used in 32 patients and a retroperitoneal approach in 11. In patients with aortic disease, a longitudinal opening of the aorta was made and extended proximally between the renal arteries (Fig 1). The endarterectomy was begun near the renal orifice with an incision into the aortic media (Fig 2). Transaortic REA was used on a total of 76 renal arteries; 10 were totally occluded. Of the 76 REAs, 5 required intraoperative revision, with implantation into an aortic graft or bypass from an aortic graft. These revisions were done because of fragility of the renal artery orifices after the procedure or because of inadequate blood flow. Two patients died within 30 days of surgery; cardiac arrest occurred in 1 patient on the first postoperative day and 1 patient died of uncontrolled coagulopathy the day after surgery. Major complications occurred in 6 patients, including renal failure requiring dialysis (2 patients), myocardial infarction (2 patients), sepsis (1 patient), and pneumonia (1 patient). Of the surviving patients, preoperative hypertension resolved in 4 of 36, 26 were improved, and 6 were unchanged. Renal function improved in 5 of 26 patients with preoperative renal dysfunction, remained stable in 15, and worsened in 6. At late follow-up (beyond 30 days of surgery), 5 additional patients died: 2 of multisystem organ failure, 1 of myocardial infarction, 1 of liver cancer, and 1 of unknown causes.

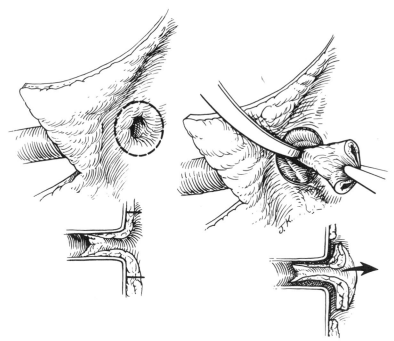

FIGURE 2.—**A,** focused en face and cross-section views demonstrate initiation of localized aortorenal endarterectomy by incision of aortic media around renal artery orifice. Once initiated, contiguous aortic plaque often requires extension of endarterectomy to adjacent aorta. **B,** elevation of aortic button with gentle traction and dissection in medial plane to free renal extension of aortic plaque by circumferential eversion of the renal artery to satisfactory tapered end point. (Courtesy of Clair DG, Belkin M, Whittemore AD, et al: Safety and efficacy of transaortic renal endarterectomy as an adjunct to aortic surgery. *J Vasc Surg* 21:926–935, 1995.)

*Conclusion.*—Transaortic renal endarterectomy was found to be a safe and effective procedure for these patients with combined aortic disease and atherosclerotic renovascular disease. Eighty-three percent of patients were found to have improved control of hypertension and improvement in preexisting renal dysfunction in 19%.

► Although these authors predictably conclude that transaortic REA is safe and effective, I am not so sure. Five of 43 patients (12%) required conversion to bypass procedure because of technical difficulties. Their clinical results were generally satisfactory, with a 30-day mortality of 4.7% and major morbidity of 14%. When we attempt transaortic visceral endarterectomy, we frequently have difficulty with a precise end point in 1 or more visceral arteries. If the plaque does not feather out cleanly, as the expression goes, "you are in deep night soil." Because we have had no recognized difficulty with renal bypass, I have not felt the need to convert to endarterectomy. I believe it to be an acceptable form of therapy, but one that I do not choose.

### Simultaneous Aortic and Renal Artery Reconstruction: Evolution of an Eighteen-year Experience

Cambria RP, Brewster DC, L'Italien G, et al (Massachusetts Gen Hosp, Boston; Harvard Med School, Boston)
J Vasc Surg 21:916–925, 1995                                              9–4

*Introduction.*—Patients who undergo aortic and renal artery construction have varied clinical and functional consequences of the lesions that can focus on aortic disease, renovascular disease, or both. Renovascular disease is found during angiographic evaluation of aortic disease in nearly 30% of patients. Surgical approach to these patients remains controversial. A conservative approach has been advocated, especially in those patients who have a clinically silent renal artery lesion. However, recent studies have found that high-grade renal artery stenosis, particularly those found during evaluation of aortic disease, frequently progress, often with clinical deterioration. The outcome, risks, and experience with patients who underwent simultaneous aortic and renal artery reconstruction were described.

*Methods.*—Medical records from 170 patients who underwent simultaneous abdominal aortic graft and renal artery reconstruction during an 18-year period were retrospectively reviewed. Demographic data, clinical outcomes, and follow-up evaluations were recorded. Surgical technique and clinical variables were better assessed by dividing the 170 patients into 2 cohorts. Group 1 had been treated between 1976 and 1989; group 2 had undergone surgery between 1990 and 1994.

*Results.*—No major differences were noted in patient demographic data between the 2 groups, with the exception of a higher rate of smoking among patients in group 2. However, the clinical profiles of the patients did differ. The incidence of coronary artery disease and associated treatments (coronary artery bypass graft/percutaneous transluminal coronary angioplasty) were significantly higher among patients in group 2, whereas patients in group 1 had a significantly higher incidence of renal dysfunction. However, the patients' clinical manifestation did not differ; 54% of patients were initially evaluated for abdominal aortic aneurysm, 17% for aortoiliac occlusive disease, and 29% for renal disease or combined aortic/ renal artery disease. A unilateral aortorenal prosthetic graft was used for renal reconstruction in 80% of all patients. Bilateral renal artery reconstruction and transaortic endarterectomy were performed significantly more frequently in patients in group 2. A retroperitoneal approach was used in 30% of patients in group 2, whereas this approach was rare in patients in group 1. The operative mortality of patients in group 1 was 9% (9 in 110) compared with 1.7% (1 in 60) for patients in group 2 (Table 3). Major complications occurred in 23.6% of patients in group 2 and in 18.3% of patients in group 1. The rates of renal artery reconstruction failure were similar between the 2 groups (1.8% for group 1 vs. 1.7% for group 2). For all patients, the cumulative 5-year survival rate was 75%.

TABLE 3.—Perioperative Results

| Factor | Group I (n = 110) | | Group II (n = 60) | | p Value |
|---|---|---|---|---|---|
| | No. | % | No. | % | |
| Operative mortality rate | 10 | 9 | 1 | 1.7 | 0.06 |
| Early renal artery reconstruction failure | 2 | 1.8 | 1 | 1.7 | NS |
| Major complications* | 26 | 23.6 | 11 | 18.3 | NS |

\* Includes major cardiac, pulmonary, and renal complications as defined in the original article.
(Courtesy of Cambria RP, Brewster DC, L'Italien G, et al: Simultaneous aortic and renal artery reconstruction: Evolution of an eighteen-year experience. *J Vasc Surg* 21:916–925, 1995.)

Multivariate analyses found a baseline creatinine of 2 mg/dL or greater to be a significant predictor of late mortality.

*Conclusion.*—The mortality rate associated with simultaneous aortic and renal artery reconstruction was found to be within the expected range for aortic surgery alone. Better detection and aggressive treatment of coronary artery disease may be an important factor in this outcome. Patients with asymptomatic renal artery lesions found during evaluation of aortic disease may be candidates for aggressive surgical intervention.

▶ Vascular surgery has reached a sufficient age that a comparison of contemporary and historical results is now popular. It is gratifying that these surgeons have reduced their elective operative mortality for combined aortic and renal reconstruction from 9% to 1.7%. How was this accomplished? The authors attribute this to more aggressive treatment of coronary artery disease in recent years. However, improved patient selection likely had an equally important role, because the authors found that preoperative renal dysfunction was the only significant predictor of perioperative and late death, and they excluded more patients with renal dysfunction in recent years.

The majority of patients in this series were found during a primary evaluation of aortic disease to have renal artery stenosis. Although most of these patients had hypertension, less than half were poorly controlled, which raises the real question of *when* to repair renal artery stenoses in combination with aortic surgery. The authors applied a criteria of 75% or more stenosis and obviously selected their patients carefully, because they employed the combined operation in less than 2% of patients undergoing aortic surgery. Unfortunately, the authors did not compare the results of their combined cases with those patients who had associated renal artery stenosis but who did not undergo renal artery reconstruction. Thus, we cannot be certain whether the addition of renal artery repair increased the survival or prevented dialysis in any of these patients. Although several studies have demonstrated that severe renal artery stenoses tend to progress to occlusion, the functional impact of this natural history in patients with limited life expectancy because of systemic atherosclerosis has yet to be established. Thus, it appears that surgeons who combine aortic and renal reconstructions should carefully select younger patients without preexisting renal dysfunction who have severe stenoses and can be certain that their own operative results are as good as those reported here. In most centers, the addition of renal artery reconstruction to aortic surgery increases mortality substantially, and this likely eliminates any benefit achieved by renal artery repair. It is no secret that excellent results require excellent patient selection. Older or higher-risk patients need evidence that renal artery repair will improve their poorly controlled hypertension for this to be worthwhile.

**J. Cronenwett, M.D.**

▶ As the Baptist preacher would say: Amen, amen, and amen.

**J.M. Porter, M.D.**

**Renal Artery Fibromuscular Dysplasia: Results of Current Surgical Therapy**
Anderson CA, Hansen KJ, Benjamin ME, et al (Wake Forest Univ, Winston-Salem, NC)
*J Vasc Surg* 22:207–216, 1995                                                      9–5

*Background.*—With the advent of potent antihypertensive agents and percutaneous treatment methods, operative intervention for renal artery (RA) fibromuscular dysplasia (FMD) has been reserved for either failure or complications of nonsurgical methods. In addition, the patient demography and variety of RA-FMD submitted to surgery has changed. Hence, current results of surgery for RA-FMD may differ from those of previous reports.

*Objective.*—Data from 40 consecutive adults with hypertension who underwent operative RA repair of FMD between 1987 and 1994 were reviewed retrospectively to describe current surgical management of this condition and to define contemporary clinical characteristics and surgical results in patients older than 21 years.

*Clinical Characteristics.*—More than half (53%) of the patients were older than 45 years (mean age 43.7 years). The mean duration of hypertension was 10.7 years (range 1–58 years), and 39 had hypertension despite medical treatment. By angiographic appearance, RA-FMD was classified as medial fibroplasia in 80%, intimal fibroplasia in 15%, or perimedial dysplasia in 3%; 28 patients had histologic confirmation of RA-FMD. Eight (20%) patients had extrarenal FMD, and 28 (70%) had branch RA-FMD, including RA dissection in 3, RA occlusion in 3, and RA macroaneurysms in 9.

*Management.*—Thirty-four patients underwent unilateral RA procedures and 6 had bilateral procedures. Renal artery reconstruction for FMD included aortorenal bypass with saphenous vein in 35 and polytetrafluoroethylene in 3. Branch RA repair was performed in 28 kidneys, including ex vivo repair in 11.

*Outcome.*—No deaths occurred perioperatively or during a mean follow-up of 29 months. There were 3 (7%) graft occlusions within 30 days

TABLE 2.—Blood Pressure Response to Operation ($n = 40$)

| | | *Preoperative* | | | *Postoperative* | |
|---|---|---|---|---|---|---|
| *Response* | *No. of patients (%)* | *Mean blood pressure (mm Hg) ± SD* | *No. of medications ± SD* | | *Mean blood pressure (mm Hg) ± SD* | *No. of medications ± SD* |
| Cured | 13 (33) | 176.1 ± 28.4/120.3 ± 23.4 | 1.6 ± 0.9 | | 126.2 ± 10.9/80.3 ± 6.9 | 0.0 ± 0.0 |
| Improved | 23 (57) | 197.8 ± 28.1/115.5 ± 18.3 | 2.0 ± 1.0 | | 141.9 ± 17.7/87.8 ± 10.2 | 1.1 ± 0.9 |
| Failed | 4 (10) | 186.7 ± 29.5/102.7 ± 14.2 | 2.0 ± 1.0 | | 150.7 ± 11.0/98.7 ± 10.1 | 1.7 ± 1.1 |

(Courtesy of Anderson CA, Hansen CK, Benjamin ME, et al: Renal artery fibromuscular dysplasia: Results of current surgical therapy. *J Vasc Surg* 22:207–216, 1995.)

of surgery and 3 graft stenoses at 1, 3, and 4 years after surgery. Initially hypertension in 33% of patients was considered cured with diastolic blood pressure of 90 mm Hg or less with no antihypertensive therapy, improved in 57%, and failed in 10 (Table 2). Despite this beneficial blood pressure response, patients older than 45 demonstrated a significantly reduced rate of cure of hypertension than younger adults (Table 4). Overall blood pressure response was not affected by the preoperative duration of hypertension. However, among patients younger than 45, duration of hypertension was significantly less in patients whose conditions were cured after surgery (average 1.7 years) compared with those whose conditions improved or failed (average 9.7 years). Although each early graft failure occurred after branch RA repair, blood pressure response after surgery was not affected by branch RA-FMD or the need for ex vivo repair. Compared with a surgical series 2 decades earlier, patients in the present study were significantly older, with longer preoperative duration of hypertension, and more frequently demonstrated branch RA involvement and extrarenal atherosclerosis. The rate of beneficial blood pressure response was similar during the 2 periods, but the present-day series demonstrated significantly lower cure rate of hypertension.

*Conclusion.*—In most selected patients, a beneficial blood pressure response is currently observed after surgical correction of RA-FMD. How-

TABLE 4.—Correlations Between Blood Pressure Response (Cured vs. Not Cured), Patient Age, and Duration of Hypertension

| *Parameter* | *BP response cured/not cured* | *Mean ± SE* | *Δ Means* | *95% CI (Δ)* | *p Value* |
|---|---|---|---|---|---|
| Patient age (yr., $n = 40$) | 13/27 | 33.9 ± 2.7/48.4 ± 3.4 | −14.5 | (−23.9, −5.1) | < 0.01 |
| Duration hypertension in all patients (yr., $n = 40$) | 13/27 | 5.4 ± 2.6/12.3 ± 2.9 | −6.8 | (−15.9, 2.3) | 0.14 |
| Duration hypertension in patients < 45 years (yr., $n = 19$) | 10/9 | 1.7 ± 0.16/9.7 ± 2.7 | −8.0 | (−14.1, −1.8) | 0.02 |

* Δ, differences of mean values.

(Courtesy of Anderson CA, Hansen CK, Benjamin ME, et al: Renal artery fibromuscular dysplasia: Results of current surgical therapy. *J Vasc Surg* 22:207–216, 1995.)

ever, compared with an earlier surgical experience, contemporary patients undergoing operative repair of RA-FMD differ in many demographic features that lessen their chance for cure of hypertension.

▶ We increasingly turn to the Bowman Gray group for the gospel on renal artery repair. The generally excellent results reported herein are noteworthy.

---

**Renal Artery Anomalies in Patients With Horseshoe or Ectopic Kidneys: The Challenge of Aortic Reconstruction**
de Virgilio C, Gloviczki P, Cherry KJ, et al (Mayo Clinic and Found, Rochester, Minn)
*Cardiovasc Surg* 3:413–420, 1995                                                      9–6

---

*Introduction.*—Renal fusion and ectopia are uncommon anomalies, but they can present special challenges during aortic surgery. A 37-year experience with 21 aortic procedures in 20 patients with horseshoe, pelvic, or crossed fused ectopic kidneys was reviewed to evaluate morbidity and to define optimal management of these anomalies. For the 16 men and 4 women aged 48–82 years, indications for surgery included aortic aneurysm in 16 procedures and aortoiliac occlusive disease in 5 (with renovascular hypertension in 2).

*Diagnosis/Management.*—A horseshoe or ectopic kidney was detected preoperatively in 13 (65%) patients using ultrasonography, IV urography, CT, and arteriography (Table 1). Arteriography revealed multiple or anomalous renal arteries in 9 of 12 (75%) patients. At surgery, 15 (75%) patients had multiple or anomalous renal arteries, including 10 with multiple renal arteries often with an aberrant origin from the lower aorta, aortic bifurcation, or common iliac artery and 5 with normal number of renal arteries but with either an anomalous early isthmic branch or an aberrant origin from the lower aorta or common iliac artery. All 3 patients with pelvic kidneys, the 1 patient with crossed fused ectopic kidney, and 11 of 16 patients with horseshoe kidneys had accessory or anomalous renal arteries.

Surgery involved infrarenal aortic aneurysm repair in 15 instances and thoracoabdominal aneurysm repair in 1. Five patients underwent aortobifemoral bypass for aortoiliac occlusive disease. Six patients required renal artery revascularization, with reimplantation of renal arteries using Carrel patches in 4, transaortic renal endarterectomy in 1, and aortorenal bypass in 1. The renal symphysis was divided in 2 patients.

*Outcome.*—There were no hospital deaths. Six (29%) patients had major complications, including bleeding requiring operation, renal failure requiring short-term dialysis, pancreatitis, gastrointestinal bleeding, pneumonia, and thrombophlebitis. Three (15%) patients had minor complications, including lymphoceles in 2 and transient azotemia in 1.

*Recommendations.*—Aortic reconstruction in the presence of a horseshoe kidney, pelvic, and crossed fused ectopic kidney requires careful

TABLE 1.—Diagnostic Procedures for Renal Fusion and Ectopia

| | No. of examinations | No. positive |
|---|---|---|
| Ultrasonography | | |
| Pelvic kidney | 2 | 0 |
| Horseshoe kidney | 6 | 3 |
| Crossed fused ectopic | 1 | 1 |
| Total | 9 | 4(44) |
| Computed tomography | | |
| Pelvic kidney | 2 | 1 |
| Horseshoe kidney | 3 | 3 |
| Crossed fused ectopic | 0 | |
| Total | 5 | 4(80) |
| Intravenous urography | | |
| Pelvic kidney | 0 | |
| Horseshoe kidney | 8 | 6 |
| Crossed fused ectopic | 0 | |
| Total | 8 | 6(75) |
| Ateriography | | |
| Pelvic kidney | 0 | |
| Horseshoe kidney | 11 | 10 |
| Crossed fused ectopic | 1 | 1 |
| Total | 12 | 11(92) |

*Note:* Values in parentheses are percentages.
(Courtesy of de Virgilio C, Gloviczki P, Cherry KJ, et al: Renal artery anomalies in patients with horseshoe or ectopic kidneys: The challenge of aortic reconstruction. *Cardiovasc Surg* 3:413–420, 1995. Reproduced with permission of *Cardiovasc Surg*; Copyright 1995 American Heart Association.)

planning. Computed tomography is the best noninvasive method to detect these renal anomalies. When they are suspected preoperatively, aortography is recommended to define the frequently associated renal artery anomalies. At surgery, the renal arteries must be identified and preserved, with reimplantation into the aortic graft if necessary. Division of the renal symphysis is rarely required. Although perioperative morbidity is increased, aortic reconstruction in patients with renal fusion or ectopia can be performed safely without increased mortality.

▶ Several truisms apply to horseshoe or ectopic kidneys in association with aortic surgery. The first truism is that you had better learn about the renal anomaly before surgery. This can be accomplished by any of the standard imaging techniques. The second is that you must obtain detailed arteriography to define the renal artery anatomy. Armed with this information, you can usually plan a successful operation. We prefer the extraperitoneal approach for these patients, and in general we do not like to divide the renal isthmus. Many, but not all, of these patients will require renal artery reimplantation or reconstruction, and this can almost always be planned from detailed preoperative studies. If there was ever a group of patients in whom you don't want to be snookered into finding the anomaly only at the time of surgery, this is it. Keep in mind the ureters run anterior to the ectopic renal mass.

### Does Concomitant Aortic Bypass and Renal Artery Revascularization Using the Retroperitoneal Approach Increase Perioperative Risk?

Darling RC III, Shah DM, Chang BB, et al (Albany Med College, NY)
*Cardiovasc Surg* 3:421–423, 1995        9–7

*Background.*—Up to 22% of patients with aortic aneurysmal and occlusive disease also have renal artery disease. Although repair of abdominal aortic aneurysms and aortoiliac occlusive disease is associated with an acceptable mortality rate of 3%, higher perioperative mortality has been reported in combined aortic and renal revascularization. Patients who had aortic procedures alone and those having combined procedures were studied to evaluate mortality and morbidity rates.

*Methods.*—Aortic procedures were performed in 785 patients with aneurysmal and occlusive disease. In 73 of these patients, 77 renal artery revascularizations were also performed. The retroperitoneal approach to the aorta and renal arteries was used. Indications for renal artery revascularization included significant stenosis or anatomical involvement, renovascular hypertension, and renal impairment.

*Results.*—Operative mortality was 2.9% in patients who had an aortic procedure alone and 3% in patients who had combined procedures. In patients who had combined procedures, complications were a stroke, a reexploration for bleeding, 2 cases of pulmonary pneumonia, and 5 cases of elevated serum creatinine levels. Of these, 2 patients died, 2 improved, and 1 had an occluded graft. One patient had early graft thrombosis and 1 had late thrombosis. Follow-up was 2 to 58 months.

*Conclusion.*—The mortality and morbidity rates for aortic bypass combined with renal artery revascularization using the retroperitoneal approach are acceptable. The main technical advantage of this approach is that the suprarenal aorta can be controlled easily and renal revascularization can also be performed easily.

▶ The authors ask the haunting question: Does combining aortic and renovascular surgery increase the operative risk? About 20 previous papers have said yes. These authors, however, describe equally excellent results in both their isolated aortic reconstruction patients and their combined aortic renal reconstruction patients. I conclude that these are superb surgeons deserving adulation.

## Miscellaneous Topics

### The Management of Splenic Artery Aneurysms: Experience With 23 Cases

Mattar SG, Lumsden AB (Emory Univ, Atlanta, Ga)
*Am J Surg* 169:580–584, 1995                                                9–8

*Objective.*—Splenic artery aneurysm (SAA) is a rare but potentially fatal lesion with its risk of rupture and hemorrhage. A 14-year experience on the diagnosis and management of SAAs was reviewed.

*Clinical Features.*—Between 1979 and 1993, 9 men and 14 women aged 10–79 years were diagnosed with SAA. The majority were asymptomatic, 2 had abdominal pain and cardiovascular collapse, and 1 described chronic left hypochondrial pain. Sixteen patients had portal hypertension, including 13 with splenomegaly. Splenic artery aneurysms were identified by angiography in 21 patients, often as part of the preoperative evaluation for treatment of portal hypertension. Nine patients had Doppler ultrasound, and 10 had abdominal CT.

*Management and Outcome.*—A total of 44 SAAs were found. Twelve patients had multiple SAAs, primarily in the distal third of the artery. Seven patients had SAAs greater than 2 cm in diameter. Only 4 patients had calcified SAAs. Two patients with ruptured SAAs underwent emergency aneurysm excision and splenectomy; 1 died. One patient underwent elective SAA excision and splenectomy. Three patients underwent aneurysm ligation, and another was treated with embolization. The remaining 16 asymptomatic patients whose aneurysms were less than 2 cm in diameter were treated expectantly for a mean of 3 years. In 4 patients who had been followed for up to 7 years, none of their SAAs had grown or altered from its quiescent state. There were no documented deaths attributable to SAA in patients treated expectantly; 6 patients died of unrelated causes.

*Recommendations.*—Treatment is indicated for lesions more than 3 cm and lesions in patients younger than 60 if there are no prohibitive factors. The present experience supports active treatment for patients who are symptomatic or those with enlarging SAAs, particularly women anticipating pregnancy or patients undergoing orthotopic liver transplantation. Expectant treatment is recommended for most other patients with SAAs.

▶ Using the time-honored method of retrospective chart review, these authors have identified 23 patients undergoing treatment of 44 SAAs during a 14-year period. Of considerable interest is the observation that 16 of these 23 patients had portal hypertension. Only a few of the 23 patients underwent surgery, because most had aneurysms less than 2 cm in diameter and were treated with observation only. Although it suffers from all of the flaws of a retrospective chart review, there is interesting information here.

### True Aneurysm of the Superior Gluteal Artery: Case Report and Review of the Literature

Schorn B, Reitmeier F, Falk V, et al (Georg-August-Univ of Göttingen, Germany)
*J Vasc Surg* 21:851–854, 1995                                    9–9

*Introduction.*—Pelvic trauma and perforating injuries are the primary causes of rare aneurysms (or pseudoaneurysms) of the superior gluteal artery (SGA). An instance of symptomatic true aneurysm of the SGA in an otherwise healthy man was reported.

*Case Report.*—Man, 43, without history of trauma, reported sciatic pain of 6 weeks' duration radiating from the left buttock into the left leg. Physiotherapy and IM injection of local anesthetics had not improved the symptoms. Physical examination revealed a tender, ill-defined pulsating mass in the left buttock. Ultrasonographically the mass (3 by 4.5 cm) appeared smooth and liquid filled and showed a pulsatile flow with color-coded duplex scanning. A solitary, saccular aneurysm of the SGA (without extravasation of contrast agent) was revealed via selective angiography of the left internal iliac artery. Computed tomography showed that the aneurysm was of extrapelvic origin; no other aneurysms were found. High flow made coil placement for superselective embolization of the feeding artery impossible. For surgery the patient was placed such that a retroperitoneal approach to the left iliac artery would be possible in the event of uncontrolled bleeding. The aneurysm was exposed with a dorsal approach (Fig 3). The aneurysm was 5 cm in diameter and lay close to the sciatic nerve. Small vessels originating from the aneurysm were ligated and separated. The left iliac common artery was temporarily occluded via a balloon catheter placed percutaneously through the ipsilateral femoral artery, and the SGA was clamped. The aneurysm was opened and endoaneurysmorrhaphy performed. Histologic evaluation confirmed typical features of a true arterial arteriosclerotic aneurysm. The patient's symptoms resolved.

*Discussion.*— Therapy is indicated for gluteal artery aneurysm if symptoms arise from displacement of adjacent structures or if risk exists of rupture or sciatic nerve damage. Potential access to the internal iliac artery during surgery is essential, because in the event of bleeding, extrapelvic access may not allow sufficient control of the feeding artery. Complete dissection of the gluteal aneurysm is indicated to provide reliable control and allow safe manipulation around the sciatic nerve. Separating the gluteus maximus muscle from the iliac crest is preferable to transverse

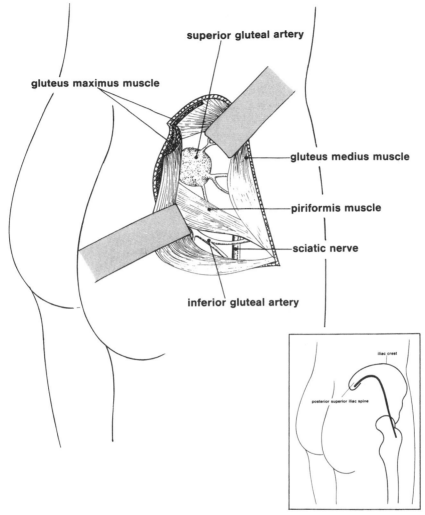

superior gluteal artery

gluteus maximus muscle

gluteus medius muscle

piriformis muscle

sciatic nerve

inferior gluteal artery

iliac crest

posterior superior iliac spine

**FIGURE 3.**—Skin incision was begun at the posterior superior iliac spine, paralleled the first third of the iliac crest, and continued toward the major trochanter. Exposure of the superior gluteal artery was accomplished by reflection of the gluteus maximus and medius muscles after dissection of the gluteus maximus muscle from the iliac crest. (Courtesy of Schorn B, Reitmeier F, Falk V, et al: True aneurysm of the superior gluteal artery: Case report and review of the literature. *J Vasc Surg* 21:851–854, 1995.)

dissection of this muscle. This surgical strategy allowed safe and successful management of the aneurysm.

▶ This case report is included because of its novelty. I have never seen such a patient and, before reading this article, would have had absolutely no idea how to approach this surgically. The very nice illustrations are noteworthy.

# 10 Leg Ischemia

## Graft Surveillance

### The Value of Pre-Discharge Duplex Scanning in Infrainguinal Graft Surveillance

Wilson YG, Davies AH, Currie IC, et al (Bristol Royal Infirmary, England)
*Eur J Vasc Endovasc Surg* 10:237–242, 1995                                    10–1

*Objective.*—There is considerable variation in protocols for duplex-based graft surveillance (GS), and it is not clear how best to detect "at risk" grafts. It is not often recommended that GS begin before discharge from hospital.

*Methods.*—Experience with early color duplex scanning was reviewed in 123 patients entering GS. Patients were initially scanned 1 week after bypass and were restudied at 6 weeks and after 3, 6, 9, and 12 months. Hemodynamic criteria of abnormality included a peak mean flow velocity (PMV) less than 45 cm/sec and focally disordered velocity with a $V_2/V_1$ ratio of 1.5 or greater. A ratio greater than 2 indicates stenosis of about 50% or greater.

*Results.*—Forty-six grafts (37%) were abnormal on initial scanning. Completion studies by arteriography, flow measurement, or both had failed to identify these abnormalities. Six grafts had occluded within 1 week of placement, and 27 had a focal increase in PMV with a mean flow velocity ratio of 2.6. There were 4 arteriovenous fistulas. Eighteen of 40 patients with patent but abnormal grafts were immediately investigated. Twenty-five patients with an abnormal velocity ratio were observed, but 8 of them have required intervention for definitive stenosis, which, on review, usually was causing hemodynamic disturbance within 1 week of surgery. A progressive increase in the flow velocity ratio indicated tightening stenosis in these cases.

*Conclusion.*—Predischarge color duplex scanning is helpful in detecting technical problems with grafts in the lower extremity. Graft abnormalities that may precede definitive stenoses may be detected in this way and closely monitored.

▶ The question posed in this paper is: Just when should the first postoperative lower extremity vein graft surveillance duplex be performed? These authors recommend performing such a study before hospital discharge, a position with which we agree. Both they and we have noted the occasional patient with distinct graft flow abnormalities less than 7 days after graft placement. Such abnormalities have led us to perform repeat arteriography and, on occasion, repeat surgery 6 or 7 days after the initial graft placement. Although one may take the position that there are some things you would rather not know, it actually makes sense to repair the graft before postoperative fibrosis makes repeat surgery extremely difficult if not untenable. I observe that we routinely arteriogram all visceral artery repairs before discharge and again have been surprised on occasion to find a few unsuspected occlusions leading to early repeat surgery. Overall we are obtaining objective duplex or arteriographic documentation of surgical patency in most of our patients before hospital discharge. On balance, I think this is a step forward.

---

### Should All in Situ Saphenous Vein Bypasses Undergo Permanent Duplex Surveillance?

Mohan CR, Hoballah JJ, Schueppert MT, et al (Univ of Iowa, Iowa City)
*Arch Surg* 130:483–488, 1995                                          10–2

---

*Objective.*—A total of 219 patients bearing 245 greater saphenous vein bypasses were examined to learn whether it is appropriate to evaluate pure in situ lower limb bypasses by color duplex surveillance (CDS) for longer than 6 months.

*Methods.*—Color duplex surveillance of the entire bypass and the inflow and outflow arteries was performed at the time of discharge, 1 month later, and then every 3 months for the first year and every 6 months in the second year. Thereafter CDS was done annually. Abnormal findings included a peak systolic velocity less than 45 cm/sec throughout the bypass and a velocity ratio (peak systolic velocity at the site of stenosis divided by that at an adjacent normal bypass segment) greater than 3.

*Results.*—Follow-up data for 6 months or longer were available for 171 bypasses, and the average follow-up of these bypasses was 30 months. At 5 years the primary patency rate was 60% and the secondary patency rate was 89%; the limb salvage rate was 92%. Fifty-four of the 171 bypasses were abnormal on CDS in the first 6 months. Arteriography confirmed abnormalities necessitating endovascular or operative intervention in 37 of 42 cases. Only 2 bypasses that appeared normal on CDS in the first 6 months were occluded or required revision subsequently, compared with 43 of the 54 abnormal bypasses.

*Conclusion.*—Color duplex surveillance for up to 6 months after construction of an in situ bypass in the lower extremity helps detect threatening lesions, but the study is much less productive after this time.

▶ Should duplex graft surveillance beyond 6 months be carried out in patients who are completely normal up to 6 months? This question has been raised by others. Without question, the number of graft abnormalities detected is greatest in the first 6 months. Nonetheless, it is our clear opinion that continued graft surveillance is mandatory. See Abstract 10–3.

---

**Do Normal Early Color-Flow Duplex Surveillance Examination Results of Infrainguinal Vein Grafts Preclude the Need for Late Graft Revision?**
Passman MA, Moneta GL, Nehler MR, et al (Oregon Health Sciences Univ, Portland)
*J Vasc Surg* 22:476–484, 1995                                                                10–3

---

*Background.*—Stenotic lesions in the vein graft and disease progression in the inflow or outflow arteries are the main causes of infrainguinal vein graft failure. Previous research has indicated that almost all vein graft stenoses occur in the first postoperative year. It has been suggested that normal findings on duplex examination during this period eliminate or reduce the need for ongoing graft surveillance. To date the optimal duration of postoperative duplex surveillance has not been adequately established. The color-flow surveillance examinations of patients who had infrainguinal reverse vein graft revisions during 4.5 years were reviewed.

*Methods and Findings.*—Four hundred forty-seven infrainguinal bypass operations were performed at 1 center between January 1990 and July 1994. Abnormal color flow duplex surveillance findings indicated the need for surgical revision in 36 grafts (8.1%). Thirty-one men and 5 women aged 43 to 86 comprised the study group. Initial duplex assessments were performed 2 weeks after graft implantation in 23 patients, between 2 weeks and 3 months in 10, and between 3 and 6 months in 3. Duplex findings indicating the need for revision included a midgraft peak systolic velocity (PSV) of 45 cm/sec or less in 11 patients, a focal PSV of 200 cm/sec or greater in 23, and a PSV between 150 and 200 cm/sec in 1. In another patient, duplex findings suggested occlusion, but angiography subsequently showed this graft to be patent. Initial abnormal duplex findings were documented within 2 weeks of graft implantation in 14% of the patients, between 2 weeks and 3 months in 22%, between 3 and 6 months in 33%, between 6 and 12 months in 17%, and after 1 year in 14%. Midgraft PSVs of 45 cm/sec or less and focal velocities of 200 cm/sec or greater were identified on the initial duplex evaluation in only 25% of the patients needing revision.

*Conclusion.*—Most duplex abnormalities prompting graft revision are found within 1 year of graft implantation but not on the first duplex examination. In the current series, 31% of duplex abnormalities prompting revision were initially found more than 6 months after surgery. Thus, discontinuing graft surveillance based on normal early findings will lead to thrombosis of some otherwise salvageable vein grafts.

▶ See also Abstract 10–2. In our experience, 31% of duplex abnormalities leading to vein graft revision were first detected more than 6 months after operation, and 14% were first detected more than 1 year after operation.[1]

Thus, clearly long-term graft surveillance is not only desirable but mandatory. Under no circumstances should graft surveillance be voluntarily discontinued after 6 or 12 months of normal findings. Early graft flow normality does not convey immortality to the graft.

*Reference*

1. Passman M, Moneta GL, Nehler MR, et al: Do normal early color-flow duplex surveillance examination results of infrainguinal vein grafts preclude the need for late graft revsion? *J Vasc Surg* 22:476–481, 1995.

## Simple Hyperaemia Test as a Screening Method in the Postoperative Surveillance of Infrainguinal *in Situ* Vein Bypasses

Nielsen TG, Sillesen H, Schroeder TV (Univ of Copenhagen)
*Eur J Vasc Endovasc Surg* 10:298–303, 1995                                        10–4

*Background.*—Intermediate failure of infrainguinal vein bypass surgery is most commonly caused by graft stenosis. Ultrasound duplex scanning is the preferred method of identification of failing grafts; however, this technique requires examination of the entire graft in detail and can be time consuming and technically difficult. The results of single-point waveform analysis at rest and during postischemic hyperemia were correlated with the findings of conventional duplex scanning and ankle-brachial index (ABI) measurements to develop a simplified surveillance protocol for infrainguinal vein bypasses.

*Methods.*—Ninety-one in situ vein bypasses were studied to determine the value of 3 Doppler waveform parameters obtained from a single point of the bypass in identifying stenoses. The presence and severity of stenoses assessed by conventional duplex scanning and ABI measurements were correlated with midgraft peak systolic velocity (PSV), pulsatility index (PI), and ratio of hyperemic and resting time-average mean velocities (TAMVs) (TAMV ratio = $TAMV_{hyperemia}/TAMV_{rest}$). Receiver operating characteristics (ROC) analysis was used to determine the optimal value of the waveform parameters in distinguishing stenotic and nonstenotic bypasses.

*Results.*—Significant stenoses were identified in 24 patients when complete duplex scanning of the entire graft revealed an increase in the peak systolic velocity by a factor of 2.5. Discrimination between normal and stenotic bypasses was poor for PSVs less than 55 cm/s and suboptimal for PIs less than or equal to 3.8. The best parameter for identification of graft stenosis was hyperemic response as assessed by TAMV ratio. Twenty-one of 24 lesions were correctly indicated by a TAMV ratio of 2.0 or less, resulting in a sensitivity of 88% and a specificity of 75%. Of the 3 bypasses with evidence of stenosis yet with TAMV ratios greater than 2.0, none failed during follow-up.

*Conclusion.*—Valuable hemodynamic information is provided by a hyperemia test based on Doppler waveform analysis of resting and hyperemic bypass velocity profiles for postoperative surveillance of infrainguinal vein bypasses. This simple technique has value as a screening test in selection of patients who require further analysis with complete duplex imaging of the entire limb.

▶ In an effort to simplify postoperative graft surveillance, these authors have devised a hyperemic screening test. After 2 minutes of manual occlusion of the in situ graft, velocity is measured distal to the point of occlusion. Normal velocity is greater than twice resting velocity. Failure to achieve greater than twice resting velocity indicates the presence of a graft lesion, in this study, with a sensitivity of 88% and a specificity of 75%. Although this may be an accurate observation, I do not identify the need for continually attempting to simplify the life of the vascular laboratory. Certainly an entire vein graft can be easily scanned in a short time. Although you may be able to save 10 minutes using this method, is it really all that helpful? In addition, I have doubts as to whether this method will accurately detect lesions distal to the point of insonation.

---

**Ongoing Vascular Laboratory Surveillance Is Essential to Maximize Long-Term in Situ Saphenous Vein Bypass Patency**
Erickson CA, Towne JB, Seabrook GR, et al (Med College of Wisconsin, Milwaukee; Zablocki V A Med Ctr, Milwaukee, Wis)
*J Vasc Surg* 23:18–27, 1996                                          10–5

---

*Introduction.*—Up to one third of infrainguinal autogenous vein bypass grafts will require intervention during follow-up because of the development of lesions that can lead to graft failure. Some grafts, including those constructed with spliced vein segments and those injured and repaired during the initial procedure, are at increased risk for subsequent problems. The records of a series of patients with autogenous vein grafts were reviewed to quantitate the value of long-term graft surveillance.

*Methods.*—From January 1981 to October 1994, 380 men and 119 women underwent 556 lower extremity autogenous vein bypasses at the study institution. The conduit used was in situ saphenous vein in 97% of cases; critical limb ischemia was the most common indication for grafting. A surveillance protocol for patient monitoring consisted of clinical evaluation and serial noninvasive hemodynamic testing. After initial postoperative studies, patients were evaluated every 3 months during the first 2 years and every 6 months thereafter. Defined abnormal findings included the presence of postoperative arteriovenous fistulas, retained valves, structural abnormalities, and blood flow patterns that suggested 50% to 75% graft diameter reduction.

*Results.*—Cumulative patient survival was 91% after 1 year, 68% after 5 years, and 37% after 10 years. Serial hemodynamic data, available for analysis in 462 grafts, revealed 450 abnormalities in 236 grafts or limbs. Most (65%) occurred within the first 2 years and involved stenosis (37%) or low-flow velocity (22%) (Table 3). With a median patient follow-up of

TABLE 3.—Abnormalities Detected During Surveillance for 462 Saphenous Vein in Situ Bypasses; 1981–1984

| Abnormality | No. of grafts (%) |
|---|---|
| Stenosis (high flow velocity) | 167 (37%) |
| Low flow velocity | 100 (22%) |
| Decreased ABI or TP | 83 (18%) |
| Arteriovenous fistula | 47 (10%) |
| Graft thrombosis | 39 (9%) |
| Retained valve | 7 (1.5%) |
| Aneurysm | 3 (1%) |
| Pseudoaneurysm | 3 (1%) |
| Distal disease | 1 (0.5%) |
| Total | 450 |

*Abbreviations: ABI*, ankle/brachial index; *TP*, toe pressure.
(Courtesy of Erickson CA, Towne JB, Seabrook GR, et al: Ongoing vascular laboratory surveillance is essential to maximize long-term in situ saphenous vein bypass patency. *J Vasc Surg* 23:18–27, 1996.)

35 months, primary patency was lost in 31% of grafts. Fifty of the 169 grafts free of abnormalities at 24 months subsequently developed at least 1 abnormality. Thirty of 67 interventions performed after 24 months involved previously unrevised grafts. The median interval from vascular surgery to detection of an abnormality varied with the location of the defect. Of 556 extremities, 169 required at least 1 intervention after the initial bypass procedure to maintain graft patency or limb viability.

*Conclusion.*—The patency of infrainguinal autogenous vein bypass grafts is at risk even years after the initial procedure. Regular surveillance can identify lesions amenable to revision and ensure the best long-term outcome.

▶ I like studies that support my long-standing biases. If you believe, as I do, that the saphenous vein is the best graft the patient is going to get, you better take care of it. Surveillance seems to be the way to do that, as shown in this paper, as well as other well-conducted studies. The news here is, however, you must continue this practice indefinitely—good advice in spite of cost concerns.

**W. Abbott, M.D.**

▶ See also Abstracts 10–2 and 10–3. Without question leg vein bypass grafts require permanent surveillance.

**J.M. Porter, M.D.**

### Intensive Surveillance of Femoropopliteal-Tibial Autogenous Vein Bypasses Improves Long-Term Graft Patency and Limb Salvage

Bergamini TM, George SM Jr, Massey HT, et al (Univ of Louisville, Ky; VA Med Ctr, Louisville, Ky)
*Ann Surg* 221:507–516, 1995                                              10–6

*Objective.*—The effect of intensive surveillance of autogenous vein bypass on graft patency and limb salvage was evaluated.

*Background.*—In patients with critical ischemia, bypasses from the femoral to the popliteal or tibial arteries can improve limb salvage. Postoperative surveillance of a bypass can improve long-term graft patency and limb salvage because stenotic lesions can be detected and repaired before thrombosis occurs. Duplex scanning is more effective than examination or ankle brachial indices at locating stenoses.

*Methods.*—In 615 patients, autogenous vein bypass was performed; 169 bypasses were to the popliteal artery and 446 were to the tibial artery. The in situ saphenous vein bypass was used in 454 patients. Indications for surgery were ischemia in 507 patients, claudication in 88 patients, and popliteal aneurysm in 20 patients. Surveillance consisted of ankle brachial index and duplex scan with graft velocities measured at 1 month, 3 months, 6 months, and every 6 months thereafter.

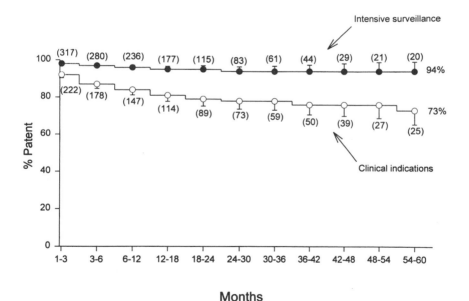

**FIGURE 2.**—Patients with grafts followed by intensive surveillance (*closed circles*) had a significantly higher (P < 0.02) limb salvage rate compared with follow-up by clinically indicated procedures (*open circles*). (Courtesy of Bergamini TM, George SM Jr, Massey HT, et al: Intensive surveillance of femoropopliteal-tibial autogenous vein bypasses improves long-term graft patency and limb salvage. *Ann Surg* 221:507–516, 1995.)

*Results.*—Of the 615 bypasses, 317 had intensive surveillance, 222 had other clinically indicated procedures, and 76 were excluded. At 5 years, primary patency was 56% for bypasses followed by intensive surveillance and 67% for those treated by other procedures. At 5 years, secondary patency was 80% for bypasses followed by intensive surveillance and 67% for those followed by other procedures. At 5 years, limb salvage was 94% for bypasses with intensive surveillance and 73% for those treated by other procedures (Fig 2). At 2 years, secondary patency was 79% for revision of patent bypasses and 55% for thrombosed bypasses.

*Conclusion.*—Intensive surveillance significantly improves the patency of long-term autogenous vein bypass and limb salvage. Intensive surveillance allows graft-threatening lesions to be detected and corrected before thrombosis can occur.

▶ As you may have noted, this year we have a gaggle of papers addressing vein graft surveillance. All authors favor surveillance; most (including all the enlightened ones) favor permanent surveillance, although at decreased intervals as time passes. I note with interest that Dr. Greenhalgh of Charing Cross Hospital has recently questioned the value of graft surveillance, pointing out that there are no relevant prospective randomized studies. Although I believe he is correct, I point out that there are no relevant randomized studies supporting the use of penicillin in pneumococcal pneumonia, and the pivotal study establishing heparin as a valuable treatment for pulmonary embolism randomized only 31 patients. Such is the stuff science is made of.

## Postoperative Edema

### Lymph Drainage and the Development of Post-Reconstructive Leg Oedema Is Not Influenced by the Type of Inguinal Incision: A Prospective Randomised Study in Patients Undergoing Femoropopliteal Bypass Surgery

Haaverstad R, Johnsen H, Sæther OD, et al (Univ Hosp of Trondheim, Norway)
*Eur J Vasc Endovasc Surg* 10:316–322, 1995                    10–7

*Objective.*—The formation of postoperative leg edema after femoropopliteal bypass surgery has been attributed to impaired lymph drainage resulting from intraoperative damage to the lymphatics. Types of groin incision were analyzed in a prospective randomized clinical trial to determine whether the type influences postoperative leg edema formation.

*Patients.*—The patient population consisted of 14 women and 10 men ages 54 to 84, 16 of whom underwent femoropopliteal bypass for intermittent claudication and 8 for critical lower limb ischemia. Of the 24 patients, 12 (group A) were randomized to receive a lateral incision and 12 (group B) to a direct medial incision over the femoral vessels in the groin. The intention of the lateral incision was to avoid lymphatic disruption, whereas no special attention was paid to the lymphatic network when the direct medial incision was used. The increase in leg volume was calculated on day 7 using the formula of a truncated cone, with the contralateral limb serving as control. At approximately 7 days after operation, all patients underwent air plethysmography or color-coded duplex scanning to exclude venous thrombosis and lymphoscintigraphy with technetium-99m–labeled human serum albumin to detect lymphatic lesions.

*Results.*—On day 7 after the bypass operation, the median increase in leg volume was 24.5% in group A and 23.3% in group B (NS). Obstruction of the lymphatics was detected in 5 patients in group A and in 3 patients in group B (NS). However, the increase in leg volume was 31.2% in the 8 patients with obstruction of the lymphatics compared with a 19.6% leg volume increase in the 16 patients in whom no or only minor lymphatic lesions were detected ($P < 0.05$).

*Conclusion.*—The type of groin incision used in patients undergoing femoropopliteal bypass surgery does not prevent lymphatic damage and the formation of postoperative leg edema. However, the higher leg volume increase in patients with lymphatic obstruction suggests that damage to the lymphatics could have a role in the formation of leg edema.

▶ After years of intense meditation, I conclude that post-bypass leg edema has 2 causes. In moderately ischemic patients, I believe the most important cause is lymphatic interruption, incident to surgery, primarily in the groin, although abetted by interruption in the superficial medial knee area. In severely ischemic limbs, I believe edema results in part from reperfusion syndrome, probably related to preexisting ischemic damage to the capillaries. The problem with this article is that the incisions in the groin did not avoid lymphatic damage. In a previous paper where lymphatic damage was actually avoided, less edema resulted.[1] On balance, I have come to accept postoperative limb edema as a normal 1- to 3-month happening after leg bypass surgery. All these people, in my experience, require compressive garments on their lower extremity. We formerly relied almost exclusively on elastic stockings, usually of the 20- to 30-mm gradient variety. However, we have found that a surprising number of old people reject these stockings and refuse to wear them despite maximal threats. In recent years we have found excellent patient acceptance of the new Circ-Aid compressive velcro device. I do recommend Circ-Aid for those of you having trouble getting patients to accept elastic stockings.

*Reference*

1. Porter JM, Lindell TD, Lakin PC: Leg edema following femoropopliteal autogenous vein bypass. *Arch Surg* 105:883–888, 1972.

## Does the Limb Swell After Revascularisation by Percutaneous Transluminal Angioplasty?

Payne SPK, Jones K, Painter D, et al (Univ of Oxford, England; Royal Berkshire Hosp, Reading, England)
*Eur J Vasc Endovasc Surg* 9:272–276, 1995                                                      10–8

*Background.*—After successful revascularization of the lower limb, it often swells. The mechanism of this postoperative swelling is not well understood but is assumed to be caused by either damage to lymphatic drainage vessels or the hyperemic response of revascularized tissue. If limb swelling was due to lymphatic damage, then it should not occur following revasularization by percutaneous transluminal angioplasty (PTA). This was investigated prospectively in 25 patients undergoing PTA for symptomatic occlusive arterial disease of the lower limb.

*Methods.*—The 25 patients had ankle–brachial pressure index (ABPI) and foot volume measurements just before angioplasty, just before discharge, and after 6 days at home to determine whether PTA-induced revascularization was associated with limb swelling.

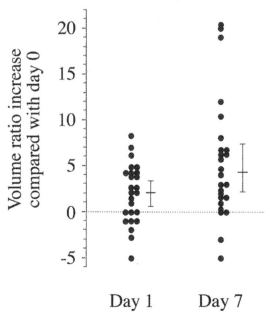

FIGURE 3.—Increase in limb volume after angioplasty. The scattergram shows changes in the ratio of revascularized limb volume to contralateral limb volume compared with preangioplasty. *Bars* depict median values and 95% confidence limits. (Reprinted from *Eur J Vasc Endovasc Surg*; vol 9; Payne SPK, Jones K, Painter D, et al; Does the limb swell after revascularisation by percutaneous transluminal angioplasty?; pp 272–276; 1995; by permission of the publisher Academic Press Limited, London.)

*Results.*—All angioplasties were successful, and all patients reported symptomatic improvement. Revascularization by PTA was associated with a significant increase in the volume of the treated limb, by 2% immediately after angioplasty, and by 4% on the seventh day compared with the contralateral limb (Fig 3).

*Conclusion.*—In 25 patients who underwent successful percutaneous transluminal angioplasty revascularization of a lower limb without damage to the lymphatic drainage system of that limb, significant postoperative swelling occurred. This implies that postoperative limb swelling is a consequence of revascularization, and the use of less invasive revascularization techniques will not eliminate it. Further research should be directed at minimizing the consequences of revascularization injury.

▶ This is an excellent follow-up to the preceding article. Clearly percutaneous transluminal angioplasty should cause minimal, if any, lymphatic disruption. I reach conclusions different from those of the authors. They claim that edema does follow angioplasty, but they measured only a maximum 4% swelling on the seventh day. The authors in the previous paper studying patients after leg bypass surgery found a 23% to 24% increase in volume. Thus, I conclude that only minimal volume changes occurred after angioplasty, compatible with the revascularization phenomenon previously discussed. My interpretation differs from that of the authors.

## Grafts From Alternative Veins

### Results of Bypass to the Popliteal and Tibial Arteries With Alternative Sources of Autogenous Vein

Gentile AT, Lee RW, Moneta GL, et al (Oregon Health Sciences Univ, Portland)
*J Vasc Surg* 23:272–280, 1996                                        10–9

*Background.*—An all-autogenous approach to infrainguinal arterial bypass necessitates many bypasses with alternative autogenous veins (AAVs) because the length of ipsilateral or contralateral greater saphenous vein (GSV) is inadequate. However, concerns have been raised about the durability and efficacy of infrainguinal vein bypasses made of venous conduits other than a single segment of greater saphenous vein (SSGSV). Bypasses with AAVs and GSVs performed between 1980 and 1994 were reviewed.

*Methods.*—The vascular surgical history, vascular disease risk factors, and life-table survival data of patients requiring bypass to popliteal or tibial arteries were compared. Surgical indications, morbidity and mortality, limb salvage rates in patients undergoing surgery for limb-salvage indications, subsequent need for revision, and life-table-assisted primary patency were compared between AAV and SSGSV procedures.

*Findings.*—A total of 919 autogenous vein bypasses were performed to the popliteal or a tibial artery. Twenty percent were done with AAVs, including whole or partial arm vein conduits in 77%. In 61% of the AAVs, vein splicing was required. Mortality among patients undergoing SSGSV passes was 2% and undergoing AAV bypasses was 1%. Because of increased wound complications, the morbidity associated with GSV was higher. Seventy-seven percent of patients with AAV bypass extremities and 20% with SSGSV bypasses had had previous ipsilateral arterial surgery. More AAV bypasses were to a tibial artery than the popliteal artery. Revisions were needed in 12% of SSGSV and 15% of AAV popliteal bypasses. The 5-year assisted primary patencies were 82% for ipsilateral SSGSV, 77% for contralateral SSGSV, and 63% for AAV femoropopliteal bypasses. The respective limb salvage rates were 91%, 86%, and 74%. Revisions were needed in 12% of the SSGSV and in 30% of the AAV tibial bypasses. The 5-year assisted primary patencies were 74% for ipsilateral SSGSV, 82% for contralateral SSGSV, and 72% for AAV femorotibial bypasses. Limb salvage rates were 84%, 92%, and 78%.

*Conclusion.*—When the ipsilateral GSV is unavailable or unsuitable, the use of AAV and contralateral GSV for infrainguinal arterial bypass is clearly justified. The authors' preference is to use the contralateral GSV first. If this is not available, arm veins can be used.

▶ In recent years, 20% of leg bypasses at our institution have been performed with other than ipsilateral or contralateral greater saphenous veins. In a significant majority of these patients, whole or partial arm vein conduits were used. In 61% of this 20%, vein splicing was required. Two thirds of the 20% had undergone prior ipsilateral arterial surgery. The autogenous veins had a diminished 5-year assisted primary patency of 63%, and a 5-year limb salvage of 74%, distinctly less than that of the saphenous vein group. Of special interest is the observation that 30% of the alternate vein conduits required surgical revision during the period of follow-up compared with 12% of single-segment saphenous veins. These differences in conduit behavior are interesting. An appropriate summary appears to be that if one is going to operate on a large number of reoperative patients, alternate vein conduits are going to be required if an all autogenous policy is deemed desirable. Furthermore, if alternate vein conduits are used, careful postoperative graft surveillance is mandatory, because as many as 30% of these patients will develop vein graft defects requiring revision during follow-up.

---

**Results of a Policy With Arm Veins Used as the First Alternative to an Unavailable Ipsilateral Greater Saphenous Vein for Infrainguinal Bypass**
Hölzenbein TJ, Pomposelli FB Jr, Miller A, et al (Harvard Med School, Boston)
*J Vasc Surg* 23:130–140, 1996                                               10–10

---

*Objective.*—In a retrospective review of 250 arm vein grafts, the performance of this graft as the primary alternative to contralateral saphenous vein was assessed in patients without a suitable ipsilateral saphenous vein.

*Patients and Methods.*—Patients consisted of 143 men and 81 women with a mean age of 68.3; 82.6% had diabetes mellitus. Bypass grafts in this

TABLE 3.—Indication for the Use of Arm Veins as an Autogenous
Conduit in 250 Grafts

|  | No. | Percent |
|---|---|---|
| Previous ipsilateral distal bypass* | 144 | 57.6 |
| Previous CABG with ipsilateral saphenous vein | 62 | 24.8 |
| Previous ipsilateral bypass and CABG* | 7 | 2.8 |
| Previous contralateral bypass* | 2 | 0.8 |
| Previous stripping | 12 | 4.8 |
| Saphenous vein unsuitable | 23 | 9.2 |
| Total | 250 | 100 |

*Referring to the extremity where the saphenous vein was used in this particular procedure.
*Abbreviation: CABG*, coronary artery bypass grafting.
(Courtesy of Hölzenbein TJ, Pomposelli FB Jr, Miller A, et al: Results of a policy with arm veins used as the first alternative to an unavailable ipsilateral greater saphenous vein for infrainguinal bypass. *J Vasc Surg* 23:130–140, 1996.)

consecutive series were divided into 3 groups according to indication for operation. Eighty-five grafts were primary, involving patients whose first distal bypass procedure was performed on this extremity. There were 103 repeat grafts in patients who had failure of a previous graft on the same leg. The remaining 62 revision grafts were in patients who had previously undergone a distal arterial reconstructive operation on the ipsilateral leg. Also examined for impact on graft patency were vein configuration and orientation of the vein graft, quality of the vein as assessed by angioscopy, frequency and location of endoluminal disease, and subsequent surgical decisions. Patients were followed for graft patency, limb salvage, and survival.

*Results.*—All but 2 procedures were performed for limb salvage. A total of 114 femorotibial-pedal, 62 jump or interposition, 41 femoropopliteal, and 33 popliteodistal grafts were constructed; 199 grafts were single vein and 51 were composite vein. The cephalic vein alone was the source in 50.4% of cases, the basilic vein alone in 14%, and both cephalic and basilic vein in 35.6%. In 97 grafts (38.8%) the contralateral saphenous vein was an available conduit. Approximately half of the procedures required interventions guided by angioscopy to "upgrade" the graft. The most common indications for use of arm veins were a previous ipsilateral distal bypass and previous coronary artery bypass grafting (CABG) with ipsilateral saphenous vein (Table 3). Early ($\leq$30 days) patency, 94.5% overall, did not differ significantly among anatomic subgroups. At 1 year, cumulative primary patency was 70.6%, secondary patency was 76.9%, and limb salvage was 88.2%. Limb salvage at 3 years was 92.4% for primary grafts, 67.1% for revision grafts, and 79.9% for repeat grafts.

*Conclusion.*—Arm veins are easily accessible and can yield excellent patency rates in patients threatened with loss of the limb and lacking an adequate ipsilateral saphenous vein. It may be necessary to explore the entire arm to find enough suitable vein segments to reach the distal target artery.

▶ These authors have had about the same experience with alternative vein conduits as reported in the previous article. On balance, alternative veins do not appear to function as well as single segment greater saphenous veins, but they certainly appear superior to any available prosthetic.

## Surgical Series

### Critical Limb Ischaemia: Management and Outcome. Report of a National Survey

The Vascular Surgical Society of Great Britain and Ireland (Royal Liverpool Univ, England)

*Eur J Vasc Endovasc Surg* 10:108–113, 1995                    10–11

*Background.*—The prevalence and outcome of critical limb ischemia (CLI) were estimated in a prospective national survey carried out in Great Britain and Ireland in 1993.

*Methods.*—A representative sample of 100 vascular surgeons was randomly selected from a national vascular surgeon registry and stratified according to the number of vascular surgical operations performed annually: group 1, 0 to10; group 2, 11 to 20; group 3, 21 to 30; and group 4, more than 30 infrainguinal reconstructions performed annually.

*Results.*—The extrapolated incidence of CLI was 21,540 in 20,000 patients (1/2,500 annually) (Table 4). Within this group of patients, 30% were diabetic. The overall mortality rate was 13.5% and the amputation rate was 21.5%. The average stay in hospital was 25 days. The majority of patients were offered some form of primary revascularization therapy, with a 75% rate of successful limb salvage. Amputation was associated with significantly higher mortality, longer hospital stay, and greater need for institutional support than revascularization. Surgeons with less annual experience with vascular disease performed significantly more amputations and had lower limb salvage rates than more experienced surgeons. There was no difference in mortality rates for patients treated by these different groups of surgeons.

*Conclusion.*—Critical limb ischemia represents a significant burden on hospital services, which is likely to increase as the population ages. The results of this survey demonstrate that successful limb salvage can be

---

TABLE 4.—Projection of National Workload Relating to Critical Limb Ischemia

| National Projection of Annual Workload | |
|---|---|
| Number patients | 20,000 |
| Number legs | 21,540 |
| Deaths | 2,760 |
| Revascularisations | 12,810 |
| Primary amputation | 3,210 |
| Total amputation | 4,860 |
| Revascularisation: primary amputation ratio | 4 : 1 |

(Reprinted from *Eur J Vasc Endovasc Surg*; vol 10; Harris PL: Critical limb ischemia: Management and outcome. Report of a national survey; pp 108–113; 1995 by permission of the publisher Academic Press Limited, London.)

performed in the majority of cases at significantly lower cost than amputation. It benefits the patient and the community to ensure that vascular surgical sevices are available. It may be advantageous to concentrate the available resources in specialized units, which have more experience and a higher success rate in the treatment of CLI.

▶ This ambitious paper purports to present an estimate of the prevalence of CLI in Great Britain and Ireland, as well as an assessment of the current standard of treatment. This is the result of an audit conducted by the Vascular Surgical Society of Great Britain and Ireland. Some extremely interesting data emerges. The incidence of critical limb ischemia appears to be 1 in 2,500 population per year, and 30% of the affected patients were diabetic. Overall mortality was 13.5%, and amputation rate, 21.5%. Not surprisingly, limb salvage rate achieved by vascular surgeons appeared superior to that achieved by other surgeons. The United Kingdom and Ireland are so homogeneous that studies such as this are actually possible. I believe that in the United States a study such as this would be extremely difficult or impossible.

---

**Critical Limb Ischaemia in Patients Over 80 Years of Age: Options in a District General Hospital**
Humphreys WV, Evans F, Watkin G, et al (Gwynedd Hosp, Bangor, UK; Univ College of North Wales, Cardiff)
*Br J Surg* 82:1361–1363, 1995                                                    10–12

---

*Background.*—As increasing numbers of elderly patients are admitted to general district hospitals with critical limb ischemia (CLI), these hospitals are beginning to perform more revascularization procedures. A comparison was made of the results of amputation and revascularization in elderly patients admitted to a general district hospital with CLI to determine whether this is justified.

*Methods.*—The results of 33 octagenarian patients who underwent primary amputation were compared with those of 82 octagenarian patients who underwent 114 reconstructions for CLI between 1984 and 1994.

*Results.*—The operative survival rate was significantly lower after amputation than after revascularization. Quality of life was little improved in amputees or those whose grafts were not patent but was significantly improved in the 62% with successful revascularizations. The total operative costs were higher for revascularization than for amputation, but this was more than offset by the high costs to the community of postamputation patient care. The total cost of revascularization was £13,546, while the total cost for amputation was £33, 095. The majority of patients who had been able to live in their own home before CLI returned there after revascularization. This was not true after amputation.

*Conclusion.*—Octagenarians with CLI who underwent primary amputation were compared with those who underwent revascularization at a general district hospital. Revascularization improved quality of life and had a substantially lower total cost than amputation when performed in this setting.

▶ These authors have analyzed a subset of CLI patients older than 80 undergoing arterial reconstruction and compared them with similar patients undergoing primary amputations. Not surprisingly, patients who had successful reconstruction had considerably improved quality of life compared with amputation patients and, interestingly, the cost of therapy was about one third that of the total cost of patients undergoing amputation. Considerable information, including some from our own institution,[1] indicates that elderly patients living independently and ambulating before the onset of severe limb ischemia tend to do well after successful reconstruction with a maintenance of independent living and ambulation. We conclude that every effort should be made to reconstruct these patients. On the other hand, patients who are nursing home dependent and nonambulatory before the onset of critical limb ischemia rarely return to either independent living or ambulation. Perhaps a persuasive case could be made for primary amputation in these select patients, but I am not convinced. The only patients in whom we do not attempt reconstruction are patients with permanent profound neurologic impairment.

*Reference*

1. Abou-Zamzam AM: Functional outcome following infrainguinal bypass for limb salvage. *ISCVS Program 1996*, p 68.

---

### Durability of Short Bypasses to Infragenicular Arteries
Shah DM, Darling RC III, Chang BB, et al (Albany Med College, New York)
*Eur J Vasc Endovasc Surg* 10:440–444, 1995                    10–13

---

*Objectives.*—The common femoral artery is traditionally used as the inflow source for distal bypass procedures in patients with limb-threatening ischemia, but the popliteal and tibial arteries are increasingly used in this application because of their durability. A 12-year experience with popliteal and tibial arteries used as alternative inflow sources was reported.

*Patients.*—Between 1981 and 1993, 95 patients with a mean age of 59.6 underwent 106 popliteal or tibial to distal artery bypass operations. The indications for bypass were claudication in 1 patient and limb salvage in the other 105 (99.1%) patients. Although only those whose angiograms showed no significant disease in the proximal arterial system were eligible for distal bypass, proximal disease was suspected at the time of surgery in 22 patients. The below-knee popliteal artery was used in 70 procedures (66.0%), the above-knee popliteal in 15 (14.2%), the anterior tibial in 11 (10.4%), and the posterior tibial in 10 (9.14%) procedures. The main reason for using distal inflow sources in these patients was to conserve autogenous veins. The outflow vessels used included the anterior tibial artery in 21.7%, the posterior tibial in 18.9%, the peroneal in 20.8%, the dorsalis pedis in 36.7%, and the plantar artery in 1.9%.

*Results.*—There were 3 perioperative deaths (2.8%). Major nonfatal complications included nonfatal myocardial infarction (3.8%), stroke (1.9%), and wound edge necrosis or infection (4.7%). The cumulative primary graft patency rate was 90.7% 1 year and 74.9% 2 to 5 years after operation, and the cumulative secondary graft patency rate was 93.8% at 1 year and 82.6% at 2 to 5 years. Five patients required major amputations; 2 of whom because of bypass occlusion and 3 because of persistent nonhealing lesions. The cumulative 5-year mortality rate was 53%. The patency rate was not significantly affected by which inflow or outflow vessel was used for the arterial repair.

*Conclusion.*—The use of popliteal or tibial arteries as alternative inflow sources for arterial bypass operations in patients who do not have significant proximal arterial disease provides excellent long-term patency.

▶ Once again we learn that the most distal unobstructed artery present should be used as the inflow site for leg bypass. I hereby proclaim this principle to be firmly established and in no need of restatement. Does anyone disagree? For boring repetition of established dogma, these authors are awarded the Honorable Mention Camel Dung Award.

---

**Preferential Use of Vein for Above-Knee Femoropopliteal Grafts**
Wilson YG, Wyatt MG, Currie IC, et al (Bristol Royal Infirmary, England)
*Eur J Vasc Endovasc Surg* 10:220–225, 1995                    10–14

---

*Background.*—The use of polytetrafluoroethylene (PTFE) is favored for above-knee grafting by many centers despite long-term inferiority of the prosthetic material. Cited advantages of PTFE include preservation of the vein for subsequent revisions, decreased wound morbidity, and simplification of the surgical procedure. At the study institution, however, vein remains the first choice graft material. Results were reported for 109 patients who underwent above-knee femoropopliteal bypass between 1983 and 1992.

*Patients and Methods.*—Vein grafts were performed in 87 patients with a mean age of 66 and PTFE grafts in 23 patients with a mean age of 71 years. The rates of diabetes mellitus, claudication, and critical ischemia were similar in the 2 groups. The vein graft and PTFE graft groups were compared for primary 3-year graft patency, limb salvage, and survival.

*Results.*—A total of 112 reconstructions were performed on the 109 patients. In cases where vein was absent or inadequate, PTFE was selected for the graft. A 6-mm unsupported prosthesis was used in all 23 patients. The initial failure rate was high in both vein and PTFE groups, and after 3 years of follow-up the difference in patency rates between the 2 groups was not significant. With a median follow-up of 64 months, occlusion had occurred in 31% of vein grafts and 48% of PTFE grafts. Amputation was eventually performed in 9 (32%) occluded vein grafts and in 6 (55%) occluded PTFE grafts. Above-knee amputation was more common in the PTFE group (80%) than in the vein group (20%). Vein was required for only 4 of 17 secondary procedures, and local ipsilateral saphenous vein was used in 2 of these cases.

*Conclusion.*—A number of studies have claimed that the results of PTFE are close enough to those achieved with vein to justify first-line use of PTFE to preserve the vein. Yet in the authors' experience, the consequences of graft failure were more disastrous in the PTFE group than in the vein group. The major amputation rate after failure of a PTFE graft was more than twice that after vein graft failure. Furthermore, preservation of the vein proved not to be an important consideration.

▶ Most people believe that vein is the best conduit for above-knee femoral-popliteal bypass, but the proof is thin. This group shows equivalent patency in a concurrent series, a higher (but not statistically so) need for amputation after PTFE graft failure, and a greater need for above-knee amputation in that group. But this is 112 grafts over 10 years, and nothing about the mode of failure is given. If this paper reflects the fact, it's important. But I'm skeptical.

**W. Abbott, M.D.**

▶ I agree with the authors that veins should be preferentially used, even in the small percentage of patients requiring an above-knee bypass, a position agreed to by almost all right-thinking people. I also agree with Dr. Abbott that this article hardly proves the point. At our institution we have a principle: Do the best operation first.

**J.M. Porter, M.D.**

**Arterial Reconstruction for Limb Salvage: Is the Terminal Peroneal Artery a Disadvantaged Outflow Tract?**
Darling RC III, Shah DM, Chang BB, et al (Albany Med College, NY)
*Surgery* 118:763–767, 1995                                             10–15

*Background.*—Many vascular surgeons avoid the distal peroneal artery for perimalleolar distal anastomosis during limb salvage procedures. The long-term limb salvage and patency rate of a series of distal peroneal artery reconstructions was evaluated to determine the usefulness of this procedure.

*Methods.*—The 2,867 infrainguinal reconstructions performed at 1 institution from 1977 to 1994 were reviewed. Of these, 159 were performed to the distal 5 cm of the peroneal artery. This population was 63% male, 65% diabetic, 64% hypertensive, and 43% smokers. The average age was 73. The in situ saphenous vein bypass was performed in 65%, excised vein bypass in 31%, and prosthetic bypass in 4% of these procedures.

*Results.*—The primary patency rate for distal peroneal bypass was 86% at 30 days, 82% at 1 year, and 69% at 5 years. The secondary patency rate was 90% at 30 days, 86% at 1 year, and 75% at 5 years. The limb salvage rate was 93% at 30 days, 91% at 1 year, and 87% at 5 years. These results were not significantly different from those reported with other perimalleolar bypasses. The mortality and morbidity rates were also similar to those for other bypass procedures.

*Conclusion.*—In this series of bypass patients, distal peroneal artery bypass had acceptable short- and long-term patency rates, excellent limb salvage rates, and acceptable morbidity. Distal peroneal artery bypass is as effective and useful as other perimalleolar bypass procedures for arterial reconstruction and limb salvage.

▶ I officially proclaim that tibial arteries are inherently interchangeable and one should use the least obstructed as the recipient for a bypass graft. The peroneal artery is officially not a disadvantaged outflow. Whoever said it was? Dare I again award another Honorable Mention CDA for sheer repetition?

## Limb-Threatening Ischemia Due to Multilevel Arterial Occlusive Disease: Simultaneous or Staged Inflow/Outflow Revascularization

Harward TRS, Ingegno MD, Carlton L, et al (Univ of Florida, Gainesville)
*Ann Surg* 221:498–506, 1995                    10–16

*Objective.*—The outcome of patients with simultaneous inflow/outflow arterial reconstruction for severe limb-threatening ischemia was reviewed.

*Background.*—Both inflow and outflow bypasses can be needed to salvage a limb in patients with limb-threatening ischemia resulting from severe multilevel arterial occlusive disease. Simultaneous inflow/outflow bypass can be used to avoid the risks associated with separate staged inflow/outflow procedures. The scope of complete revascularization is great, and therefore the morbidity and mortality of simultaneous inflow/outflow bypass may be extreme.

*Methods.*—From a review of medical records of patients who had lower extremity arterial reconstruction, 54 patients who had simultaneous aortoiliac and infrainguinal bypasses were identified. Of these, 24 had significant cardiac disease, 53 had a history of smoking, and 15 had diabetes mellitus. The mean age of patients was 65. Indications for surgery were limb-threatening ischemia in 89% of patients and severe short-distance claudication in 11%.

*Results.*—To correct inflow disease, direct aortoiliac reconstruction was performed in 28 patients, and other extra-anatomical bypasses were performed in 26 patients. Outflow revascularization was achieved by infrainguinal bypass to the infragenicular arteries in 46 patients, profundaplasty in 26 patients, and a composite bypass conduit in 14 patients. At 30 days, limb salvage was 97%, morbidity was 61%, and mortality was 19%. The

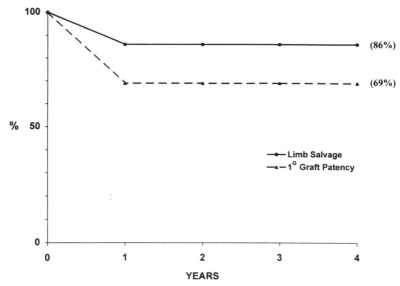

**FIGURE 2.**—Cumulative primary outflow bypass graft patency and limb salvage in limbs undergoing simultaneous inflow/outflow arterial revascularization. (Courtesy of Harward TRS, Ingegno MD, Carlton L, et al: Limb-threatening ischemia due to multilevel arterial occlusive disease: Simultaneous or staged inflow/outflow revascularization. *Ann Surg* 221:498–506, 1995.)

1-year primary patency rate for outflow bypass grafts was 69% (Fig 2). Most complications and deaths occurred in patients who had aortic inflow and complex outflow procedures; in this group, morbidity was 84% and mortality was 47%. In patients with all other inflow/outflow procedures, morbidity was 46% and mortality was 2.9%. Blood loss and operative times were significantly greater for complex procedures.

*Conclusion.*—In patients with severe, multilevel arterial occlusive disease, simultaneous inflow/outflow arterial revascularization is safe and effective. However, when complex outflow procedures are combined with direct aortoiliac reconstruction, a staged procedure is recommended because of the potential for lower morbidity and mortality.

▶ How the authors can conclude from the presented data that simultaneous inflow/outflow arterial revascularisation is safe escapes me. By comparison with other series that they quote, they have shown otherwise, and they give no data of their experience with staged procedures for comparison. Admittedly their patients showed a high incidence of comorbidity, but there is little comfort in a limb salvage rate of 97% if morbidity is 61% and mortality already 19% by 30 days, and presumably still rising. Their message is important that unplanned operations are bad, hemorrhage is bad, and long operations are bad. Careful selection should reduce the need for multilevel reconstruction from the authors' 12% to less than 4%; and if it has to be done, 2 teams of surgeons should share the workload and the responsibility for that decision, particularly in patients suffering from claudication. See also Abstract 8–4.

**A.E.B. Giddings, M.D.**

---

**Femorotibial Bypass for Claudication: Do Results Justify an Aggressive Approach?**
Conte MS, Belkin M, Donaldson MC, et al (Harvard Med School, Boston)
*J Vasc Surg* 21:873–881, 1995                                                10–17

---

*Introduction.*—The role of infrainguinal arterial reconstructive surgery for claudication remains controversial. During the last 16 years, Brigham and Women's Hospital has liberally used femorotibial bypass procedures in a select group of patients with disabling claudication as part of an aggressive approach to limb salvage. A retrospective review of these procedures was conducted to define a role for tibial bypass in the management of severe claudication.

*Patients.*—From 1977 to 1993, 53 patients underwent 57 femorotibial reconstructions for claudication, representing 5% of all infrainguinal vein reconstructions. All reconstructions were performed with autogenous vein conduit, 70% of which involved the greater saphenous vein in situ. Distal anastomoses were constructed to the tibioperoneal trunk in 12%, anterior tibial in 18%, posterior tibial in 47%, and peroneal artery in 23%. Mean follow-up for 45 grafts was 30 months.

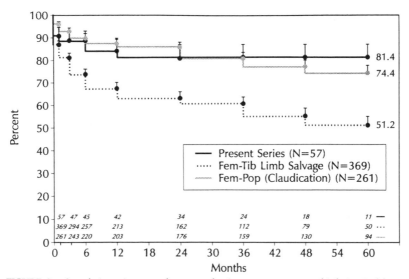

FIGURE 2.—Cumulative primary graft patency for 3 concurrent groups of infrainguinal bypasses (1976–1993). *Abbreviations: Fem-Tib,* femorotibial; *Fem-Pop,* femoropopliteal. (Courtesy of Conte MS, Belkin M, Donaldson MC, et al: Femorotibial bypass for claudication: Do results justify an aggressive approach? *J Vasc Surg* 21:873–881, 1995.)

TABLE 4.—Comparative 5-Year Results of Infrainguinal Vein Bypass, 1976–1993

| | This Series (n = 57 grafts) | FT/LS (n = 369 grafts) | FP/CLAUD (n = 261 grafts) |
|---|---|---|---|
| Survival (%) | 54 ± 15 | 61 ± 4 | 78 ± 3* |
| Limb loss (%) | 0 | 25 ± 2† | 3 ± 1† |
| 1° Patency (%) | 81 ± 6 | 51 ± 4† | 74 ± 3 |
| 2° Patency (%) | 86 ± 5 | 61 ± 4† | 81 ± 3 |
| Cumulative palliation (3 yrs) (%) | 71 ± 9 | — | 78 ± 3 |

*Abbreviations: FT*, femorotibial; *LS*, limb salvage; *FP*, femoropopliteal; *CLAUD*, claudication.
(Courtesy of Conte MS, Belkin M, Donaldson MC, et al: Femorotibial bypass for claudication: Do results justify an aggressive approach? *J Vasc Surg* 21:873–881, 1995.)

*Outcome.*—There were no perioperative deaths, and major complications occurred in 9%. Overall 5-year survival was 54%, and no limbs were lost. At 5 years cumulative primary graft patency was 81% (Fig 2), and secondary graft patency was 86%; and these rates were significantly better than those achieved in a concurrent series of tibial bypasses for limb salvage and equivalent to those achieved with femoropopliteal bypass for claudication (Table 4). Furthermore, cumulative successful palliation at 3 years did not differ significantly from that observed for femoropopliteal bypass for claudication. Follow-up interviews indicated that patients reported improved walking distance, reduced claudication, and high degree of overall satisfaction with their operation.

*Conclusion.*—Patients at low risk who are severely limited by claudication and with available autogenous vein and suitable tibial outflow to the ischemic muscular bed should be considered for revascularization. Femorotibial bypasses performed for claudication have patency rates equivalent to those of femoropopliteal bypass and superior to those obtained for limb salvage.

▶ The authors ask the haunting question: Should one do a tibial bypass for claudication? Over a 16-year period they performed 57 such bypasses without a death and with a 5-year primary patency of 81% and 5-year patient survival of 54%. They accurately conclude that with results this good by all means tibial bypasses should be offered to selected patients for claudication indications. I agree—another pseudosurgical principle laid to rest.

## The Impact of Gender on the Results of Arterial Bypass With in Situ Greater Saphenous Vein

Belkin M, Conte MS, Donaldson MC, et al (Harvard Med School, Boston)
*Am J Surg* 170:97–102, 1995                                                    10–18

*Objective.*—The effect of gender on in situ infrainguinal bypass was evaluated.

*Background.*—Most studies have not addressed the effect of gender on short- and long-term results of infrainguinal bypass surgery. Studies that have addressed the effect of gender on surgical results have reported conflicting findings. By the year 2040, it is estimated that 20% of the population will be older than 65, two thirds of them women. It is also estimated that in the next century, the majority of patients with peripheral vascular disease will be women.

*Methods.*—During a 10-year period, in situ saphenous vein bypass was performed in 244 women and 338 men. The mean patient age was 70.9 years for women and 66.8 years for men. Women had a higher incidence of hypertension than men. Women had a lower incidence of coronary artery disease, history of smoking, and chronic obstructive pulmonary disease. For both men and women, the primary indication for surgery was limb salvage. Bypass to the tibial level was performed in 52.5% of men and 42.2% of women.

*Results.*—Perioperative mortality was lower in women. The incidence of major complications was similar for men and women. The incidence of significant wound complications was higher in women. At 10 years, there were no significant differences between men and women for primary graft patency, secondary patency, limb salvage, or patient survival. Patency rates were slightly lower in women for bypasses to the tibial arteries. The 5-year primary patency rates were slightly lower in women for bypasses performed for limb salvage. Secondary patency rates for bypasses performed for limb salvage were similar for both men and women.

*Conclusion.*—Overall patency, limb salvage, and survival after infrainguinal bypass surgery were the same for men and women. Treatment of infrainguinal occlusive disease should not be based on perceived differences in surgical results in men and women.

▶ This paper shows that if the same people do the same operation for the same indication (30% claudicants) on the same subjects, similar men and similar women will have similar results. It raises intriguing questions about gender-related bias in manifestation, referral, and intervention. Longevity, equity, and a rising proportion of female smokers (at least in England) is likely to increase significantly the demand for vascular services within our lifetime.

**A.E.B. Giddings, M.D.**

▶ I am pleased these authors confirmed our prior report of similar bypass outcome in men and women.[1]

**J.M. Porter, M.D.**

*Reference*

1. Harris EJ, Taylor LM, Moneta GL, et al: Outcome of infrainguinal arterial occlusive disease in women. *J Vasc Surg* 18:627–636, 1993.

## Progression of Atherosclerosis in Arteries Distal to Lower Extremity Revascularizations

McLafferty RB, Moneta GL, Masser PA, et al (Oregon Health Sciences Univ, Portland; Portland Veterans Affairs Hosp, Ore)
*J Vasc Surg* 22:450–456, 1995                10–19

*Objective.*—The progression of atherosclerotic occlusive disease in the lower extremities after revascularization was studied.

*Background.*—Thousands of lower extremity revascularizations are performed every year to treat lower extremity atherosclerosis. Anatomical progression of atherosclerosis has been studied directly only in carotid, coronary, and renal arteries. Almost all studies of progression of lower extremity atherosclerosis have been indirect. Information on progression is needed to properly design studies of treatments for lower extremity atherosclerosis, and to determine the effect of revascularization on progression of arterial disease.

*Methods.*—In 150 patients who underwent revascularization for atherosclerotic occlusive disease, duplex scanning or angiography was performed to determine progression of disease. Presurgical and follow-up arteriograms were compared. The state of superficial femoral and popliteal arteries were classified as 50% stenosis or less, 50% to 99% stenosis, or occluded. Tibial arteries were classified according to continuous visibility

TABLE 2.—Number (Percent) of Arteries With Detectable Progression of Arterial Occlusive Disease in Examinations Performed After Lower Extremity Infrainguinal or Suprainguinal Revascularization

| | Observation Interval | | |
| Groups | 6 months–2 years | 2–4 years | >4 years |
| --- | --- | --- | --- |
| Infrainguinal | | | |
| Group 1 | | | |
| Superficial femoral | 6/23 (26) | 5/12 (41) | 5/9 (56) |
| Popliteal | 5/26 (19) | 3/14 (21) | 3/11 (27) |
| Tibial (Ant. and Post.) | 9/40 (23) | 4/24 (13) | 2/23 (9) |
| Group 4 | | | |
| Tibial (Ant. and Post.) | 9/78 (12) | 8/64 (13) | 23/62 (37) |
| Totals | 29/167 (17) | 20/114 (18) | 33/105 (31) |
| Suprainguinal | | | |
| Group II | | | |
| Superficial femoral | 4/15 (27) | 2/17 (12) | 2/10 (20) |
| Popliteal | 1/16 (6) | 1/20 (5) | 2/15 (13) |
| Tibial (Anterior and Posterior) | 0/24 (0) | 6/40 (15) | 2/15 (13) |
| Group III | | | |
| Superficial femoral | 7/35 (20) | 6/40 (15) | 16/50 (32) |
| Popliteal | 2/16 (7) | 2/40 (5) | 4/41 (4) |
| Tibial (Anterior and Posterior) | 4/62 (6) | 22/80 (28) | 8/88 (9) |
| Totals | 18/182 (10) | 39/237 (16) | 34/219 (16) |

Note: Group I, nonoperated contralateral extremity in a patient with a femoral popliteal bypass; group II, donor extremity in a patient with a femoral to femoral bypass; extremities contralateral to an iliac artery balloon angioplasty; group III, extremities revascularized with a suprainguinal bypass or angioplasty; and group IV, extremities revascularized with a femoral popliteal bypass.

(Courtesy of McLafferty RB, Moneta GL, Masser PA, et al: Progression of atherosclerosis in arteries distal to lower extremity revascularizations. *J Vasc Surg* 22:450–456, 1995.)

from the popliteal trifurcation to the ankle. Progression was defined as increase in 1 category of stenosis.

*Results.*—There was progression of atherosclerotic occlusive disease in 18% of native arteries, 39% of extremities, and 52% of patients at a mean follow-up of 4.8 years. Overall progression was seen in 21% of arteries in patients who had infrainguinal bypass and 14% of arteries in patients who had suprainguinal bypass (Table 2). Progression was noted more often in examinations done 4 years or more after baseline arteriography than in those done 6 months to 2 years or 2 to 4 years after baseline arteriography. Progression was noted in 30% of superficial femoral arteries; 32% of these with 50% stenosis or greater became occluded. Superficial femoral, popliteal, and tibial artery progression was similar in revascularized and nonrevascularized extremities after suprainguinal bypass. Tibial artery progression was similar in operated and nonoperated limbs after femoropopliteal artery bypass.

*Conclusion.*—Progression of atherosclerotic occlusive disease is common in patients requiring revascularization. Progression is more common in patients requiring femoropopliteal artery bypass than suprainguinal bypass. Progression of atherosclerotic occlusive disease in patients who have vascular surgery is associated with lower extremity ischemia but is not adversely affected by arterial reconstruction.

▶ We need much more data coming from studies such as this to best be able to direct our shrinking resources to patient groups who really need treatment by virtue of knowing they are destined to need it.

**W. Abbott, M.D.**

## Miscellaneous Topics

### Exercise Rehabilitation Programs for the Treatment of Claudication Pain: A Meta-Analysis

Gardner AW, Poehlman ET (Univ of Maryland, Baltimore; Baltimore Veterans Affairs Med Ctr, Md)

*JAMA* 274:975–980, 1995                                                      10–20

*Introduction.*—Intermittent claudication occurs at an annual incidence of 20 per 1,000 individuals 65 years or older. Disabling symptoms are expected to occur in 1.3 million elderly individuals every 2 years over the next 50 years. Treatment for claudication consists of drug therapy, which is expensive and minimally effective, and surgery, which has risks of cardiovascular complications. Exercise rehabilitation is a noninvasive, inexpensive, and effective method of treating symptoms of intermittent claudication. Components of exercise rehabilitation programs most effective in providing improvements in claudication pain symptoms were identified in a meta-analysis.

*Methods.*—A search of English language literature was conducted to locate published studies on exercise rehabilitation programs for patients with intermittent claudication. To be considered for inclusion, studies had to use treadmill testing before and after an exercise program as part of the assessment. Studies were excluded if times or distances walked before onset of pain and maximal pain were not reported. Duration and mode of exercise, program length, pain end point used during the exercise session, and level of supervision were recorded for each study. Patient characteristics, walking times and distances to onset of pain, and treadmill protocol intensity were also recorded.

*Results.*—Twenty-one studies met the criteria for study inclusion; 18 were noncontrolled and nonrandomized and 3 were randomized trials. For the 18 noncontrolled trials, mean duration of exercise was 39.1 minutes per session (3.1 sessions per week) and mean duration of program length was 21.8 weeks. For the randomized trials, mean duration of exercise was 30 minutes per session (3 sessions per week) for 30.3 weeks. In the nonrandomized trials, a significant increase from baseline in the distance walked to onset of pain was noted, as was a significant increase in the distance to maximal pain. For the randomized trials, patients in exercise groups also experienced significant increases in distance to onset of pain and to onset of maximal pain compared with control patients. Individual components of the exercise programs were evaluated for their independent effects on claudication pain. Exercise duration of 30 minutes or longer, exercise frequency of 3 sessions or more per week, programs 26 weeks or longer, walking as the exercise used, and near-maximal pain as an end point for each training session were each found to result in significantly greater improvements in distance to onset of pain and distance to maximal pain. A large percentage of the variance observed in increases in distance to onset and to maximal pain could be explained by use of pain as an end point during exercise, program length, or type of exercise used. Age was found to correlate with improvement, with older patients experiencing greater increases compared with younger patients.

*Conclusion.*—Participation in exercise rehabilitation programs resulted in increases of 120% to 180% in distance to onset and to maximal claudication pain in patients with peripheral vascular disease. Use of near-maximal pain as an end point during exercise sessions, program duration of 6 months or more, and use of walking as the exercise were found to be the components of the rehabilitation program most responsible for patients' improvements.

▶ Although we all think we know that exercise is effective treatment for claudication, many details remain ethereal. For example, how far should we ask patients to walk, how often, and for how many months? What type of improvement can we reasonably expect? This interesting meta-analysis, which suffers from all the defects of this form of autoeroticism, suggests that walking exercise is better than any alternate exercise, patients should exercise more than 3 sessions per week, and that exercise duration should be longer than 30 minutes. Total duration of training should be approximately 6 months. On this program you can expect about a doubling of pain free walking. It appears important to have the patients walk to near-maximal pain, not merely to the onset of pain. The only difference that I identify in our own approach is that we ask our patients to walk a total of 1 mile daily in interrupted sessions. In a majority of patients this will certainly be more than 30 minutes. On balance, I find this article provides important practical information helping us direct exercise therapy in our claudicating patients. A sobering fact, however, is that only 30% to 40% of claudicants are able to perform substantial walking exercise, the remainder having sufficient co-morbid conditions to make it impossible. See also Abstract 8–1.

---

**Reduction of Requirement for Leg Vascular Surgery During Long-Term Treatment of Claudicant Patients With Ticlopidine: Results From the Swedish Ticlopidine Multicentre Study (STIMS)**
Bergqvist D, Almgren B, Dickinson JP (Univ Hosp, Uppsala, Sweden)
*Eur J Vasc Endovasc Surg* 10:69–76, 1995                                    10–21

---

*Objective.*—The value of long-term treatment with ticlopidine in preventing the need for vascular surgery in patients with claudication was studied.

*Background.*—Antiplatelet treatment can lower the risk of acute thrombotic events. It is not known if antiplatelet treatment can reduce the need for peripheral vascular surgery in high-risk patients. Risks for vascular surgery and amputation in the management of patients with claudication were reported.

*Methods.*—Ticlopidine (250 mg) or placebo was administered twice daily to 687 patients with claudication. Vascular surgery events were recorded for 7 years. Risks for leg vascular surgery were calculated using drug treatment and 11 risk factors for vascular disease.

*Results.*—Per annum, 2.4% of patients overall had a first operation. The effect of the drug was maintained through the treatment period of 7 years (Fig 1). More than 50% of procedures were in the aortoiliac region. Additional operations were required in 25% of patients who underwent operation during the study period. The need for amputation was rare. The need for vascular reconstructive surgery was reduced by 50% by treatment with ticlopidine. This was true in intention-to-treat and on-treatment analyses. The only risk factor for surgery was male gender. The strongest predictor of need for surgery was prior peripheral arterial surgery. There were no statistically significant associations between the risk factors examined and effect of ticlopidine treatment.

*Conclusion.*—Treatment with ticlopidine for platelet inhibition may have a role in preventing the need for vascular surgery in patients with intermittent claudication. There was no evidence that hyperglycaemia altered the risk for surgery affecting the blood supply above the groin vs. below the groin (Table 4).

▶ Another late discovery from the Swedish study of the last decade is that claudicants who have already had 1 cardiovascular event have a marginal

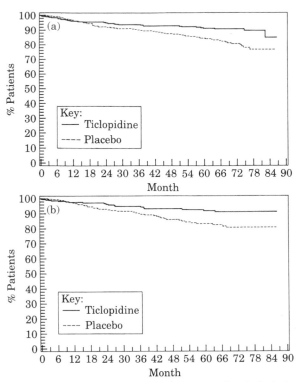

FIGURE 1.—Kaplan-Meier plots of the proportion of patients (ordinate) who had not undergone leg vascular surgery (types 1, 2, 3, 4, or 6) at each time after randomization (abscissa). **A,** all events occurring up to the determined end of study medication (31.12.1978 or prior death—intention-to-treat analysis). **B,** events occurring and patients at risk only while taking study medication (on-treatment analysis). (Reprinted from *Eur J Vasc Endovasc Surg;* vol 10; Bergqvist D, Almgren B, Dickinson JP: Reduction of requirement for leg vascular surgery during long-term treatment of claudicant patients with ticlopidine: Results from the Swedish ticlopidine multicentre study [STIMS]; pp 69–76; 1995; by permission of the publisher Academic Press Limited, London.)

TABLE 4.—Surgery and Glycemia

| | Normoglycemic Patients* | | Hyperglycemic Patients* | |
|---|---|---|---|---|
| | Placebo | Ticlopidine | Placebo | Ticlopidine |
| Total patients | 273 | 280 | 49 | 49 |
| Type 1 surgery—aortofemoral region: number of operations | 29 | 13 | 4 | 2 |
| Type 2 surgery—femorodistal region: number of operations | 10 | 5 | 2 | 1 |

* Fasting blood glucose as measured at study entry: normoglycemic, fasting blood glucose < 5.8 mmol/L; hyperglycemic, fasting blood glucose ≥ 5.8 mmol/L. Five events of type 1 or 2 were recorded for the 36 patients for whom a prestudy fasting glucose value was not recorded.
(Reprinted from *Eur J Vasc Endovasc Surg;* vol 10; Bergqvist D, Almgren B, Dickinson JP: Reduction of requirement for leg vascular surgery during long-term treatment of claudicant patients with ticlopidine: Results from the Swedish ticlopidine multicentre study [STIMS]. pp 69–76; 1995, by permission of the publisher Academic Press Limited, London.)

benefit from ticlopidine; bear in mind, however, that one third of the patients dropped out of this twice-daily treatment program, and the real effect may be no greater than that of once-daily low-dose aspirin in reducing cardiovascular mortality. The validity of their conclusions concerning vascular surgery is difficult to assess because there was no control of leg status on entry to the trial and no control of the indications for further surgery. The most significant message for this group of claudicants having mainly proximal reconstruction is that 1 operation tends to lead to another. There are no data here from critically ischemic or IDDM patients, and for claudicants there is more convincing evidence elsewhere that antiplatelet drugs may be of benefit.

**A.E.B. Giddings, M.D.**

---

**Propionyl-L-Carnitine in Intermittent Claudication: Double-Blind, Placebo-Controlled, Dose Titration, Multicenter Study**
Brevetti G, Perna S, Sabbá C, et al (Univ Federico II, Naples, Italy; Univ of Bari, Italy)
*J Am Coll Cardiol* 26:1411–1416, 1995                                    10–22

---

*Background.*—Carnitine is a naturally occurring compound that plays an important role in regulating energy flow in skeletal muscle. In patients with intermittent claudication, administration of carnitine increases carnitine muscle content and improves exercise capacity. The efficacy, safety, and tolerability of treatment with oral propionyl-L-carnitine were evaluated in a large series of patients with intermittent claudication in a multicenter, double-blind, placebo-controlled trial.

*Methods.*—After maximal walking distance was recorded, 245 patients with intermittent claudication were randomly assigned to receive either propionyl-L-carnitine or placebo. The initial dose of 500 mg twice daily was increased at 2-month intervals up to 3 g/day in patients who were not responsive. The 2 treatment regimes were compared on day 180.

*Results.*—The patients receiving treatment had significantly more improvement in their exercise capacity than those in the placebo group. There were no adverse effects of treatment as monitored by ECG or routine biochemical and hematologic test results. Propionyl-L-carnitine was well tolerated. The majority of patients responded significantly to a dose of 2 g/day.

*Conclusion.*—In a series of patients with intermittent claudication, treatment with propionyl-L-carnitine, at a dose of 2 g/day, appeared to be effective in improving exercise capacity, safe, and well tolerated.

▶ This study is essentially a repeat of a prior publication by the same authors.[1] Multicenter study of the use of propionyl-L-carnitine in claudication in Europe has significantly reached a positive conclusion, namely, that propionyl-L-carnitine does appear to improve walking in claudicants and that the improvement is statistically significant. Carnitine is an intermediate in the energetic metabolism of muscle. The authors have elsewhere presented relatively convincing evidence that patients with claudication have a relative deficiency of this essential metabolic cofactor. This drug has the marvelous advantage of being cheap and, as far as anyone knows, totally safe. Several important studies are ongoing, and 1 major study has just turned up positive. I believe we will hear more about this drug in the future.

*Reference*

1. Brevetti G, Chiariello M, Ferulano G, et al: Increases in walking distance in patients with peripheral vascular disease treated with L-carnitine: A double-blind, cross-over study. *Circulation* 77:767–773, 1988.

**Carnitine-Related Alterations in Patients With Intermittent Claudication: Indication for a Focused Carnitine Therapy**
Brevetti G, di Lisa F, Perna S, et al (Univ Federico II, Naples, Italy; Univ of Padua, Italy)
*Circulation* 93:1685–1689, 1996                                                10–23

*Background.*—Patients with peripheral arterial disease have altered carnitine metabolism. Taking L-carnitine supplements may correct the abnormalities of carnitine metabolism and lead to better walking performance. The response to L-carnitine therapy in terms of plasma acetylcarnitine and walking performance was evaluated in patients with peripheral arterial disease.

*Methods.*—The study included 22 patients with peripheral arterial disease and claudication and 8 normal controls, all of whom underwent measurement of plasma carnitine and its esters at rest and after maximal exercise. The patients were then randomized to receive either placebo or L-carnitine, 500 mg intravenously in a single bolus, and the carnitine measurements were repeated. The metabolic effects of treatment were measured, as was the patients' posttreatment walking performance.

*Results.*—Ten patients, designated group IC1, had a normal mean plasma acetylcarnitine level of 3.7 μmol/L at rest, which increased significantly with maximal exercise. The remaining 12 patients, designated group IC2, had an elevated mean plasma acetylcarnitine at rest and a significant decrease with exercise (Fig 2). Patients in group IC1 had better walking performance than those in group IC2. Treatment with L-carnitine was associated with a significant increase in plasma acetylcarnitine level during exercise for most patients with group IC2, along with a significant improvement in walking performance. For patients in group IC1, L-carnitine treatment produced no change in acetylcarnitine levels or improvement in walking performance. The improvements in walking capacity with L-carnitine treatment were affected exclusively by the exercise-induced changes in plasma acetylcarnitine level, and stepwise multiple regression analysis is suggested.

| Normal subjects | Group IC 1 | Group IC 2 |
|---|---|---|

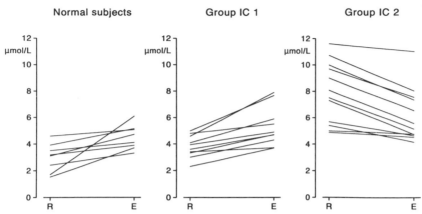

FIGURE 2.—Individual values of plasma acetylcarnitine at rest and at peak exercise in normal subjects and in IC1 and IC2 patients. *Abbreviations: R*, rest; *E*, peak exercise; *IC1*, intermittent claudication group 1; *IC2*, intermittent claudication group 2. (Brevetti G, di Lisa F, Perna S, et al: Carnitine-related alterations in patients with intermittent claudication: Indication for a focused carnitine therapy. *Circulation* 1996; 93:1685–1689; Reproduced with permission of *Circulation*. Copyright 1995 American Heart Association.)

*Conclusion.*—Among patients with peripheral arterial disease, L-carnitine treatment appears to improve walking ability only for those who have an abnormal plasma acetylcarnitine response to exercise. Measuring plasma acetylcarnitine levels at rest and after exercise can help in identifying patients who are likely to benefit from carnitine supplementation. This treatment may play a key role in removing excess acetyl-coenzyme A and improving oxidative metabolism in patients with peripheral arterial disease.

▶ See also Abstract 10–22. In this interesting biochemical study, blood acetylcarnitine levels were measured at rest and after exercise in 22 claudicants and 8 normal subjects. The authors suggest herein that they can predict which patients will respond to exogenous carnitine by analyzing serum acetylcarnitine levels after exercise before treatment. Responding patients have a decrease in acetylcarnitine levels with exercise, whereas nonresponding patients have the normal increase in levels. Exogenous carnitine favorably affected the claudication distance only in those patients who had a decrease with exercise, again suggesting the relative deficiency mentioned in the prior abstract. I have always been impressed with the carnitine data.

## Intravenous Pentoxifylline for the Treatment of Chronic Critical Limb Ischaemia: The European Study Group

Bergqvist D (Univ Hosp, Uppsala, Sweden)
*Eur J Vasc Endovasc Surg* 9:426–436, 1995                                    10–24

*Objective.*—The efficacy and safety of IV pentoxifylline in patients with chronic critical limb ischemia were assessed.

TABLE 6.—Change in Pain Assessment at Final Visit in Patients With Peripheral Pressures at Baseline 60 mm Hg or Less

| | Number (%) of Patients | |
|---|---|---|
| | Pentoxifylline (n = 100) | Placebo (n = 101) |
| *Pain score (no. of patients)* | | |
| Decrease by 3 points | 4 (4%) | 0 |
| Decrease by ≥2 points | 28 (28%) | 15 (15%) |
| Increase by ≥2 points | 3 (3%) | 4 (4%) |
| Increase by 3 points | 1 (1%) | 0 |
| *Visual analogue scale (mm)* | | |
| Baseline, median (IQR) | 40 (26–60) | 39 (21–60) |
| Final visit, median (IQR) | 11 (0–33) | 27 (4–49) |
| Difference (IQR) | −20 (−43–0) | −5 (−27–4) |

*Abbreviation: IQR, interquartile range.*
(Reprinted from *Eur J Vasc Endovasc Surg*; vol 8; Bergqvist D: Intravenous pentoxifylline for the treatment of chronic critical limb ischaemia: The European study group. pp 426–436; 1995; by permission of the publisher Academic Press Limited, London.)

*Background.*—Chronic critical limb ischemia is an advanced stage of peripheral vascular disease. Current treatment is usually surgical. Vascular reconstruction is performed in approximately 60% of patients, and primary amputation is performed in 20% of patients; another 20% of patients receive other temporary treatment. Current treatments are associated with significant morbidity and mortality, as well as poor long-term prognosis. Pharmacotherapy may be an alternative for those who are not eligible for surgery.

*Methods.*—Intravenous pentoxifylline infusion (600 mg) or placebo was administered twice daily to 314 patients with chronic critical limb ischemia. After 7 days, each patient's condition was reviewed, and treatment was extended for another 14 days if the patient had not deteriorated. Pain was assessed, and consumption of analgesic was measured.

*Results.*—There were significantly positive results in favor of pentoxifylline in intention-to-treat and per protocol analyses. With the use of the pain intensity score system, 28% of patients receiving pentoxifylline and 15% of patients receiving placebo had an improvement of 2 points or more (Table 6). Diabetes mellitus, eligibility for surgery, and extremely impaired peripheral hemodynamics did not affect treatment response.

*Conclusion.*—The use of IV pentoxifylline to treat rest pain in patients with chronic critical limb ischemia is supported. There is a need for effective, conservative management of patients who are ineligible for vascular reconstruction, as well patients who are eligible but are being prepared for intervention.

▶ Chronic critical limb ischemia as defined in this paper means rest pain, distal foot gangrene, or both. Pentoxifylline was administered intravenously to the study patients. Although the study showed positive results in favor of pentoxifylline, the end points were not particularly persuasive, primarily consisting of pain assessment. Secondary end points were walking capacity and assessment of global clinical impression by the physician and the patient. Interestingly, the improvement in walking was not statistically significant in favor of the drug. The only conclusion that can be reached by this ambitious study is that pentoxifylline provides superior pain relief in patients with severe limb ischemia than does placebo. I suppose a small victory beats a major defeat.

## Failure of Foot Salvage in Patients With End-Stage Renal Disease After Surgical Revascularization

Johnson BL, Glickman MH, Bandyk DF, et al (Eastern Virginia School of Medicine, Norfolk; Univ of South Florida, Tampa)

*J Vasc Surg* 22:280–286, 1995                                                   10–25

*Background.*—Patients with end-stage renal disease (ESRD) and critical lower limb ischemia are being recomended for lower limb revascularization in the hopes of improving their quality of life. Unfortunately, the complication and failure rates are high for this procedure. A role for primary amputation has been considered, but the patient cohort for whom this would be beneficial has not been defined. The factors responsible for failure of foot salvage in ESRD patients with critical lower limb ischemia who had infrainguinal bypass grafting were examined in a retrospective analysis.

*Methods.*—A retrospective review was performed of the records of 69 infrainguinal bypass grafts performed between November 1983 and December 1994 in 53 ESRD patients with critical lower limb ischemia. This group included 37 on hemodialysis, 10 who had kidney transplants, 6 on peritoneal dialysis, 28 feet with gangrene, 25 with nonhealing ulcers, and 16 with ischemic pain at rest. Diabetes mellitus was present in 81% of these patients. Survival, limb salvage, and graft patency were the end points examined in this study.

*Results.*—In this series of ESRD patients undergoing distal arterial reconstructions, the 30-day operative mortality rate was 10% and the 2-year

TABLE 4.—Cumulative Limb Salvage Rates

| Interval (mo.) | No. of Limbs at Risk | No. of Limbs Lost | No. Withdrawn | Interval Limb Loss | Cumulative Salvage (%) | SE (%) |
|---|---|---|---|---|---|---|
| 0–1 | 69 | 6 | 8 | .91 | 100 | 0 |
| 1–3 | 55 | 6 | 3 | .89 | 91 | 3.7 |
| 3–6 | 46 | 3 | 8 | .93 | 81 | 5.2 |
| 6–12 | 35 | 4 | 8 | .87 | 75 | 6.3 |
| 12–18 | 23 | 1 | 4 | .95 | 65 | 8.0 |
| 18–24 | 17 | 1 | 5 | .93 | 62 | 9.3 |
| 24–30 | 11 | 0 | 1 | 1.00 | 57 | 11.3 |

*Abbreviation: SE*, standard error.

(Courtesy of Johnson BL, Glickman MH, Bandyk DF, et al: Failure of foot salvage in patients with end-stage renal disease after surgical revascularization. *J Vasc Surg* 2:280–286, 1995.)

TABLE 6.—Clinical Failure After Revascularization in 53 End-Stage Renal Disease Patients (69 Procedures)

| | | Failure of Foot Salvage | | |
|---|---|---|---|---|
| Postoperative Time | Perioperative Death | Graft Thrombosis | Foot Amputation* | Clinical Failure Rate (%) |
| 1 month | 7 | 2 | 5 | 20 |
| 1 year | 7 | 8 | 13 | 41† |

* Foot lost with patent bypass graft.
† Minimum failure rate because not all patients were monitored for 1 year (2 patients lost to follow-up, 7 patients monitored <1 year).
(Courtesy of Johnson BL, Glickman MH, Bandyk DF, et al: Failure of foot salvage in patients with end-stage renal disease after surgical revascularization. *J Vasc Surg* 2:280–286, 1995.)

survival rate was 38%. Primary graft patency was 96% at 1 month, 72% at 1 year, and 68% at 2 years. The cumulative limb salvage rate was 91% at 1 month and 57% at 2 years (Table 4). After 1 month, 20% of the procedures could be considerd failures (Table 6). Within 2 months, 11 foot amputations were performed and 22 were performed within 14 months. Limb loss resulted from graft failure in 9, foot ischemia despite a patent bypass in 8, and uncontrolled infection in 5 cases. In the group of patients who required amputations, 59% were performed despite a patent bypass. The limb salvage rate was 74% in patients without gangrene and 51% in patients with gangrene.

Conclusion.—There is a high failure rate of foot salvage in ESRD patients with critical lower limb ischemia who undergo infrainguinal bypass. This patient record review demonstrated that failure resulted from wound healing problems rather than graft thrombosis. Earlier referral for revascularization would improve the success rate of this procedure. Primary amputation should be considered in patients with foot gangrene.

▶ Everyone knows that ESRD patients have a bad outcome with leg surgery.[1-4] For yet another restatement of what every vascular surgeon on the planet already knew, I award these authors the coveted Camel Dung Award. Wear it proudly!

*References*

1. Edwards JM, Taylor LM, Porter JM: Limb salvage in end stage renal disease. *Arch Surg* 123:1164–1168, 1988.
2. 1994 YEARBOOK OF VASCULAR SURGERY, p 267.
3. 1995 YEARBOOK OF VASCULAR SURGERY, p 244.
4. 1996 YEARBOOK OF VASCULAR SURGERY, p 272.

### Effects of Spinal Cord Stimulation (SCS) in Patients With Inoperable Severe Lower Limb Ischaemia: A Prospective Randomised Controlled Study

Jivegård LEH, Augustinsson L-E, Holm J, et al (Östra Hosps, Göteborg, Sweden; Sahlgrenska Hosp, Göteborg, Sweden)
*Eur J Vasc Endovasc Surg* 9:421–425, 1995          10–26

*Background.*—Severe chronic lower limb ischemia, if left untreated, leads to pain, ulcerations, and gangrene. Unfortunately, revascularization is not always possible. Electrical spinal cord stimulation (SCS) has been reported to reduce pain, promote ulcer healing, and increase circulation in ischemic limbs. A prospective, randomized controlled clinical trial was performed to determine whether SCS improved limb salvage in patients with inoperable lower limb ischemia.

*Methods.*—Diabetic or atherosclerotic patients were included in this study if they had severe chronic lower limb ichemia with pain at rest or ischemic ulcers and if vascular reconstruction was impossible. Patients were excluded if ischemia was rapidly progressing; gangrene, extensive infection, or nonhealing ulcers were present, or SCS was contraindicated. Patients were scheduled for follow-up 2, 6, 12, and 18 months after randomization.

*Results.*—The SCS group consisted of 25 patients, and the analgesic, or control, group consisted of 26 patients. Macrocirculatory parameters were not different between these 2 groups during the follow-up period (Fig 1). Significant long-term pain relief was reported only in the SCS group (Fig

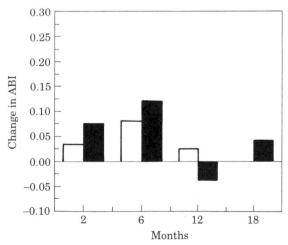

FIGURE 1.—Change in ankle-brachial index during follow-up compared with the randomization value: control (*open boxes*); spinal cord stimulation (*filled boxes*). There were no significant changes in either group (Wilcoxon's rank sum test). *Abbreviation: ABI,* ankle-brachial index. (Reprinted from *Eur J Vasc Endovasc Surg;* vol 9; Jivegard LEH, Augustinsson L-E, Holm J, et al: Effects of spinal cord stimulation (SCS) in patients with inoperable severe lower limb ischemia: A prospective randomized controlled study; pp 421–425; 1995; by permission of the publisher Academic Press Limited, London.)

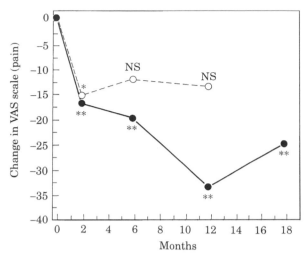

FIGURE 3.—Change in VAS score for pain during follow-up: control (*open circles*); spinal cord stimulation (*solid circles*). There were too few (<5) observations at 18 months in the control group for analysis. Abbreviations: *VAS, Visual Analogue Scale; NS,* * *P* < 0.05; * * *P* < 0.01. (Reprinted from *Eur J Vasc Endovasc Surg;* vol 9; Jivegard LEH, Augustinsson L-E, Holm J et al: Effects of spinal cord stimulation (SCS) in patients with inoperable severe lower limb ischemia: A prospective randomized controlled study; pp 421–425, 1995; by permission of the publisher Academic Press Limited, London.)

3). The limb salvage rate was 62% in the SCS group and 45% in the control group at 18 months. This difference was not significant. There was significantly less tissue loss in the SCS group. Among patients without arterial hypertension, there was a significantly lower amputation rate in the SCS than in the control group.

*Conclusion.*—In patients with inoperable severe lower limb ischemia, electrical SCS provided long-term pain relief, but salvage was not significantly improved at 18 months follow-up. These results also suggest that SCS may improve limb salvage in patients without hypertension, but larger studies are required to examine the significance of this effect.

▶ I believe I have heard about all the information concerning SCS in patients with limb ischemia that I can benefit from. I conclude that this modality has the potential to relieve pain but does not substantially improve blood flow and does not improve limb salvage. In the overall big picture I see little or no clinical use for this treatment. There are only 2 things we can reliably do to relieve ischemic limb pain: revascularization or amputation. I do not identify any pressing need for long-term treatment of chronically painful ischemic limbs with anything other than surgery.

## The Protective Effect of Vein Cuffed Anastomoses Is Not Mechanical in Origin

Norberto JJ, Sidawy AN, Trad KS, et al (George Washington Univ, Washington, DC)

*J Vasc Surg* 21:558–566, 1995                10–27

*Background.*—After arterial injury, intimal hyperplasia (IH), in other words, proliferation of vascular smooth muscle cells, is particularly likely to occur at the outflow anastomoses of prosthetic bypass grafts. The resulting stenosis can lead to graft flow reduction and thrombosis. Previous studies have shown that interposing a vein cuff between an expanded polytetrafluoroethylene (ePTFE) graft and artery at the site of distal anastomoses can decrease IH formation at the arterial outflow. In clinical studies, placing an interposition vein cuff at the distal anastomosis of ePTFE grafts to infrageniculate arteries has been shown to improve long-term patency rate. Mechanical factors that could be involved in the protective effects of cuffed anastomoses, including the expansibility of the vein cuff and the angle of the cuffed anastomosis, were examined in dogs.

*Methods.*—Platelet aggregation studies were performed to select compatible dogs for the study. Group A consisted of 9 dogs in which 4-mm e-PTFE grafts were placed, along with a 1-cm interposition vein cuff at the distal anastomosis, in the left carotid artery. An identical procedure was carried out on the left side, with the addition of an ePTFE jacket to prevent vein cuff expansion with arterial pulsation (Fig 1).

In another 5 dogs, comprising group B, a 4-mm ePTFE graft was placed in both carotid arteries. On the left side, the distal anastomosis between the graft and artery was made at an acute angle, as is typical in bypass graft placement. On the right side, a 1-cm long, 6-mm diameter e-PTFE segment

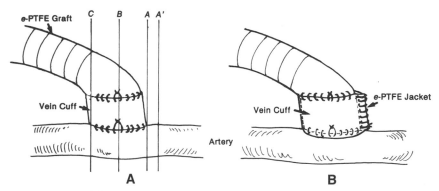

FIGURE 1.—A, left side distal anastomosis in group A. Vein cuff is interposed between e-PTFE graft and carotid artery. A', A, B, and C denote sectioning levels for intimal hyperplasia thickness measurements. The same levels were used for the right side. B, right-side distal anastomosis in group A. Vein cuff is snugly encircled by e-PTFE jacket, which is incorporated in graft/cuff anastomosis. *Abbreviation: e-PTFE,* expanded polytetrafluoroethylene. (Courtesy of Sidawy AN, Trad KS, Sidawy MK, et al: Effect of vein cuff and e-PTFE on the development of outflow intimal hyperplasia. *Surg Forum* 42:345–346, 1991. From Norberto JJ, Sidawy AN, Trad KS, et al: The protective effect of vein cuffed anastomoses is not mechanical in origin. *J Vasc Surg* 21:556–558, 1995.)

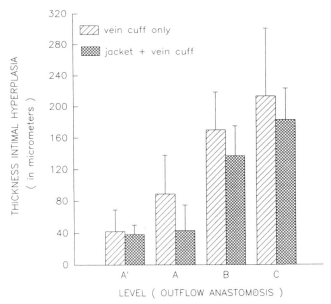

FIGURE 5.—Comparison of thickness of intimal hyperplasia at outflow anastomosis between jacketed and control groups. All units are in micrometers, x ± standard error of the mean (n = 8). A', 1 mm distal to toe of anastomosis; B, midportion of anastomosis; C, heel of anastomosis. (Courtesy of Norberto JJ, Sidawy AN, Trad KS, et al: The protective effect of vein cuffed anastomoses is not mechanical in origin. *J Vasc Surg* 21:556–558, 1995.)

was interposed perpendicularly between the artery and graft, mimicking the angle of anastomosis between a vein cuff and artery. The grafts were harvested for microscopic assessment of IH 10 weeks later.

*Results.*—One animal in group A had bilateral graft thrombosis. In the remaining 8 dogs, there was no significant difference in the thickness of IH between the jacketed and nonjacketed anastomoses (Fig 5). In group B, 4 of the 5 animals had bilateral graft thrombosis.

*Conclusion.*—The ability of vein cuffed anastomoses to protect against IH does not appear mechanical in origin. The protective effect results from neither vein cuff expansibility nor a perpendicular anastomotic angle.

▶ I really don't know if a distal anastomotic cuff in prosthetic leg grafts improves patency. Available data are controversial and inconclusive. These authors believe that the cuff probably does help but that any derived benefit is not related to increased anastomotic compliance. On those rare occasions when we are forced to use a prosthetic to a tibial artery (about 2 times per year), I do attempt to include a Taylor patch at the distal anastomosis. My anecdotal experience indicates these grafts still fail, although perhaps slightly later than they would have failed without the Taylor patch.

## Re-Endothelialisation in Autogenous Vein Grafts

Ishikawa M, Sasajima T, Kubo Y (Asahikawa Med College, Japan)
*Eur J Vasc Endovasc Surg* 11:105–111, 1996                    10–28

*Introduction.*—Progressive intimal hyperplasia is the main cause of late vein graft failure, and it occurs mainly within the first 2 years after implantation. The mechanism and prevention of intimal hyperplasia is not clear. Endothelial cell injury during preparation of grafts and vein graft quality may be important factors in the development of intimal hyperplasia. The course of reendothelialization in an entire graft after implantation was clarified, and the effects of heparinized autogenous blood and heparinized saline solution immersion on the preservation of the endothelial cell were compared.

*Methods.*—Autogenous femoral veins of dogs were immersed in heparinized saline solution or heparinized autogenous blood. The veins were implanted into the ipsilateral femoral artery and removed 1 day to 4 to 8 weeks after implantation. The silver staining method was combined with scanning electron microscopy and staining for Factor VIII–related antigen to confirm the presence of endothelial cells.

*Results.*—Almost all of the endothelial cells fell away from the luminal surface of the graft in the earlier period after implantation. Endothelial cells regenerated multifocally and irregularly on the luminal surface of the vein graft. For grafts immersed in heparinized saline solution, the percentage area of endothelial cell coverage was 44.3% before implantation, 6.2% at 1 day, 14.5% at 1 week, and 81.3% at 4 weeks. For grafts immersed in heparinized autogenous blood, the values were 73.5% before implantation, 20.6% at 1 day, 79.2% at 1 week, and 95.5% at 4 weeks. However, the relatively rapid speed of reendothelialisation slowed down considerably 1 week after implantation in the latter grafts.

*Conclusion.*—Heparinized autogenous blood is superior to heparinized saline solution for the preservation of endothelial cells in autogenous vein grafts in dogs. Thus, heparinized autogenous blood is strongly recommended as preparation media for autogenous vein grafts. Reendothelialisation is incomplete even at 8 weeks after surgery, suggesting that these areas may develop into intimal hyperplasia.

▶ I suppose these authors are correct that soaking an autogenous vein graft in heparinized blood preserves endothelium better than soaking the graft in heparinized saline solution. The real question, however, is whether preservation of vein graft endothelium during grafting conveys any benefit to the recipient. I conclude it is not a simple 1-to-1 relationship. It is my belief that almost all autogenous vein grafts are severely denuded of endothelium at the time of reimplantation or shortly thereafter. Over a course of weeks, the endothelium returns, and most of these grafts do well. I am not convinced that the details of graft handling during implantation have any substantial influence on graft patency. Nonetheless, we continue to prepare our vein grafts with the use of chilled autologous heparinized blood, and I suppose we will continue to do so.

## A Comparative Evaluation of Externally Supported Polytetrafluoroethylene Axillobifemoral and Axillounifemoral Bypass Grafts

Mohan CR, Sharp WJ, Hoballah JJ, et al (Univ of Iowa, Iowa City)
*J Vasc Surg* 21:801–809, 1995                                    10–29

*Background.*—The axillofemoral bypass for lower extremity revascularization was first performed in 1962. The addition of a femorofemoral crossover limb can be added to permit revascularization of both lower extremities. Axillounifemoral (AxUF) or axillobifemoral (AxBF) bypass has been used for high-risk patients or for patients requiring removal of an infected aortic graft, but it is not known whether addition of the femorofemoral limb improves late patency. A series of externally supported polytetrafluoroethylene (PTFE) AxBF and AxUF bypass grafts were analyzed for patency after 2 years of follow-up to determine if patency can be improved in this way.

*Methods.*—Between January 1988 and June 1994, 36 AxBF and 22 AxUF bypass grafts were performed at 1 institution. Graft patency was evaluated at 1 month, 6 months, and then at yearly intervals for 2 years.

*Results.*—There was no significant difference in the 30-day operative mortality between these 2 procedures. The primary patency rate was 80% and the secondary patency rate was 89% for the whole group at 3 years (Fig 1). There was no significant difference between the primary or secondary patency rates for the 2 procedures at 2 years.

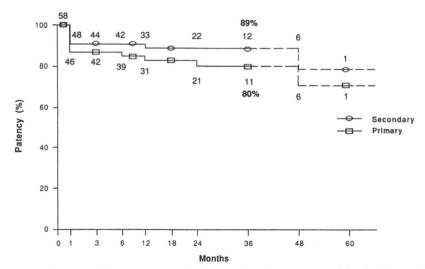

FIGURE 1.—Cumulative patency rate of axillofemoral grafts. (Courtesy of Mohan CR, Sharp WJ, Hoballah JJ, et al: A comparative evaluation of externally supported polytetrafluoroethylene axillobifemoral and axillounifemoral bypass grafts. *J Vasc Surg* 21:801–809, 1995.)

*Conclusion.*—In this series of patients undergoing bypass grafting, there was no difference in the patency of externally supported PFTE AxBF and AxUF bypass grafts up to 2 years after the procedure. The addition of the femorofemoral limb to the AxUF bypass does not improve patency and is not necessary unless both limbs are ischemic.

▶ These authors report an excellent 3-year primary patency of 80% and secondary patency of 89% in axillofemoral grafting. They found no difference in the patency performance of the AxBF vs. the AxUF grafts. The message I take away from this paper is that in the modern world, axillofemoral grafts are giving patency comparable with aortofemoral grafts. A much wider use of axillofemoral grafts appears fully justified, especially in our rapidly aging vascular population. The excellent results reported here are similar to our axillofemoral results recently reported. See Abstract 8–3.

---

**Deep Vein Thrombosis Associated With Lower Extremity Amputation**
Yeager RA, Moneta GL, Edwards JM, et al (Oregon Health Sciences Univ, Portland; Portland Veterans Affairs Med Ctr, Ore)
*J Vasc Surg* 22:612–615, 1995                                   10–30

---

*Background.*—Though patients undergoing lower extremity amputation are thought to have an increased risk of deep vein thrombosis (DVT), there is little documentation of this. The prevalence of DVT among a large cohort of patients undergoing vascular surgery and lower extremity amputation was studied prospectively.

*Methods.*—Seventy-one men and 1 woman having surgery over a recent 28-month period were included in the study. Mean patient age was 68. Forty-one below-knee and 31 above-knee amputations were performed. Duplex scanning for DVT was done perioperatively.

*Findings.*—Nine patients (12.5%) were found to have DVT. The thromboses were bilateral in 1 patient, ipsilateral in 4, and contralateral to amputation in 4. The risk of developing DVT was significantly greater in patients with a history of venous disease. Thrombi were detected at or proximal to the popliteal vein in 8 patients and isolated to the tibial veins in 1. Thromboses were found before surgery in 6 patients and afterward in 3. Heparin anticoagulation was used to treat DVT. None of the patients had clinical symptoms suggesting pulmonary embolism.

*Conclusion.*—Lower extremity amputation was associated with DVT at or proximal to the popliteal vein in 11% of the patients in this cohort. Patients with a history of venous disease and with preexisting amputation seemed to be at greatest risk for DVT. Diabetes mellitus, sepsis, and malignancy may also predispose patients requiring lower extremity amputation to the development of DVT.

▶ I used to believe that DVT was sufficiently rare in vascular patients as to be of little importance. First we were informed by the group at the Cleveland

Clinic that 18% of patients suffered acute DVT after aortic aneurysm surgery.[1] In the article reported here, we learn that DVT occurred in 12.5% of patients undergoing major lower extremity amputation. Interestingly, a significant majority of these patients had their DVT before the performance of limb amputation. Without question, major limb amputation patients should receive DVT prophylaxis surrounding the time of limb amputation. Perhaps other vascular patients should also.

*Reference*

1. 1995 YEAR BOOK OF VASCULAR SURGERY, p 381.

---

**Effects of Compression and Type of Bed Surface on the Microcirculation of the Heel**
Abu-Own A, Sommerville K, Scurr JH, et al (Univ College, London; Middlesex Hosp, London)
*Eur J Vasc Endovasc Surg* 9:327–334, 1995                               10–31

---

*Background.*—It is not uncommon for pressure ulcers to develop on the heel. The level of compression necessary to reduce perfusion in the heel to the level where ischemia and tissue necrosis may begin was examined using a specially designed laser Doppler fiberoptic system.

*Methods.*—A device consisting of a stand with an adjustable pivoted arm mounted on it was designed to compress the heel (Fig 1). A standard 5-cm diameter pressure–applying acrylic indenter with a slot to accommodate a low-profile laser Doppler probe was used to apply a force of 50g to 1,500g to the heel. The pressure applied was measured by an interface pressure sensor. The pressures were applied with the subject supine in

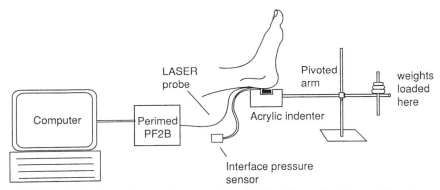

FIGURE 1.—Experimental system for compression of the heel. An acrylic indenter with a slot to accommodate a low profile laser Doppler probe is used to compress the heel. The laser Doppler fluxmeter is logged to a computer for data recording. The compression applied to the skin of the heel is measured by an interface pressure sensor. (Reprinted from *Eur J Vasc Endovasc Surg*; vol 9; Abu-Own A, Sommerville K, Scurr JH, et al: Effects of compression and type of bed surface on the microcirculation of the heel; pp 327–334, 1995.)

either a regular hospital bed or a Frameless Air Support Therapy (FAST) low air–loss system, with the system chamber pressure at 5, 10, 20, or 30 mm Hg. The study group consisted of 10 older patients at risk of developing an ulcer, 10 age- and sex-matched controls, and 10 young, healthy volunteers. Patients with diabetes mellitus were excluded from the study.

*Results.*—The resting laser Doppler flux (LDF) was significantly lower in the patient group than in either control group. Compression of the heel with the apparatus caused a progressive decrease in heel LDF in all groups. Compression of greater than 50 mm Hg on a standard hospital bed reduced the LDF to a value of zero. When a subject lay on the FAST system with the pressure set for 5 mm Hg, the LDF values were significantly higher than in the standard hospital bed. If the pressure was raised to more than 5 mm Hg, the LDF was reduced to zero in the FAST system also.

*Conclusion.*—In a standard hospital bed, pressure on the vulnerable heel area is high enough to decrease circulation and encourage the development of a pressure ulcer in an at-risk patient. If the patient lies on a low air–loss system, such as the FAST system, with the heel chamber inflated to 5 mm Hg, heel microcirculation is maintained. If the chamber pressure is inflated higher, microcirculation is once again lost. If pressure ulcers are to be prevented in vulnerable patients, interface pressure under the heel must be maintained as low as possible, not exceeding 30 mm Hg.

▶ We are increasingly encountering limb ischemia patients with significant pressure ulcers of the heel. Without question, large ischemic heel ulcers are 1 of the most difficult lesions in vascular surgery in which to achieve a satisfactory outcome. Muscle flaps haven't been very good at covering this in our experience. Partial calcanectomy and primary closure seems to work sometimes but at the expense of significant alterations in foot mechanics. Clearly we should do all that is possible to prevent the development of heel ulcers in our limb ischemic patients when they are immobilized. I have found the use of 1 of the variety of large "space boots" to be beneficial. When properly used, these boots completely relieve heel compression with the patient in the supine position. The data presented in this paper indicate that the microcirculation of the heel is quite vulnerable to compression, even more so in patients than in normal controls.

# 11 Upper Extremity Vascular and Hemoaccess

## Angioaccess

### The Percutaneous Treatment of Angioaccess Graft Complications
Katz SG, Kohl RD (Huntington Mem Hosp, Pasadena, Calif)
*Am J Surg* 170:238–242, 1995                                    11–1

*Background.*—Percutaneous methods are being used increasingly in patients with angioaccess graft complications. However, the role of these techniques and their outcomes in patients on hemodialysis are still not clear. One experience with percutaneous treatment of angioaccess fistula was reviewed to investigate its role in patients receiving maintenance hemodialysis.

*Methods.*—Forty-five patients undergoing 55 percutaneous procedures for failed or failing angioaccess grafts during a 3-year period were included in the review. The ages of the 23 women and 22 men ranged from 22 to 86.

*Findings.*—Thirty-four thrombolysis procedures were attempted, of which 32 were successful. Forty-nine of 51 balloon dilations were technically satisfactorily. The patency rates of grafts not requiring thrombolysis were significantly higher than those of grafts requiring thrombolysis. In addition, patency was significantly higher in grafts undergoing angioplasty of sites remote from the venous anastomosis than in grafts undergoing venous anastomotic dilation.

*Conclusion.*—Percutaneous methods appear to be most effective for failing but patent angioaccess grafts, especially those with stenoses remote from the venous anastomosis. The benefit of such techniques decreases significantly in grafts that have progressed to occlusion. Early lesions amenable to balloon angioplasty can be detected through rigorous access surveillance programs that monitor grafts for increased venous pressure and recirculation.

▶ The role of interventional therapy in the treatment of failing or failed angioaccess remains both undefined and controversial. These authors conclude that interventional therapy is not very good for occluded grafts and is not very good for venous anastomotic stenoses. It appears better for venous stenosis remote from the anastomosis. In general, the results of interventional therapy on these grafts is poor. The 12-month patency was only about 45% for a dilatation of venous anastomotic stenoses compared with 92% for nonanastomotic stenoses. On balance, I find dealing with arteriovenous access a maddening experience. I don't think interventional therapy is all that good, but I suppose it is occasionally preferable to reoperative surgery.

---

**The Gracz Arteriovenous Fistula Evaluated: Results of the Brachiocephalic Elbow Fistula in Haemodialysis Angio-Access**
Bender MHM, Bruyninckx CMA, Gerlag PGG (Saint Joseph Hosp, Veldhoven, The Netherlands)
*Eur J Vasc Endovasc Surg* 10:294–297, 1995                                                11–2

---

*Background.*—The relative value of the elbow fistula and the graft fistula as alternatives for angioaccess is debated. The fistula patency and

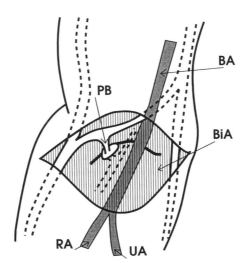

FIGURE 1.—The cephalic vein and the median cubital vein are dissected, locating the perforating branch. The cicipital aponeurosis is incised. *Abbreviations: PB*, perforating branch; *BiA*, bicipital aponeurosis; *BA*, brachial artery; *RA*, radial artery; *UA*, ulnar artery. (Reprinted from *Eur J Vasc Endovasc Surg*; vol 10; Bender MHM, Bruyninckx CMA, Gerlag PGG: The Gracz arteriovenous fistula evaluated: Results of the brachiocephalic elbow fistula in haemodialysis angio-access; pp 294–297; 1995; by permission of the publisher Academic Press Limited, London.)

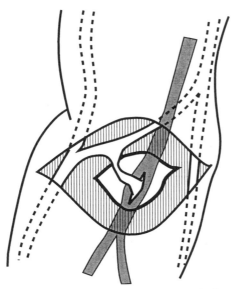

FIGURE 3.—The Gracz fistula. The brachial artery is anastomosed side to end to the perforating branch, using the excised part of the deep vein as a venous patch. (Reprinted from *Eur J Vasc Endovasc Surg;* vol 10; Bender MHM, Bruyninckx CMA, Gerlag PGG: The Gracz arteriovenous fistula evaluated: Results of the brachiocephalic elbow fistula in haemodialysis angio-access; pp 294–297; 1995; by permission of the publisher Academic Press Limited, London.)

complication rates in braciocephalic elbow fistulas of the Gracz and side-to-side configuration were reported.

*Methods.*—Seventy-three elbow fistulas created between 1988 and 1993 were included in the retrospective review. Fifty were Gracz fistulas, and 23 were side-to-side elbow fistulas.

*Findings.*—The elbow fistulas had a cumulative patency of 84% at 1 year and 78% at 3 years. Revision and failure rates associated with the Gracz fistula were not significantly different from those of the side-to-side fistula. Thrombosis was the most common indication for revision, occurring in 4 Gracz fistulas only. Two of these complications were caused by venous stenosis, and 2 were of unknown causes. Stenosis with low flow occurred in 2 Gracz fistulas and in 1 side-to-side fistula. An aneurysm and venous hypertension occurred in 1 Gracz fistula each. Overall the complications rates were 9% for the side-to-side fistulas (Fig 1) and 18% for the Gracz fistulas (Fig 3).

*Conclusion.*—The elbow fistula has a long patency with few complications. It performs as well as wrist fistulas and better than the graft fistulas previously reported. The outcomes of the Gracz elbow fistula are comparable with those of the side-to-side elbow fistula. Graft fistulas should be done only as tertiary procedures.

▶ The authors make a plea that graft fistulas should be reserved for tertiary procedures only, with the primary procedure being the Brescia-Cimino fistula at the wrist and the secondary procedure being autogenous arteriovenous anastomoses in the region of the elbow using either the Gracz configuration or the side-to-side configuration. In general, I believe their conclusions are correct. I hope the nice illustrations of the Gracz fistula will be of some assistance.

## Dialysis Access Grafts: Anatomic Location of Venous Stenosis and Results of Angioplasty

Kanterman RY, Vesely TM, Pilgram TK, et al (Washington Univ, St Louis)
*Radiology* 195:135–139, 1995                                                     11–3

*Background.*—Maintaining adequately functioning vascular access can be difficult in long-term hemodialysis. The development of neointimal hyperplastic stenoses is the most common cause of graft failure. These stenoses typically occur at the native vein-graft anastomosis. The distribution of stenoses and angiographic findings in patients with similar forearm dialysis polytetrafluoroethylene (PTFE) grafts were investigated.

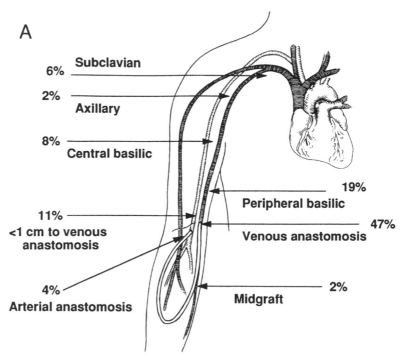

FIGURE 1.—**A,** schematic drawing demonstrates anatomical distribution and percentage stenosis (93 stenoses in 67 patients in whom an initial dialysis fistulogram was obtained). (Courtesy of Kanterman RY, Vesely TM, Pilgram TK, et al: Dialysis access grafts: Anatomic location of venous stenosis and results of angioplasty. *Radiology* 195:135–139, 1995. Radiological Society of North America.)

*Methods and Findings.*—Diagnostic radiographs of fistulas in 125 patients were analyzed. Ninety-five patients met the study criteria, having similar unrevised forearm PTFE loop dialysis grafts. Ninety-three stenoses were identified on initial fistulograms in this group. Forty-seven percent were at the venous anastomosis, and 11% were within 1 cm of the anastomosis. According to life-table analysis, the patency rates for the first angioplasty in a given graft were 63% at 6 months and 41% at 12 months. For the second angioplasty, the patency rates were 50% at 6 months and 25% at 12 months (Fig 1, A).

*Conclusion.*—Serial venous angioplasty procedures may be beneficial in prolonging the life of a graft. However, patency rates decrease with subsequent procedures.

▶ I am always worried when I encounter an interventional article in the radiology literature. Interestingly, 47% of detected stenoses occurred at the venous anastomosis, 27% in the proximal veins, and 8% in the proximal brachiocephalic veins. Only 4% of stenoses detected were arterial. Angioplasty generally functioned rather poorly, although once again appeared better than a poke in the eye with a sharp stick. I continue to be amazed at the amount of clinical attention required for preservation of functioning arteriovenous access grafts.

---

**Early Experience With Stretch Polytetrafluoroethylene Grafts for Haemodialysis Access Surgery: Results of a Prospective Randomised Study**
Tordoir JHM, Hofstra L, Leunissen KML, et al (Academic Hosp, Maastricht, The Netherlands)
*Eur J Vasc Endovasc Surg* 9:305–309, 1995                                    11–4

---

*Background.*—Expanded polytetrafluoroethylene (ePTFE) grafts implanted as an arteriovenous (AV) conduit are considered an acceptable alternative to autogenous Brescia/Cimino fistulas at the wrist created for hemodialysis access when fistula failure occurs or when direct AV anatomosis cannot be performed in patients with insufficient superficial arm veins. The complication and patency rates of stretch ePTFE prostheses were compared prospectively with those of standard ePTFE grafts implanted for hemodialysis vascular access.

*Methods.*—Seventeen stretch and 20 standard ePTFE graft AV fistulas were created in 37 patients during a 2-year period. Duplex examinations were performed regularly to detect stenoses in the fistula circuit.

*Findings.*—Thrombotic events occurred in 40% of the patients with standard grafts and in 12% with stretch grafts. The groups had a similar incidence of puncture complications. Patients with stretch ePTFE grafts had a cumulative primary patency rate of 59% at 1 year, which was significantly higher than in patients with standard ePTFE grafts, with a rate of 29%. Duration of puncture site bleeding was comparable in the 2 groups. Significantly more stenoses were demonstrated on duplex examination in the standard ePTFE graft group.

*Conclusion.*—The longitudinal stretch properties of the new PTFE prosthesis may result in better primary patency rates than are possible with standard ePTFE graft AV fistulas. In this study, graft performance during and after dialysis did not differ between groups. Further research is needed to characterize the mechanical behavior of the stretch ePTFE prosthesis.

▶ These authors have found that the new stretch ePTFE grafts function significantly better than standard ePTFE grafts. In fact, the 12-month patency was twice as good with the new grafts. Fewer stenoses were detected with duplex scanning. I take this as a clear testimonial in favor of the new graft. Confirmatory data are awaited.

## Brachiocephalic Arterial Reconstruction

### Carotid-Axillary Artery Bypass: A Ten-Year Experience
Criado FJ, Queral LA (Union Mem Hosp, Baltimore, Md)
*J Vasc Surg* 22:717–723, 1995                    11–5

*Background.*—Extrathoracic bypass is the preferred treatment for revascularization in patients requiring operative repair of symptomatic occlusion of the proximal subclavian arteries. A 10-year experience with

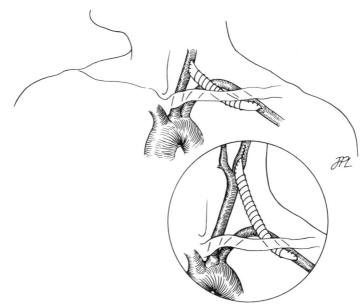

**FIGURE 2.**—Carotid-axillary bypass with ringed expanded polytetrafluoroethylene graft tunneled under clavicle. *Inset,* technical variant when concomitant carotid endarterectomy is necessary. (Courtesy of Criado FJ, Queral LA: Carotid-axillary artery bypass: A ten-year experience. *J Vasc Surg* 22:717–723, 1995.)

carotid-axillary artery bypass in patients with occlusive lesions of the proximal subclavian artery was reported.

*Methods.*—Twenty-six carotid axillary bypasses were performed between March 1984 and November 1994 (Fig 2). The patients were 16 men and 10 women aged 56 to 82. All had symptomatic lesions of the proximal subclavian artery. Only 3 patients were lost to follow-up, between 12 and 38 months.

*Findings.*—None of the patients died perioperatively. Two had small cervical wound hematomas. Transient symptoms of brachial plexus irritation, which resolved spontaneously, were documented in another 2 patients. There were no permanent nerve or lymphatic complications. Carotid-axillary bypass graft patency was 96% at a mean 47 months after surgery. Eighty-eight percent of the patients were symptom free in the long term.

*Conclusion.*—The axillary artery seems to be a useful alternative to the subclavian artery for constructing a cervical bypass in patients with symptomatic proximal stenosis or occlusion of the subclavian artery. Ringed Dacron and expanded polytetrafluoroethylene graft conduits tunneled under the clavicle both performed well in the current series. Long-term patency and symptom relief appear to be excellent.

▶ I agree that the carotid-axillary bypass is a useful alternative to direct subclavian reconstruction, and we use it frequently. However, I strongly disagree with 2 of the authors' points, namely, that this surgery is best performed with a prosthetic bypass and that it is best performed with retroclavicular tunneling. We routinely use the vein bypass tunneled subcutaneously from the carotid artery in the preclavicular plane to either the axillary or the brachial artery based on anatomical circumstances. This has come to be our procedure of choice for symptomatic subclavian-axillary stenosis or occlusion. We find it preferable to direct surgical repair of these vessels, especially in reoperative surgery. I find preferential use of a prosthetic conduit in this setting abhorrent, and I find retroclavicular tunneling to be making something difficult out of something that is inherently easy. I hope my position is clear.

---

## Extrathoracic Reconstruction of Arterial Occlusive Disease Involving the Supraaortic Trunks

Owens LV, Tinsley EA Jr, Criado E, et al (Univ of North Carolina, Chapel Hill)
*J Vasc Surg* 22:217–222, 1995                                                                     11–6

---

*Background.*—Arterial occlusive disease of the supra-aortic trunks can involve the subclavian, common carotid, or innominate arteries. One experience with supra-aortic trunk revascularizations was reviewed to compare various types of extrathoracic reconstruction procedures.

*Methods.*—Forty-seven extrathoracic bypass procedures of the supraaortic trunks were performed in 44 consecutive patients between July 1975 and May 1994. The procedures were done to correct symptomatic subclavian (SCA), common carotid (CCA), or innominate (INA) artery occlusive disease. Subclavian artery stenosis, occurring in 27 patients, was associated with upper extremity claudication in 55%, vertebrobasilar insufficiency in 15%, and both in 30%. Common carotid artery stenosis, present in 14 patients, was associated with hemispheric symptoms in 86% and global ischemia in 14%. Innominate artery stenosis, seen in 3 patients, was accompanied by transient ischemic attacks in 2 and right arm ischemia in 1.

*Findings.*—Of those undergoing SCA revascularization, 19 had carotid-subclavian or carotid-axillary bypass; 8, axilloaxillary bypass; and 3, subclavian-carotid transposition. Among those undergoing CCA reconstruction, 13 had subclavian-carotid bypass, and 1 had carotid-carotid bypass. Axilloaxillary bypasses were done in the 3 patients having INA procedures. Six patients also had a carotid endarterectomy. Concomitant vertebral artery transpositions were performed in 3 patients.

Intraluminal shunts were not performed routinely. Prosthetic grafts were used in most procedures—Dacron in 23 and polytetrafluoroethylene in 16. In the remaining 5, vein was used. The mean postoperative ICU stay was 1 day, and mean length of hospitalization was 5 days. Forty-three patients were available for follow-up, which was an average of 26.2 months. One patient undergoing an axilloaxillary procedure died perioperatively, for a death rate of 2.2%. Five of 18 grafts occluded after axillary artery procedures compared with only 1 of 29 thromboses occurring when surgery was limited to the supraclavicular fossa. All patients with patent grafts experienced relief of symptoms. No perioperative strokes occurred. One patient

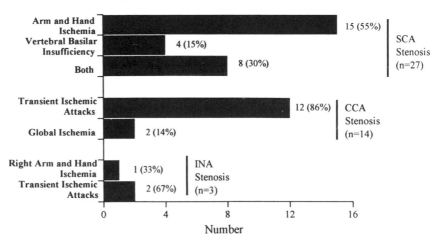

FIGURE 1.—Clinical manifestations in 44 patients with supra-aortic trunk arterial occlusive disease. (Courtesy of Owens LV, Tinsley EA Jr, Criado E, et al: Extrathoracic reconstruction of arterial occlusive disease involving the supraaortic trunks. *J Vasc Surg* 22:217–222, 1995.)

undergoing axilloaxillary bypass had a brachial plexus neuropraxia, and 4 patients had phrenic nerve neuropraxia (Fig 1).

*Conclusion.*—Extrathoracic bypasses limited to the supraclavicular fossa are excellent surgical options for patients with symptomatic supra-aortic trunk disease (except for those with occlusive disease of the innominate artery). The morbidity and mortality associated with these procedures are low, and long-term reduction of ipsilateral vascular events can be achieved.

▶ This large, rambling retrospective series reports a 20-year experience with 44 patients undergoing 47 extrathoracic bypass procedures of the supra-aortic trunks for correction of either subclavian, carotid, or innominate occlusive disease. I generally agree with the conclusions. We have come to prefer the carotid-subclavian transposition operation for subclavian revascularization when possible. It is not feasible in all cases. We almost never perform an axilloaxillary bypass but, as stated in Abstract 11–5, have come to depend on the carotid-axillary or carotid-brachial saphenous vein bypass graft. We find occasional use of a pretracheal carotid-carotid bypass. Generally the permutations of supra-aortic brachiocephalic reconstructions are limited only by the imagination of the surgeon. One must, however, take pains to assure that the donor vessel is relatively free of occlusive disease.

---

## Upper-Limb Arterial Disease in Women Treated for Breast Cancer

Taylor PJ, Cooper GG, Sarkar TK (Aberdeen Royal Infirmary, Scotland)
*Br J Surg* 82:1089–1091, 1995                                                                 11–7

---

*Background.*—Subclavian and axillary arterial disease is a well-documented, seemingly rare complication of radiotherapy for breast cancer. However, no cohort studies have established the prevalence of clinical and subclinical upper limb arterial disease after treatment for breast cancer.

*Methods.*—A 5-year cohort of 665 patients treated for breast cancer 15 to 19 years earlier was investigated to determine the prevalence of symptoms and objective evidence of circulatory insufficiency in the upper limbs. Of the 187 survivors, 102 were evaluated. Fifty of these had undergone radiotherapy along with surgery. The irradiated and nonirradiated groups were similar in age, extent of axillary dissection, and vascular risk factors. Vascular lab examination included segmental pressures and hyperemia testing. Doppler ultrasound waveform analysis, pulse volume recording, and venous outflow air plethysmography performed in both arms in each patient. The contralateral arm then served as a control.

*Findings.*—Among patients undergoing radiotherapy, 7 ipsilateral arms (14%) were symptomatic compared with 4 (8%) among those treated with surgery alone. Two contralateral control arms (2%) were symptomatic. Twenty-two percent of the ipsilateral arms of patients undergoing radiotherapy, and 4% of those of patients undergoing surgery alone showed evidence of arterial disease. Symptoms and evidence of arterial disease were unassociated. There was no evidence of abnormal venous function.

*Conclusion.*—These patients had a high prevalence of abnormal arterial physiology. Radiotherapy in the treatment of axillary disease is associated with adverse effects. Because the axillary artery is so close to the lymphatic drainage, some degree of arterial injury may be impossible to avoid.

▶ This remarkable epidemiologic survey examines the vascular status of the upper extremities in 187 15- to 19-year survivors of breast cancer. Fifty of 187 had received radiotherapy in addition to surgery. The patients who received radiation therapy had a statistically higher incidence of symptomatic occlusive disease of arm arteries than the patients who had surgery alone without radiation therapy. This once again points to a long-term adverse effect of radiation therapy for breast cancer. See also Abstract 4–11. It is noted that all patients entered in this study had their radiation therapy many years ago. Hopefully modern techniques have improved, and we will see fewer arterial occlusive problems after future radiation therapy than we have in the past.

# 12 Carotid and Cerebrovascular Disease

## Prevalence

**Carotid Artery Stenosis in Peripheral Vascular Disease**
Alexandrova NA, Gibson WC, Norris JW, et al (Univ of Toronto)
*J Vasc Surg* 23:645–649, 1996                                      12–1

*Introduction.*—Peripheral vascular disease is associated with a high probability of carotid atherosclerosis, and screening for carotid artery disease has been advocated using duplex ultrasonography for patients with peripheral vascular disease to identify those at risk of stroke. In patients with peripheral vascular disease, the prevalence and severity of symptomatic and asymptomatic carotid artery disease were studied so that operable carotid artery stenosis could be predicted.

*Methods.*—During 2 years, 372 consecutive patients with peripheral vascular disease (mean age 70 ± 10 years) were studied. They were screened for the presence of carotid atherosclerosis with color-coded duplex ultrasonography. A vascular surgeon and radiologist graded the carotid artery stenosis. A questionnaire was used to record preexisting risk factors such as sex, age, diabetes mellitus, hypertension, history of smoking, coronary artery disease, and prior stroke or transient ischemic attacks.

*Results.*—In this group, 71% had a history of smoking, 47% had coronary artery disease, 43% had hypertension, and 21% had diabetes mellitus. Carotid artery duplex scanning detected 30% or greater carotid artery stenosis in 211 (57%) of patients. Symptoms of ischemic cerebral events were found in 67 (32%) of patients, of whom 22 had potentially operable carotid artery stenosis (70%–99%). Stenosis of 60% to 99% was found in 71 of 144 symptom-free patients (Table 1). The strongest predictors of peripheral vascular disease were male sex and prior stroke or transient ischemic attack; however, all the risk factors were associated significantly with peripheral vascular disease.

TABLE 1.— Distribution of Severity of Carotid Artery Stenosis in Patients With and Without Symptoms

| Patients | No. | 0%–29% | 30%–59% | % Stenosis 60%–69% | 70%–99% | 100% |
|---|---|---|---|---|---|---|
| With symptoms | 87 | 20(23%) | 28(32%) | 6(7%) | 22(25%) | 11(13%) |
| Without symptoms | 286 | 142(50%) | 62(22%) | 22(8%) | 50(17%) | 10 (3%) |

*Conclusion.*—The study found that 25% of the group with category I or greater peripheral vascular disease, 22 with symptoms and 72 without symptoms, were potential surgical candidates after using routine carotid ultrasound screening.

▶ A significant number of patients with at least mild peripheral arterial occlusive disease underwent screening for the presence of carotid stenosis using color flow duplex. The majority of patients had detectable carotid disease, including 22 of 67 symptomatic patients who had 70% to 99% stenosis. Fifty percent of the 144 patients who were symptom free had 60% to 99% stenosis. Remarkably this study concludes that 25% of the entire cohort were candidates for carotid surgery. Although the overall number of afflicted patients is similar in the following paper, the number of patients who are potential candidates for surgery appears to be about twice as high in this paper. I am impressed by our medical colleagues.

## Prevalence of Asymptomatic Carotid Stenosis in Patients Undergoing Infrainguinal Bypass Surgery

Gentile AT, Taylor LM Jr, Moneta GL, et al (Oregon Health Sciences Univ, Portland)
*Arch Surg* 130:900–904, 1995                12–2

*Background.*—Some clinicians have recommended screening for asymptomatic carotid stenosis and prophylactic carotid endarterectomy (CEA) before major surgery. However, the prevalence of carotid stenosis in discrete patient groups is unknown. Carotid artery duplex examination was performed in asymptomatic patients undergoing infrainguinal revascularization for low extremity ischemia.

*Methods.*—Three hundred fifty-two patients undergoing infrainguinal bypass between 1987 and 1993 at 1 center were included in the prospective study. The patients were 117 men and 108 women (mean age 67). Surgery was indicated for limb salvage in 67% and claudication in 33%. Routine carotid duplex scanning was performed to detect asymptomatic carotid stenosis.

*Findings.*—Hemodynamically significant asymptomatic carotid artery stenosis or occlusion was detected in 28.4% of the patients needing lower extremity revascularization. Stenosis was 60% or greater in 12.4%. Based on duplex findings, 8 patients, with stenosis of 80% or more, had elective

CEA. None of the 225 patients undergoing leg bypass had postoperative neurologic events. In a multivariate logistic regression analysis, carotid stenosis of 50% or greater was associated with carotid bruit and rest pain.

*Conclusion.*—Duplex screening for carotid stenosis is indicated in patients requiring lower extremity revascularization. Significant numbers of patients with stenosis are missed when screening is limited to patients with carotid bruit, limb salvage indications for surgery, advanced age, or combination thereof.

▶ See Abstract 12–1. This paper differs significantly from the previous in that only patients undergoing infrainguinal bypass surgery are included here. This would appear to be a more severely diseased population than that described in the previous paper. Of the screened patients, 12.5% had stenosis leading to consideration of carotid surgery. Using regression analysis, we found that the presence of a carotid bruit or the presence of lower extremity rest pain was significantly associated with high-grade carotid stenosis. Unfortunately, limiting screening to just these patients would exclude significant numbers of patients with stenosis. This and the preceding paper bring up the contentious issue of the appropriateness of carotid screening tests. I continue to worry about the Health Care Financing Administration (HCFA) prohibition of screening studies of all types, which most assuredly should include carotid screening test. Although the HCFA policy may save money in the short haul, I do believe it is short sighted.

## Is Routine Carotid Screening for Coronary Surgery Needed?

Walker WA, Harvey WR, Gaschen JR, et al (Univ of Tennessee, Memphis; VA Med Ctr, Memphis, Tenn)
*Am Surg* 62:308–310, 1996                                                     12–3

*Background.*—The link between carotid artery disease and coronary artery disease is well known. At many hospitals this prompts routine preoperative duplex scanning of the carotid arteries in all patients undergoing coronary surgery. However, this practice has the potential to delay surgery and increase costs. The necessity of performing routine carotid screening before coronary surgery was evaluated in a 2-phase study.

*Retrospective Review.*—The first part of the study was a review of 308 consecutive patients undergoing coronary surgery at 1 hospital. Of these patients, 210 underwent preoperative duplex screening. One hundred fourteen patients were suspected of having possible carotid disease on the basis of a history and physical examination finding of transient ischemic attack or resolving ischemic neurologic deficit, cerebrovascular accident, arteriosclerotic peripheral vascular disease, abdominal aortic aneurysm, neck bruit, or previous carotid surgery. Thirty-two percent of patients in this group had a positive duplex scan compared with just 3% of patients without a positive history and physical examination.

*Prospective Study.*—In a subsequent prospective study, 83 cardiac surgery patients were classified on the basis of a positive history and physical examination into "carotid disease" and "no carotid disease" groups including 33 patients in the former and 50 patients in the latter. Twenty-seven percent of patients in the "carotid disease" group had positive duplex scans compared with none of those in the "no carotid disease" group.

*Conclusion.*—Preoperative carotid artery scans are indicated for coronary surgery patients who have a history of peripheral or cerebral vascular disease or a neck bruit on physical examination. This approach is recommended over routine duplex screening for all patients undergoing cardiac surgery, which delays surgery and increases costs.

▶ It seems to me that the criteria of carotid positivity was set too low in this study. A peak velocity of only 150 cm/sec was required, and I suspect this is in the range of 40% to 50% diameter reduction in most patients. Nonetheless, these authors found that positive findings were significantly limited only to patients who had carotid symptoms, a cervical bruit, or established peripheral vascular arterial disease, hardly a surprising conclusion. See the previous abstracts.

## Aspirin Treatment

### The Warfarin-Aspirin Symptomatic Intracranial Disease Study

Chimowitz MI, Kokkinos J, Strong J, et al (Univ of Michigan, Ann Arbor; Case Western Reserve Univ, Detroit; Tufts–New England Med Ctr, Boston; et al)
*Neurology* 45:1488–1493, 1995                                    12–4

*Objective.*—The effectiveness of warfarin was compared with that of aspirin for preventing ischemic stroke, myocardial infarction, and sudden death in patients having symptomatic stenosis of a major intracranial artery in a retrospective multicenter study.

*Patients.*—Seven centers enrolled 151 patients in the study, all of whom had at least 50% stenosis of the carotid, vertebral, or basilar artery or 1 of the major cerebral vessels. In addition, all patients had transient ischemic attacks (62 patients) or stroke (89 patients) in the territory of the stenotic artery. Patients with occlusion of an intracranial vessel or extracranial internal carotid stenosis of 50% or greater proximal to an intracranial stenosis were excluded.

*Treatment.*—The local physician selected treatment with either 325 mg of aspirin daily or warfarin, the latter adjusted to maintain the prothrombin time at 1.2 to 1.6 of control. Eighty-eight patients received warfarin, and 63 received aspirin. The 2 groups were comparable with respect to age, degree of stenosis, and vascular risk factors.

*Results.*—Major vascular events occurred at a rate of 18 per 100 patient-years of follow-up in aspirin-treated patients and at a rate of 8 per 100 patient-years in the warfarin group. The relative risk of stroke, myocardial infarction, or sudden death in warfarin-treated patients was 0.46.

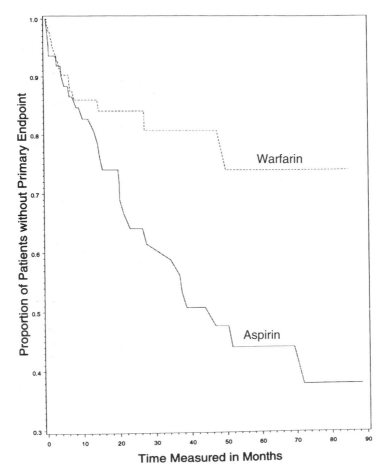

FIGURE.—Graph shows Kaplan-Meier estimates of proportion of patients remaining free of ischemic stroke, myocardial infarction, or sudden death in those treated with warfarin (*upper curve*) or aspirin (*lower curve*). (Reprinted from *Neurology* 45:1488–1493, 1995, by permission of Little, Brown and Company [Inc.].)

There were no major hemorrhagic complications in the aspirin group, but 3 warfarin-treated patients had such complications and 2 of them died.

*Conclusion.*—Warfarin may prevent major vascular events more effectively than aspirin in patients with symptomatic stenosis of a major intracranial artery (Fig). The present findings warrant a prospective randomized trial.

▶ This is a retrospective study of patients with symptomatic intracranial arterial occlusions or stenoses treated either with warfarin or aspirin at the preference of their local physician. The remarkable positivity of this study in favor of warfarin is noted and appears to directly conflict with the volumes of data favoring aspirin. The remarkable therapeutic benefits in favor of warfarin lead these authors to recommend a prospective randomized study, a position with which I am in agreement. I also favor motherhood and apple pie.

### Aspirin in Ischemic Cerebrovascular Disease: How Strong Is the Case for a Different Dosing Regimen?
Patrono C, Roth GJ (Univ of Chieti "G D'Annunzio," Italy; Univ of Washington, Seattle)
*Stroke* 27:756–760, 1996                                                                 12–5

*Background.*—Aspirin is prescribed for patients with coronary heart disease to help prevent myocardial infarction, stroke, and death from vascular causes. In this group of patients, it is widely agreed that the proper dose is between 75 and 160 mg. However, there is no such agreement as to the best dose of aspirin for patients with cerebrovascular disease, for whom recommendations range from 30 to 1,300 mg/day. Arguments were presented in favor of a lower dose of aspirin from patients with ischemic cerebrovascular disease.

*Arguments for Low-Dose Aspirin.*—Some authors recommend high doses of aspirin for patients with cerebrovascular disease, on the order of 650 to 1,300 mg. However, this recommendation is based on indirect data, such as selective comparisons of the results of different trials, mini–meta-analyses, or subgroup analyses of different trials. There have been no randomized clinical trials directly comparing the effects of low- and high-dose aspirin of adequate size to demonstrate a moderate difference in efficacy between the 2 doses. Lacking such evidence, the authors question the biological rationale for using a higher dose of aspirin in patients with cerebrovascular disease (i.e., aspirin "failure" or "resistance"). From a risk-benefit standpoint, the only way to determine the practical consequences of using high-dose aspirin is a direct, randomized comparison of the 2 competing approaches.

*Conclusion.*—Evidence to support the recommendation that patients with cerebrovascular disease should receive higher doses of aspirin is insufficient. Until such evidence is available, the lowest effective dose of aspirin (75 mg/day) should be used for the prevention of stroke and death in patients with ischemic cerebrovascular disease.

▶ These authors conclude that available information indicates that good clinical practice dictates the use of the lowest possible dose of aspirin in patients with ischemic cerebrovascular disease. The authors specifically recommend 75 mg daily (1 baby aspirin). It is noted that in an editorial in the same journal, Dr. Barnett of NASCET fame takes significant exception to this recommendation. Despite Dr. Barnett's reservations, I believe the authors are entirely correct that a single low-dose aspirin daily is adequate.

## Contralateral Occlusion

### Carotid Endarterectomy in the Presence of a Contralateral Occlusion: A Review of 315 Cases Over a 27-Year Experience

Adelman MA, Jacobowitz GR, Riles TS, et al (New York Univ)

*Cardiovasc Surg* 3:307–312, 1995                                        12–6

*Background.*—Many researchers have reported a high risk of stroke in patients with occlusion of 1 internal carotid artery (ICA) and stenosis of the other. Though patients undergoing carotid endarterectomy for repair of the stenotic carotid artery appear to have better outcomes, surgery in patients with a contralateral occlusion has been associated with a very high risk of perioperative stroke or death. The perioperative complication rate for such patients reportedly ranges from 2.8% to 14.3%. A 27-year experience with carotid endarterectomy was reviewed.

*Methods.*—One hundred eighty patients undergoing endarterectomy of the stenotic contralateral internal carotid artery (ICA) between 1965 and 1984 (group 1) were compared with 135 operated on between 1985 and 1991 (group 2). All had occlusion of 1 ICA. The groups were comparable in age, sex, incidence of coronary artery disease, hypertension, diabetes, and history of smoking. Group 2 had significantly more patients who were neurologically symptom free before surgery.

*Findings.*—Patients in group 2 had a significantly lower combined perioperative stroke or death rate than those in group 1. In group 2 patients, there was more frequent placement of intra-arterial shunt and increased use of general anesthesia. However, shunt alone did not explain the improved outcomes; equally important were the lower incidences of postoperative thrombosis, embolization, and intracerebral hemorrhage.

*Conclusion.*—In patients with ICA stenosis and contralateral occlusion, complications from carotid endarterectomy cannot be attributed to a single technical problem. The high incidence of perioperative stroke or death that has been reported in these patients reflects the increased risk that any ischemic insult may result in a neurologic event. The operative risks can be reduced through better patient selection and careful attention to cerebral perfusion and reconstruction of the carotid artery after endarterectomy.

▶ Numerous studies have demonstrated both an increased postoperative stroke rate and an increased shunt requirement when carotid endarterectomy is performed contralateral to an internal carotid occlusion. Thus, the perioperative stroke and death rate of only 0.7% achieved by the New York University (NYU) group since 1985 is truly outstanding. As is the current fashion, they then compared their recent results with their worst results prior to 1985 (6.7% stroke rate) and attempted to explain this improvement. In their more recent experience, the authors used carotid shunts more frequently, employed general anesthesia more often, and, more important, had many more asymptomatic patients. However, because only 11 strokes occurred in this entire experience and most of these had nothing to do with the contralateral carotid occlusion, the authors were unable to determine whether any of these changes had affected their results. Thus, they could conclude only that perioperative stroke associated with carotid endarterectomy has multifactorial causes, hardly a novel conclusion.

The most interesting fact in this article was that 25% of awake patients without a fixed neurologic deficit required shunting because of symptoms that developed during test clamping. This is the gold standard for shunt requirement and is a much higher percentage than reported for patients without contralateral carotid occlusion. The NYU group elected to shunt all patients with both contralateral occlusion and a preoperative fixed neurologic deficit, assuming that this group would have even less tolerance for global cerebral ischemia. This finding reinforces my bias that patients with contralateral carotid occlusion should be shunted during ipsilateral endarterectomy unless the patient is awake and an accurate assessment of shunt requirement can be made. The current article, however, was unable to prove (or disprove) the logic of this conclusion.

**J. Cronenwett, M.D.**

## Carotid Endarterectomy Contralateral to an Occluded Carotid Artery: A Retrospective Case-Control Study

Cao P, Giordano G, de Rango P, et al (Univ of Perugia, Italy)
*Eur J Vasc Endovasc Surg* 10:16–22, 1995                    12–7

*Background.*—The indication for carotid endarterectomy (CEA) has yet to be defined for patients with carotid stenosis and occlusion of the contralateral internal carotid artery (ICA). Contralateral occlusion was further explored to determine whether it is an additional perioperative risk factor in CEA.

*Methods.*—Group 1 consisted of 55 patients with carotid stenosis and contralateral occlusion undergoing CEA, and group 2 consisted of 100 patients without contralateral occlusion chosen from 367 patients with a

TABLE 7.—Perioperative Death and Stroke Rate

| | Group I (n = 55) | | Group II (n = 110) | | O.R. | 95% C.I. | p value |
|---|---|---|---|---|---|---|---|
| | Patients | % | Patients | % | | | |
| Stroke* | 0 | 0 | 2† | 2 | | | |
| Death | 0 | 0 | 1‡ | 1 | | | |
| Total | 0 | 0 | 3 | 2.7 | 0 | 0–4.85 | 0.5 |

\* Only major disabling stroke.
† One contralateral stroke.
‡ Fatal stroke.
*Abbreviations:* O.R., odds ratio; C.I., confidence interval.
(Reprinted from *Eur J Vasc Endovasc Surg*; vol 10; Cao P, Giordano G, de Rango P, et al: Carotid endarterectomy contralateral to an occluded artery: A retrospective case-control study; pp 16–22: 1995; by permission of the publisher Academic Press Limited, London.)

TABLE 9.—Late Death

| | Group I (n = 55) | | Group II (n = 110) | | O.R. | 95% C.I. | p value |
|---|---|---|---|---|---|---|---|
| | Patients | % | Patients | % | | | |
| Vascular death (cardiac + cerebral) | 8 | 14 | 7 | 6 | 2.50 | 0.77–8.25 | 0.1 |
| Cardiac | 5 | 9 | 6 | 5 | 1.73 | 0.40–7.16 | 0.5 |
| Stroke | 3 | 5 | 1 | 1 | 6.29 | 0.49–333 | 0.1 |
| Other | 2 | 4 | 2 | 2 | 2.04 | 0.14–28.69 | 0.6 |
| Total | 10 | 18 | 9 | 8 | 2.49 | 0.86–7.26 | 0.1 |

*Note:* Crude rate: mean 38.4 mo.
*Abbreviations:* O.R., odds ratio; C.I., confidence interval.
(Reprinted from *Eur J Vasc Endovasc Surg*; vol 10; Cao P, Giordano G, de Rango P, et al: Carotid endarterectomy contralateral to an occluded artery: A retrospective case-control study; pp 16–22; 1995; by permission of the publisher Academic Press Limited, London.)

patent contralateral artery. The groups were matched for gender, age, and ipsilateral symptoms. Mean follow-up was 38 months.

*Findings.*—The 30-day perioperative stroke and death rate was 0% in group 1 and 2.7% in group 2. Eleven percent of group 1 patients and 5% in group 2 had minor complications. The survival rates of patients free from stroke were 79.4% in group 1 and 83.3% in group 2. Stroke-free rates were 92.8% in group 1 and 94.3% in group 2. Patients with and without contralateral obstruction had the same incidence of late stroke, fatal or not. However, 14% of those in group 1 died of late vascular complications compared with only 6% in group 2 (Tables 7 and 9).

*Conclusion.*—In this series of patients with contralateral occlusion, CEA was unrelated to increased perioperative morbidity and mortality. The greater (though nonsignificant) incidence of vascular death in the late follow-up of patients with contralateral carotid occlusion may indicate more severe systemic vascular disease.

▶ See also Abstract 12–6. We have been swamped in recent years by an avalanche of articles reporting the safety of CEA opposite a carotid occlusion.[1-4] This monumental list of recent publications has established for all time that patients with contralateral occlusion can safely undergo ipsilateral endarterectomy. I hereby issue the following warning: Anyone publishing 1 more time that patients with a contralateral carotid occlusion can safely undergo an ipsilateral endarterectomy will assuredly receive the CDA.

*References*

1. 1994 YEARBOOK OF VASCULAR SURGERY, p 302.
2. 1994 YEARBOOK OF VASCULAR SURGERY, p 303.
3. 1995 YEARBOOK OF VASCULAR SURGERY, p 311.
4. 1995 YEARBOOK OF VASCULAR SURGERY, p 312.

## Surgical Series

### Evolution of Carotid Endarterectomy in Two Community Hospitals: Springfield Revisited: Seventeen Years and 2243 Operations Later

Mattos MA, Modi JR, Mansour MA, et al (Southern Illinois Univ, Springfield)
J Vasc Surg 21:719–728, 1995                                          12–8

*Background.*—A 1977 report disclosed a very high incidence of complications of carotid endarterectomy (CEA) at 2 community hospitals in 1 city. The hospitals' subsequent experience was reviewed to see if there had been any improvement in this problem.

*Methods and Results.*—The review included 1,981 patients undergoing a total of 2,243 CEA procedures over a 17-year period. Operative mortality improved from 6.6% to 1.6%, operative stroke rate from 14.5% to 5.3%, and combined stroke-mortality rate from 21.1% to 6.3%. Significant declines in nonfatal stroke rate were observed for patients with asymptomatic carotid artery disease, from 18.2% to 2.9%; transient ischemic attack, 17.8% to 3.9%; and previous stroke, 15.2% to 8.0%. Though patients with all types of surgical indications showed improvement in their combined stroke-mortality rate, the change was significant only for the patients with transient ischemic attack and previous stroke.

A total of 31 surgeons performed the operations; the number of procedures per surgeon ranged from 1 to 236. There was no significant relationship between the number of procedures performed and the results achieved by each individual surgeon. However, operative stroke rate was 4.1% for surgeons who did more than 12 CEAs per year vs. 7.2% for those who did fewer procedures. Vascular surgeons had lower stroke rates and combined stroke-mortality rates than surgeons without additional vascular training, though many of the nonvascular surgeons achieved results comparable to those of the vascular surgeons.

*Conclusion.*—In the 17 years since the initial report, the 2 hospitals studied showed dramatic improvements in the rate of complications associated with CEA. However, these rates remain suboptimal and have shown little change since the early 1980s. This situation is unlikely to change until CEA privileges are restricted to surgeons who have demonstrated low complication rates.

▶ Who says things haven't gotten better in Springfield? Community data such as these are important in allowing all of us to objectively assess our operative results. I wonder how many vascular surgeons have similar hard data for their entire community. I'll bet very few. I congratulate the Springfield group on taking the time to tabulate this information. Individual performers who are not reaching the standards for the community will hopefully use this information as a stimulus for improvement or cessation.

### Endarterectomy for Asymptomatic Carotid Artery Stenosis

Executive Committee for the Asymptomatic Carotid Atherosclerosis Study
(Wake Forest Univ, Winston-Salem, NC)
*JAMA* 273:1421–1428, 1995                                                     12–9

*Background.*—In 1987, the Asymptomatic Carotid Atherosclerosis Study (ACAS) was initiated to determine whether the addition of carotid endarterectomy (CEA) to aggressive reduction of modifiable risk factors and treatment with aspirin would decrease the incidence of cerebral infraction in patients with asymptomatic carotid artery stenosis. Study findings are reported herein.

*Patients and Methods.*—Thirty-nine clinical sites in the United States and Canada participated in this 6-year, prospective, randomized trial. A total of 1,662 patients (mean age 67) with asymptomatic carotid artery stenosis of 60% or greater reduction in diameter were enrolled. Of these, 1,659 were available for follow-up. All patients received treatment with daily aspirin and medical risk factor management, and 825 also were randomly assigned to CEA. Transient ischemic attack or cerebral infarction in the distribution of the study artery and any transient ischemic attack, stroke, or mortality observed perioperatively comprised the initial main outcome measures. During the last 9 months of the study, these were changed to cerebral infarction in the distribution of the study artery or any stroke or mortality occurring perioperatively. Median follow-up was 2.7 years.

*Results.*—Baseline risk factors for stroke were comparable between the medical and surgical treatment groups. During the perioperative period, 2.3% of the CEA patients had a stroke or died compared with 0.4% of the patients receiving medical treatment only. At median follow-up, the aggregate risk over 5 years for ipsilateral stroke and any stroke or mortality occurring perioperatively was approximately 5.1% for patients assigned to CEA and 11.0% for those receiving medical treatment only. Although not statistically significant because of small sample size, similar trends were observed for all subgroups considered, including deciles of stenosis, and for secondary cerebrovascular end points. When restricted to patients receiving the assigned treatment, results were essentially the same and nearly identical for patients without previous contralateral symptoms or endarterectomy.

*Conclusion.*—Carotid endarterectomy performed with less than 3% perioperative morbidity and mortality, combined with aggressive management of modifiable risk factors, can help reduce 5-year risk of ipsilateral stroke in patients with asymptomatic carotid artery stenosis of 60% or greater reduction in diameter. Patient's overall health status also should be considered when candidates are selected for CEA.

▶ This remarkable publication of the ACAS Committee has received deservedly widespread attention among vascular surgeons and others. You all are familiar with the overall reduction of 6% in the stroke rate occurring in operated patients with stenotic disease in excess of 60% diameter reduction. This benefit was significant in large part due to the very admirable 2.3% stroke death rate in the surgical series. Two findings in this publication have attracted considerable attention from the nay sayers. First, no benefit was shown for women, possibly because of small numbers, and, second, there appeared to be no increased risk for the higher degrees of carotid stenosis. Interestingly, a significant percentage of the surgical complication was attributable to arteriography. Women also appeared to have a higher perioperative complication rate. This study will provide food for thought for generations to come. We currently recommend prophylactic carotid surgery in good risk patients with 70% or greater stenosis measured by ACAS criteria. We most assuredly do not extend this recommendation to the very elderly or to patients with significant comorbid conditions.

---

### Direct Transposition of the Distal Cervical Vertebral Artery Into the Internal Carotid Artery

Koskas F, Kieffer E, Rancurel G, et al (La Salpétriè, Paris)
*Ann Vasc Surg* 9:515–524, 1995                                    12–10

---

*Background.*—In revascularization of the vertebral arteries (VAs), it is often possible to directly transpose the V3 segment of the VA into the ipsilateral internal carotid artery (ICA). This procedure can avoid the need for grafting and offers some important theoretical hemodynamic advantages. An experience with direct transposition of the V3 segment into the ICA was reported.

*Methods.*—The 13-year experience included 92 revascularization procedures in 91 patients in which the V3 segment of the VA was directly transposed into the ICA. Direct transposition was performed in 15% of vertebral revascularizations and 39% of distal vertebral revascularizations performed during the study period. Sixty-three percent of the patients were women, and the mean age was 59. Ninety-five percent of patients had vertebrobasilar ischemic symptoms before revascularization. Of 4 asymptomatic patients, 3 had spinal tumors involving the vertebral foraminal canal and 1 had severe occlusion of multiple vessels. Significant carotid occlusion was present in about one third of patients. Twenty-six percent of patients underwent endarterectomy of the ICA at the same time as direct transposition of the distal V3 segment of the VA was performed.

*Results.*—None of the patients died or had a stroke, though 2 experienced transient ischemic attacks. Early follow-up studies showed complete occlusion of the transposed VA in 9% of cases. Ninety percent of arteries were patent (Fig 1). One-month cure rate among the patients with vertebrobasilar insufficiency was 51%; another 36% of patients were in improved condition and 14% showed no change. Most patients with the latter result had occlusion or stenosis of the distal transposition by the time they left the hospital. Five-year primary patency rate was 89%, and cure rate among the patients with vertebrobasilar insufficiency was 58%.

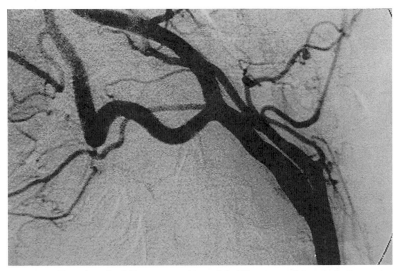

FIGURE 1.—Typical result of direct transposition of the V3 segment of the vertebral artery into the internal carotid artery as seen on an early digital subtraction angiogram. (Courtesy of Koskas F, Kieffer E, Rancurel G, et al: Direct transposition of the distal cervical vertebral artery into the internal carotid artery. *Ann Vasc Surg* 9[6]:515–524, 1995.)

Twenty-nine percent of these patients were in improved condition, 2% were unchanged, 2% had had a relapse, and 9% had varying degrees of vertebrobasilar symptoms.

*Conclusion.*—Revascularization of the distal cervical VA can be safely and reliably performed by direct transposition of the V3 segment into the ICA. Direct transposition should be considered for patients who do not have an available autograft and in whom the V3 vertebral segment can be easily freed from the atlas or axis.

▶ Dr. Kieffer's experience with VA surgery is legendary. Herein he and his colleagues report a remarkable 92 transpositions of the high cervical VA directly into the ICA. He modestly notes that this represents 15% of his personal series of 610 vertebral revascularizations. His experience is remarkable, his results are excellent, and I am sure I will draw on his experience if I have to operate on 1 of these infrequently encountered patients in the United States.

### Cranial Nerve Injuries After Carotid Artery Surgery: A Prospective Study of 663 Operations

Forssell C, Kitzing P, Bergqvist D (Malmö Univ, Sweden; Univ Hosp, Uppsala, Sweden)

*Eur J Vasc Endovasc Surg* 10:445–449, 1995                    12–11

*Objective.*—The frequency and cause of cranial nerve damage after carotid artery surgery in a large population were determined in a prospective study.

*Methods.*—During a 10-year period, 656 of 689 patients who underwent carotid artery operations were examined before and after surgery for ninth, tenth, and eleventh cranial nerve function. Voice recordings, stroboscopic light examination of the vocal cords, and examinations of the cranial nerves were made.

*Results.*—Injury to 1 or more of the examined cranial nerves was noted in 11.4% (75) of the 656 patients studied. The hypoglossal nerve was injured in 70 cases (10.7%), the recurrent laryngeal nerve was damaged in 8 (1.2%) cases, and the glossopharyngeal and superior laryngeal nerves were each injured in 2 cases (0.3%). Only 2 of the cranial nerve injuries were permanent, and the remainder recovered within 6 months. The injury to cranial nerves was more frequent in operations performed with a shunt, with patch closure, and by a junior surgeon.

*Conclusion.*—The incidence of cranial nerve injury after carotid surgery was significant. The time from arteriotomy to completion of the suture line may be a critical factor influencing the number of nerve injuries. The majority of injuries noted were reversible, and many could be avoided by having detailed knowledge of the surgical anatomy, careful handling of the tissues, precise bipolar electrocautery, and careful placement of ligatures.

▶ The incidence of detected cranial nerve injury after 609 carotid endarterectomies was 11.4% at the Malmo University Hospital. By far the most frequent injury was a hypoglossal, with recurrent laryngeal, glossopharyngeal, and superior laryngeal nerves a distant second, third, and forth. Although we have not methodically searched for cranial nerve injuries postopertively (some things you would rather not know), we infrequently recognize these injuries. Although the occasional recurrent laryngeal or hypoglossal injury does cause the patient moderate distress, by far the most distressing injury in my experience is the glossopharyngeal. These patients seemed to have a distressing problem with swallowing, which is very slow to resolve. I am convinced, on balance, that this is one area where careful surgical technique clearly leads to a reduction in complications.

## Carotid Artery Shortening: A Safe Adjunct to Carotid Endarterectomy

Coyle KA, Smith RB III, Chapman RL, et al (Emory Univ, Atlanta)
*J Vasc Surg* 22:257–263, 1995                                   12–12

*Introduction.*—Some patients with atherosclerotic involvement of the internal carotid artery have kinking and coiling of the extracranial carotid artery system. A number of techniques for straightening redundant or kinked vessels have been described, usually for use in patients undergoing carotid endarterectomy. The value of performing a carotid artery shortening procedure in addition to carotid endarterectomy was assessed in a 10-year review.

*Methods.*—The review included 107 patients who underwent concurrent carotid endarterectomy and ipsilateral carotid artery shortening from 1983 to 1992. There were 54 men and 53 women aged 47 to 89. The surgical indication was high-grade asymptomatic stenosis in 47% of patients, transient ischemic attacks in 28%, stroke in 18%, and amaurosis fugax in 7%. The patients underwent various carotid artery shortening procedures at the end of their endarterectomies (Fig 1 ).

Follow-up included contact with the patient or primary care physician and, when available, carotid artery duplex scans. The analysis focused on perioperative mortality and stroke-morbidity rates or late restenosis.

*Results.*—There were 2 postoperative deaths and 1 stroke in the study series, for a combined 30-day mortality and stroke morbidity rate of 2.7%. This compared favorably with a 4.0% combined 30-day mortality and stroke morbidity rate in 1,072 carotid endarterectomies performed during

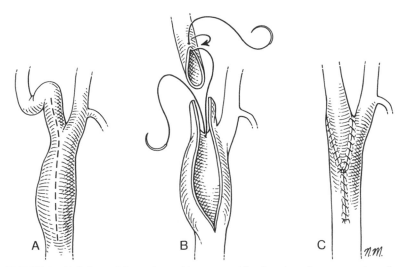

**FIGURE 1.**—Technique of internal carotid artery straightening. **A,** endarterectomy is performed through longitudinal arteriotomy. **B,** internal carotid artery is transected obliquely at its origin, then rotated 180 degrees before reanastomosis. **C,** completed anastomosis with previous back wall of internal carotid artery advanced onto arteriotomy as in situ patch. (Courtesy of Coyle KA, Smith RB III, Chapman RL, et al: Carotid artery shortening: A safe adjunct to carotid endarterectomy. *J Vasc Surg* 22:257–263, 1995.)

the same period. None of the patients undergoing carotid artery shortening had an ipsilateral stroke, recurrent symptoms, or significant restenosis during follow-up.

*Conclusion.*—Carotid artery shortening procedures can safely be added to carotid endarterectomy, with no increase in morbidity and mortality. The vascular surgeon should be familiar with these procedures, because they can be helpful in patients with carotid artery kinks and coils.

▶ The Emory group has a large and enviable experience with carotid artery surgery. After long consideration of their illustrations, I wonder why they do not obliquely transect the internal carotid in the opposite direction, eliminating the need for 180-degree rotation. At any rate, this is another in a series of useful maneuvers for carotid artery shortening. Usually we simply transect, remove the offending segment, and reanastomose, always including a generous patch across the anastomotic site.

## Stroke

**Stroke Incidence, Prevalence, and Survival: Secular Trends in Rochester, Minnesota, Through 1989**
Brown RD Jr, Whisnant JP, Sicks JD, et al (Mayo Clinic and Mayo Found, Rochester, Minn)
*Stroke* 27:373–380, 1996                                                      12–13

*Background.*—Though many studies have reported the incidence rates of stroke in various parts of the world, there are few data on trends in stroke incidence and mortality over time. The unique nature of the health care provided to the population of Rochester, Minnesota, presents an opportunity to evaluate long-term trends in the incidence and mortality of stroke. Incidence rates, mortality, radiologic imaging, and prevalence of stroke in Rochester from 1985 through 1989 were reported, including an evaluation of stroke trends from 1955 through 1989.

*Methods.*—Medical records of all Rochester residents with a potential diagnosis of stroke from 1985 through 1989 were screened and reviewed to determine the type of stroke. Yearly age- and sex-adjusted incidence rates for stroke and the various types of stroke in 5-year periods from 1955 to 1989 were calculated, and the prevalence of stroke was determined. The influence of multiple variables were analyzed using Poisson regression, and trends in short- and long-term stroke survival were evaluated using Cox proportional hazards modeling.

*Results.*—The most recent 5-year period included 496 incidence cases of stroke, for an annual age- and sex-adjusted stroke incidence rate of 145/100,000 population. This rate was similar to that from 1980 to 1984 but 13% higher than that from 1975 to 1979. Compared with the incidence rates from the 1970s, the incidence of stroke increased in all population groups older than 54 and in both sexes. Analysis of the long-term trends suggested that patient survival after cerebral infarction depended on age and calendar year. The annual incidence rate of intraparenchymal hemorrhage was double that of subarachnoid hemorrhage.

*Conclusion.*—Incidence rates of stroke during the 1980s were higher than those observed in the 1970s. The incidence rate of stroke remains higher than reported during the decline in stroke incidence during the 1960s and 1970s, even though rates of untreated hypertension have been stable or decreasing. The recent increase in stroke incidence rates probably reflects the availability of radiologic imaging studies, an increased contribution of patients with ischemic heart disease, and identification of patients with milder strokes, in addition to other, unknown factors.

▶ Are we coming to the end of the gratifying decline in stroke incidence so widely reported during the past 25 years? Using the captive audience of Rochester, Minnesota, these authors investigated the incidence of stroke during 5-year periods from 1955 to 1989. Between 1985 and 1989, the stroke incidence appeared unchanged from that reported in 1980 to 1984 and was 13% higher than the rate determined in the period 1975 to 1979. This leads these authors to conclude the decline in stroke incidence has stopped, and we are seeing a small but detectable increase. I hope they are wrong, but I bet they are correct.

---

## Low-Molecular-Weight Heparin for the Treatment of Acute Ischemic Stroke

Kay R, Wong KS, Yu YL, et al (Prince of Wales Hosp, Shatin, Hong Kong; Queen Mary Hosp, Hong Kong; Kwong Wah Hosp, Hong Kong; et al)
*N Engl J Med* 333:1588–1593, 1995                                12–14

---

*Background.*—Though the safety and efficacy of antithrombotic agents have been questioned, these agents are used frequently in patients with acute ischemic stroke. Low–molecular weight heparin, which can be given only once or twice daily subcutaneously, may be more effective and safer than standard, unfractionated heparin.

*Methods.*—Three hundred twelve patients with ischemic stroke were randomized in a double-blind, placebo-controlled comparison of 2 dosages of low–molecular weight heparin and placebo. Within 28 hours of symptom onset, patients were given high-dose nadroparin, low-dose nadroparin, or placebo treatments subcutaneously. Treatment duration was 10 days. The main outcome measure was death or dependence in activities of daily living 6 months after treatment initiation.

*Findings.*—Data on 306 patients were evaluable at 6 months. Death or dependence at 6 months was documented in 45% of patients given high-dose nadroparin, 52% given low-dose nadroparin, and 65% given placebo. A significant dose-dependent effect was noted in favor of active treatment.

*Conclusion.*—Low–molecular weight heparin improved 6-month outcomes in this series of patients with ischemic stroke when begun within 48 hours of symptom onset. Additional research is needed to establish optimal dosage and treatment duration.

▶ As assessed by death or neurologic dependency at 6 months, high-dose was more effective than low-dose low–molecular weight heparin, which was, in turn, more effective than placebo in this study. The significant dose-dependent effect noted makes it much more likely that the effects are real. These results lead one to conclude that low–molecular weight heparin is really effective in improving outcome in patients suffering ischemic stroke who have treatment within 48 hours of the onset of symptoms. It is noteworthy that the duration of treatment was only 10 days.

**Plaque Ulceration and Lumen Thrombus Are the Main Sources of Cerebral Microemboli in High-Grade Internal Carotid Artery Stenosis**
Sitzer M, Müller W, Siebler M, et al (Heinrich-Heine-Univ, Düsseldorf, Germany)
*Stroke* 26:1231–1233, 1995                                                    12–15

*Background.*—Patients with recent symptoms show higher rates of cerebral microemboli downstream from high-grade internal carotid artery stenoses than do patients without symptoms. After carotid endarterectomy, rate of microembolism declines. Forty patients either without symptoms or with recent symptoms who were undergoing carotid endarterectomy for internal carotid artery stenoses of 70% to 95% were prospectively evaluated to determine the relationship between rate of microembolism and pathoanatomical features of the carotid plaque.

*Methods.*—Rates of cerebral microemboli of the ipsilateral middle cerebral artery were assessed preoperatively via transcranial Doppler monitoring with automated emboli detection. After endarterectomy, specimens were evaluated histologically for presence of plaque fissuring, intraplaque hemorrhage, intraluminal thrombosis, or plaque ulceration.

TABLE 1.—Number of Asymptomatic or Symptomatic Patients With High-Grade Internal Carotid Stenosis in the Three Microembolic Tertiles

|  | Degree of Stenosis (Mean), % | Microemboli per Hour | | |
|---|---|---|---|---|
|  |  | 0 | ≤5 | >5 |
| Asymptomatic | 70–95 (84.6) | 10 | 0 | 2 |
| Symptomatic | 70–95 (82.5) | 3 | 14 | 11 |

Note: $\chi^2$ statistics: $P < 0.001$; degrees of freedom = 2.
(Sitzer M, Müller W, Siebler M, et al: Plaque ulceration and lumen thrombus are the main sources of cerebral microemboli in high-grade internal carotid artery stenosis. *Stroke* 26:1231–1233. Reproduced with permission of *Stroke*, Copyright 1995, American Heart Association.)

TABLE 2.—Relationships Between Preoperative Microembolic Rates and 4 Pathoanatomical Features in 39 Carotid Endarterectomy Specimens From 39 Patients With High-Grade Internal Carotid Artery Stenosis

| | Microemboli per Hour | | | |
| | 0 (*n* = 13) | ≤5 (*n* = 14) | >5 (*n* = 12) | P* |
|---|---|---|---|---|
| Plaque fissure | 7 | 7 | 5 | .82 |
| Intraplaque hemorrhage | 1 | 3 | 4 | .28 |
| Plaque ulceration | 1 | 8 | 8 | .005† |
| Lumen thrombus | 3 | 10 | 12 | .0003† |

Note: Values are numbers of patients/specimens. Patients were subdivided into tertiles according to individual microembolic rates per hour (0, ≤5, >5).
*$\chi^2$ statistics; degrees of freedom = 2.
† Significant after α-adjustment.
(Sitzer M, Müller W, Siebler M, et al: Plaque ulceration and lumen thrombus are the main sources of cerebral microemboli in high-grade internal carotid artery stenosis. *Stroke* 26:1231–1233. Reproduced with permission of *Stroke*, Copyright 1995, American Heart Association.)

*Results.*—Rates of microembolism were significantly higher among patients with symptoms (Table 1). Downstream cerebral microemboli were significantly associated with plaque ulceration and intraluminal thrombosis but not with plaque fissuring or intraplaque hemorrhage (Table 2). Plaque ulceration and intraluminal thrombosis were also related both to each other and to recent ischemic symptoms.

*Conclusion.*—In patients with high-grade internal carotid artery stenosis, the main sources of ipsilateral microembolism of the middle cerebral artery are internal carotid artery plaque ulceration and intraluminal thrombosis. Transcranial Doppler ultrasonography is the first noninvasive method capable of evaluating these 2 significant pathoanatomical features of unstable internal carotid artery stenosis. The data suggest that these features may also play a key role in symptom development.

▶ These authors conclude that cerebral microemboli from carotid atherosclerosis is more likely when there is plaque ulceration or intraluminal thrombus. I'll bet you could search the world over and find not one soul who would disagree with this conclusion. Dare I suggest a CDA for confirmation of what everyone already knew?

## Stroke Rate Is Markedly Reduced After Carotid Endarterectomy by Avoidance of Protamine

Mauney MC, Buchanan SA, Lawrence WA, et al (Univ of Virginia, Charlottesville)
*J Vasc Surg* 22:264–270, 1995                                        12–16

*Background.*—Carotid endarterectomy (CEA) is now the most common peripheral vascular operation done in the United States. However, neurologic injury continues to be a significant risk associated with this procedure. Such injury results from embolization of debris and formation of thrombus on the newly endarterectomized surface. Primary CEAs were reviewed to determine whether the risk of postoperative neurologic injury may be lower in patients not receiving protamine for heparin anticoagulation reversal.

*Methods.*—Three hundred forty-eight consecutive primary CEAs performed since 1986 were reviewed. Protamine had been given to 193 patients after surgery was completed.

*Findings.*—All patients survived to hospital discharge. The stroke rate among patients given protamine was 2.6% compared with 0% in the patients receiving no protamine. One percent of the patients in the protamine group and 1.9% in the no-protamine group had hematoma requiring reexploration. Intraoperative shunting was done in 84% of the patients not receiving protamine and in 67% of those receiving it. Patch angioplasty was done in 35% of the patients given protamine and in 15% of those not given it. However, stroke rates were not influenced significantly by shunting or patching.

*Conclusion.*—Carotid endarterectomy without reversal of heparin anticoagulation appears to be associated with a decreased stroke rate after surgery with no significant increase in morbidity. However, additional research involving greater numbers of patients from multiple centers is needed to verify these findings.

▶ Studies such as this have the remarkable potential to confuse more than clarify. This retrospective study was certainly not randomized, and, in fact, apparently all or most of the no-protamine patients were included in 1 senior surgeon's series. I reject the authors' conclusion that this study indicates that reversal of heparin anticoagulation with protamine is associated with a higher stroke rate. They simply cannot reach this conclusion from these data. At best these retrospective data could be used as an hypothesis seeking exercise, indicating the need for a prospective randomized study that avoids the pitfalls inherent in this retrospective review. For reaching such dogmatic conclusions from such data, I hereby award these authors the CDA. For additional information concerning reversal of heparin by protamine, see also Abstract 5–1.

## Thrombolysis for Stroke

### Tissue Plasminogen Activator for Acute Ischemic Stroke

Marler JR (Natl Inst of Neurological Disorders and Stroke rt-PA Stroke Study Group, Bethesda, Md)
*N Engl J Med* 333:1581–1587, 1995                                    12–17

*Background.*—Initial trials of thrombolytic therapy for patients with acute ischemic stroke were associated with high rates of intracerebral hemorrhage. These results prompted careful evaluation of the risks and benefits of recombinant human tissue plasminogen activator (t-PA) for cerebral arterial thrombolysis. Recent results have suggested that t-PA treatment is beneficial when given within 3 hours after the onset of stroke. A 2-part, randomized trial was done to evaluate the benefits of IV t-PA for patients with ischemic stroke.

*Methods.*—The first part of the trial, which included 291 patients, sought to determine whether t-PA had clinical activity in patients with ischemic stroke. This outcome was defined as a 4-point improvement over baseline in the National Institutes of Health Stroke Scale (NIHSS) score or by resolution of the neurologic deficit within 24 hours after stroke onset. The second part of the study, which involved 333 patients, was designed to determine whether t-PA treatment had sustained clinical benefit at 3 months. The results were assessed by 4 outcome measures addressing differing aspects of stroke recovery: the Barthel index, modified Rankin scale, Glasgow Coma Scale, and NIHSS. The results of the 2 parts were pooled and stratified to gain a complete picture of the effectiveness of t-PA.

*Results.*—In the first part of the study, the t-PA and placebo groups were not significantly different in the percentage of patients with neurologic improvement 24 hours after stroke onset. In the second part, however, patients receiving t-PA had significant improvement on all 4 measures. The results of part 1 predicted long-term clinical benefit in part 2, with a 1.7 global odds ratio for a favorable outcome. Patients in the t-PA group were 30% or more likely to be left with minimal or no disability at 3 months' follow-up. Six percent of patients in the t-PA group had symptomatic intracerebral hemorrhage within 36 hours after stroke onset compared with 0.6% of the placebo group. Three-month mortality was 17% for the t-PA group and 21% for the placebo group.

*Conclusion.*—For patients with acute ischemic stroke, giving IV t-PA within 3 hours after the onset of stroke appears to produce significantly better 3-month clinical outcomes than placebo. This benefit holds even though t-PA treatment carries a higher risk of symptomatic intracerebral hemorrhage. Outcomes are better with t-PA than placebo regardless of the type of stroke diagnosed at baseline.

▶ This controversial study purports to show minimal benefit at 3 months in stroke patients receiving t-PA within 3 hours of the onset of symptoms. No benefit was apparent at 24 hours. At 3 months drug patients were at least 30% more likely to have minimal or no disability compared with placebo patients. Unfortunately, this modest benefit was purchased at the expense of symptomatic intracranial hemorrhage in 6.4% of the patients receiving drug. Mortality at 3 months was equal in the 2 groups. These authors conclude that t-PA appears to improve clinical outcome at 3 months. The improvement, however, is small and is purchased at a price. See also Abstract 12–18.

### Intravenous Thrombolysis With Recombinant Tissue Plasminogen Activator for Acute Hemispheric Stroke: The European Cooperative Acute Stroke Study (ECASS)

Hacke W, Kaste M, Fieschi C, et al (Univ of Heidelberg, Germany; Univ of Helsinki; Univ of Rome; et al)

JAMA 274:1017–1025, 1995                                                12–18

*Objective.*—The European Cooperative Acute Stroke Study (ECASS) was designed as a prospective, randomized, double-blind, placebo-controlled trial of IV thrombolysis in patients with acute ischemic stroke. A total of 620 adult patients with at least moderate neurologic deficit from hemispheric stroke but no major early signs of infarction on CT examination were recruited at 75 hospitals in 14 European countries. Patients with existing neurologic conditions causing disablement or concomitant medical disorders were not included.

*Management.*—Patients were randomized to receive either recombinant tissue plasminogen activator (rt-PA) or placebo intravenously. The dose of rt-PA was 1.1 mg/kg up to 100 mg. A bolus consisting of 10% of the total dose was given over 1 to 2 minutes, followed by a 1-hour infusion of the rest of the dose. Data were available for 247 actively treated patients and 264 placebo recipients.

*Efficacy.*—After 3 months there was no significant difference in Barthel Index scores between the patients given rt-PA and those given placebo. Rankin Scale scores were somewhat better in actively treated patients in an intention-to-treat analysis. Mortality 1 month after stroke was greater in the actively treated patients but not significantly so. Neurologic scores did not improve significantly in the rt-PA group within the first week after stroke. Those surviving patients who received active treatment spent less time in hospital than those assigned to placebo.

*Survival and Safety.*—In both intention-to-treat (ITT) analysis and the target population (TP), case fatality rates were consistently higher in patients given rt-PA. Intracranial hemorrhage was comparably frequent in the 2 groups. In the ITT analysis, 40% of patients had some degree of intracranial bleeding.

*Implications.*—Although IV rt-PA does provide for neurologic improvement in some patients with acute ischemic stroke, it is difficult to identify those patients who are likely to respond. Because ineligible patients who are treated have an unacceptably increased risk of hemorrhagic complications and death, this treatment cannot be recommended for use in an unselected patient population.

▶ This European study randomized 620 patients within 6 hours of the onset of stroke to rt-PA vs. placebo. Using a bit of a convoluted analysis, these authors conclude that IV thrombolysis with rt-PA in acute ischemic stroke does appear effective in improving some functional measures at 90 days. Benefit appeared limited to patients with moderate to severe neurologic deficit without extended infarct signs on the initial CT scan. The plasminogen activator treatment of ineligible patients (those with early major CT signs of early infarction) appeared associated with an unacceptable increase of hemorrhagic complications and death. Thus, there appears to be a very narrow therapeutic window, based both on the time of manifestation and the CT scan results if benefit is to be derived from rt-PA in the treatment of acute ischemic strokes. These data do not appear to warrant the widespread use of this modality. See also Abstract 12–17.

**Randomised Controlled Trial of Streptokinase, Aspirin, and Combination of Both in Treatment of Acute Ischaemic Stroke**
Multicentre Acute Stroke Trial–Italy (MAST-I) Group (Istituto di Clinica, Milano, Italy)
*Lancet* 346:1509–1514, 1995                                                12–19

*Introduction.*—The benefits of thrombolytic drugs administered within 6 hours after acute myocardial infarction (MI) have been conclusively demonstrated. Although early administration of thrombolytic drugs after ischemic stroke increases the early recanalization rate of the intracerebral arteries, the clinical effects are still unknown. Streptokinase, given alone or with aspirin, and aspirin, given alone or with streptokinase, were studied in a controlled, multicenter clinical trial to determine whether they would have clinical benefits in patients with acute ischemic stroke similar to those observed in patients with acute MI.

*Patients.*—Of 622 patients admitted to the hospital within 6 hours of experiencing symptoms of acute ischemic stroke, 157 were randomized to receive a 1-hour infusion of 1.5 MU of streptokinase, 153 were allocated to receive 300 mg of buffered aspirin daily for 10 days, 156 to receive streptokinase infusion plus aspirin for 10 days, and 156 to receive neither drug. All patients were observed during the first 10 days after randomization and were reassessed by telephone interview at 6 months.

*Results.*—The 10-day case fatality was 19% for streptokinase alone, 34% for streptokinase plus aspirin, 10% for aspirin alone, and 13% for the control group. Thus, streptokinase combined with aspirin significantly increased the risk of early death. Streptokinase alone, with aspirin, or aspirin alone reduced the odds of death and severe disability at 6 months after randomization, but the differences did not reach statistical significance. Increasing evidence of an early hazard from thrombolytic therapy led to the interruption of the trial in January 1995. The available data were analyzed to help decide whether the trial should continue.

*Conclusion.*—Thrombolytic therapy administered within 6 hours of an acute ischemic stroke confers a marginal reduction in severe disability after the first 6 months but also increases the risk of early death. Although streptokinase and aspirin remain potentially beneficial treatments for this indication, their use in routine practice cannot be recommended at this time.

▶ A number of patients in this trial were randomized within 6 hours of stroke to receive streptokinase, aspirin, or a combination or placebo. Not only did the streptokinase result in no patient benefit, but there was a significant increase in early case fatality associated with this treatment. These authors conclude that, on balance, thrombolytic therapy with streptokinase is unattractive. Because streptokinase appears bad and the marginal benefit of tissue plasminogen activator appears small, I do not believe the total experience defines a new therapeutic principle in the treatment of early stroke patients. At best, I believe we should reserve judgment as to the efficacy of the early thrombolytic treatment of ischemic stroke.

## Miscellaneous Topics

### Appropriate Frequency of Carotid Duplex Testing Following Carotid Endarterectomy

Ouriel K, Green RM (Univ of Rochester, New York)
*Am J Surg* 170:144–147, 1995                                              12–20

*Background.*—Carotid artery duplex scanning is of recognized value in the diagnosis of occlusive disease of the carotid bifurcation. However, relatively little is known about its use after carotid endarterectomy. The use and timing of duplex ultrasound for postoperative follow-up after carotid endarterectomy were studied.

*Methods.*—Two hundred twenty-two patients who underwent a total of 281 carotid endarterectomies were studied. Duplex ultrasound scans were obtained at the initial postoperative clinic visit and every 6 months thereafter. The serial scans were analyzed to identify critical restenotic carotid lesions exceeding 80% diameter reduction. The incidence of subsequent carotid occlusion and neurologic symptoms was assessed as well.

*Results.*—During follow-up, 9% of arteries developed critical restenoses and 4% developed occlusion. The restenosis rate was 5% in the first year after carotid endarterectomy, declining thereafter to an annual incidence of about 2% per year. The rate of carotid occlusion was about 1% per year. The mean time for known restenoses to progress to occlusion was 11 months. One fourth of critical restenoses that became occluded did so within 6 months of identification, whereas two thirds became occluded within 1 year. Stroke developed in 4% of patients with critical restenoses compared with 33% of those with occlusion.

*Conclusion.*—In patients who have undergone carotid endarterectomy, duplex scanning every 6 months appears to offer the best chance of identifying critical carotid restenoses before they progress to occlusion and stroke. The number of occlusions could be decreased even more if scanning were performed every 3 months, but this may be impractical. The rate of neurologic symptoms after carotid endarterectomy is low, even for patients with critical restenoses.

▶ Perhaps a better question is should postoperative carotid duplex testing be done at all? This has been questioned by many. With a mean follow-up of 32 months with 281 carotid endarterectomies and frequent vascular laboratory follow-up, the authors noted critical restenosis in 25 arteries (8.9%) and occlusions in 12 arteries (4%). The longitudinal development of these problems over the entire period of follow-up leads the authors to conclude that semiannual duplex testing appears reasonable. I wonder.

**Brain Edema After Carotid Surgery**
Breen JC, Caplan LR, DeWitt LD, et al (Tufts Univ, Medford, Mass)
*Neurology* 46:175–181, 1996                                                12–21

*Background.*—The postoperative hyperperfusion syndrome consists of an abrupt rise in blood flow with a loss of autoregulation in patients undergoing surgical reperfusion of the brain. Manifestations include severe headache, transient ischemia, seizures, and intracerebral bleeding.

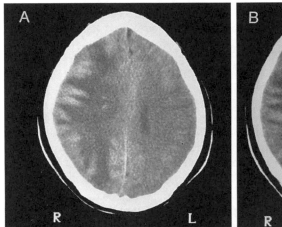
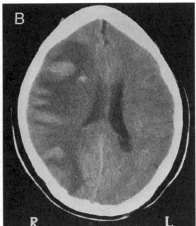
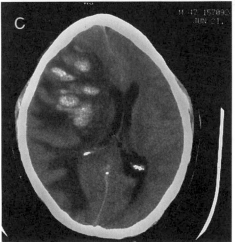

FIGURE 1.—A and B, noncontrast head CT performed on postoperative day 5 showing diffuse white matter edema throughout the right frontal and parietal lobes. B, small hyperdensity in the right frontal lobe represents a small hemorrhage. A midline shift is more evident. C, repeat noncontrast head CT performed several hours after scans in A and B showing areas of hemorrhage within the deep white matter of the right frontal lobe and more extensive shift of the midline structures. (Reprinted from *Neurology* 46:175–181, 1996, by permission of Little, Brown and Company [Inc.].)

Hypertension, which is common after carotid artery surgery, often plays a role in the pathophysiology of this syndrome. Five patients with severe white matter edema after carotid surgery, a finding not previously reported, were described.

> *Case Reports.*—Hypertension, headache, hemiparesis, seizures, and aphasia or neglect from severe white matter edema ipsilateral to the carotid surgery developed in all patients 5 to 8 days after carotid surgery and hospital discharge. A small hemorrhage was found in the edematous area in 1 patient (Fig 1). Four patients had severe hypertension, and 1 had moderate hypertension. Ultrasound or angiography demonstrated patent carotid arteries in all patients after surgery. Increased velocities ipsilateral to surgery in 2 patients and bilaterally in 1 were demonstrated on transcranial Doppler examination. Antihypertensive and anticonvulsant treatment resulted in a resolution of CT abnormalities and neurologic signs in 4 patients. The last patient died of herniation caused by massive edema.

*Conclusion.*—The hyperperfusion syndrome appears to be more common than has been appreciated. The clinical definition should include focal neurologic signs associated with white matter edema. Brain edema must be distinguished from thromboembolic stroke, because the causes and treatments of these entities are different. White matter edema has probably been overlooked in some patients in the past because the changes were slight and the resolution of earlier generation CT scanning was lower.

▶ These authors describe apparent post-CEA hyperperfusion syndrome in 5 patients, all of whom had already been discharged from the hospital. In each patient, imaging studies showed definite white matter edema. These authors suggest that brain edema, as well as focal neurologic signs, should be included as serious but potentially reversible components of the postoperative hyperperfusion syndrome. I suppose they are correct. We all have come to recognize this condition, which occurs distinctly infrequently. In a majority of patients, however, it occurs within the first few days. However, we too recognize an occasional patient with the onset of symptoms days after carotid artery surgery. Sedation and control of blood pressure appear to be the most important therapeutic modalities. We must treat this condition with extreme seriousness, because strokes and death have been well reported with the post-CEA hyperperfusion syndrome.

## Carotid Plaque Regression on Oestrogen Replacement: A Pilot Study

Akkad A, Hartshorne T, Bell PRF, et al (Univ of Leicester, England)
*Eur J Vasc Endovasc Surg* 11:347–348, 1996          12–22

*Background.*—Animal studies suggest that estrogen treatment can prevent or even reverse atheroma formation. The effects of estrogen replacement therapy on carotid plaques were evaluated in menopausal women.

*Methods.*—The pilot study included 17 women with natural or surgical menopause and known carotid plaque disease. All underwent duplex ultrasound scanning of the carotid arteries before and after 3 and 6 months of unopposed estrogen replacement therapy. Measurements included internal thickness (IMT), plaque length (PL), and plaque thickness.

*Results.*—Follow-up data were obtained on 22 carotid plaques. Nonsignificant reductions of 5% after 3 months and 6% after 6 months of estrogen treatment were seen in mean IMT. However, PL was decreased significantly by 8% at 3 months and 28% at 6 months. Plaque thickness was significantly decreased by 18% at 6 months.

*Conclusion.*—Estrogen replacement therapy may be associated with carotid plaque regression in menopausal women. The results of this pilot study are consistent with the findings of previous studies in animals.

▶ See also Abstracts 1–57 and 2–67. I am fascinated by recent data that not only detect sex hormone receptors in the vascular endothelium but suggest that carotid plaque regression may be related to estrogen replacement. I doubt if the protective effects of anything, including estrogen, will ever fully explain the relative atherosclerosis protection enjoyed by premenopausal women, but this does open fascinating avenues of new research.

## Socioeconomic Status and Carotid Atherosclerosis

Lynch J, Kaplan GA, Salonen R, et al (California Dept of Health Services, Berkeley; Univ of Kuopio, Finland)
*Circulation* 92:1786–1792, 1995          12–23

*Background.*—Lower socioeconomic status (SES) is associated with increased cardiovascular morbidity and mortality. However, the relationship between SES and early manifestations of atherosclerotic vascular disease is uncertain. The association between SES and ultrasound measured carotid artery intima-media thickness (IMT) was examined in a population-based sample of Finnish men.

*Methods.*—Of the 1,516 men (aged 42, 48, 54, or 60 years) recruited, sufficient data were available on 1,140 to include them in the study. B-mode ultrasonographic scanning of the common carotid arteries and carotid bifurcation/bulb areas was used to assess IMT. Questionnaires included 3 measures of SES: highest educational attainment, current income, and lifetime occupation.

*Results.*—Significant, inverse, graded differences between SES and IMT were found. The age-adjusted mean IMT for men with a primary school or less education was 0.96 mm, for men with some high school was 0.94 mm, and for those who completed high school was 0.82 mm. The difference in IMT between the highest and lowest education levels corresponds to a 15.4% increased risk for myocardial infarction in the lowest educational level men. Even after adjustment for attenuating risk factors, similar patterns were found for the other measures of SES (income and lifelong occupation). The graded, inverse association between SES and IMT persisted in the subgroup of men who had no carotid artery stenosis (or plaque) or apparent cardiovascular disease. When multivariate models were used, variables that were significant predictors of IMT were age, systolic blood pressure, smoking, plasma fibrinogen level, serum apolipoprotein B level, treatment for hyperlipidemia, education, and diabetes mellitus.

*Conclusion.*—The strong association of lower socioeconomic status with increased risk for atherosclerosis is evident early in the natural history of atherosclerosis. This association is mediated by known risk factors and is apparent even in healthy men.

▶ This study from Finland concludes that there is a strong association between socioeconomic status and atherosclerosis. The authors, thankfully, conclude that this association is explained entirely by known atherosclerotic risk factors, which are far more prevalent in the lower socioeconomic group. These findings appear intuitively obvious to most vascular surgeons. We infrequently treat healthy, slender, exercising, nonsmoking patients.

# 13 Grafts and Graft Complications

## Graft Healing

**Definitive Proof of Endothelialization of a Dacron Arterial Prosthesis in a Human Being**
Wu MH-D, Shi Q, Wechezak AR, et al (Univ of Washington, Seattle)
*J Vasc Surg* 21:862–867, 1995                                                          13–1

*Background.*—Until now, there has been no definitive proof that endothelialization of synthetic arterial grafts occurs in humans, beyond the limited zone of pannus ingrowth. Such proof is offered in an investigation of a replaced Dacron arterial prosthesis.

*Methods.*—A 67-year-old man required removal and replacement of a 10-mm woven Dacron axillofemoral bypass graft because of a large seroma surrounding the entire length of the graft, which had been in place for 26 months. Representative tissue blocks were obtained from along the entire graft length for study by light microscopy with hematoxylin and eosin and Masson trichrome staining, scanning electron microscopy, transmission electron microscopy, and immunocytochemical staining.

*Results.*—Stating of paraffin-embedded sections with smooth muscle cell α-actin showed smooth muscle cells in the pseudointima. In addition, Ham 56 staining demonstrated macrophages. Human endothelial cells were found on the flow surface by endothelial factor VIII/von Willebrand's factor and *U. europaeus* agglutinin (Fig 4, E–H). Endothelial cells were demonstrated in sites far from the anastomoses of graft to native vessels.

*Conclusion.*—Neoendothelialization can occur on porous synthetic arterial grafts implanted in humans. The mechanisms of endothelialization remain unclear, however. With further study of graft specimens removed from patients, it might be possible to gain insight into these mechanisms and to identify techniques to promote healing and endothelialization of vascular prostheses.

▶ Clearly there were at least "spots" of smooth muscle and endothelium on this Dacron graft removed some 24 months after placement. Unfortunately, the authors are not able to tell us what percentage of the surface was covered by this tissue, and the observation that this graft resided within a huge seroma does not make it especially attractive as a model. All this paper really seems to prove is that spots of endothelium appear to be possible in Dacron graft in humans. On the other hand, I thought they had already proved that.[1]

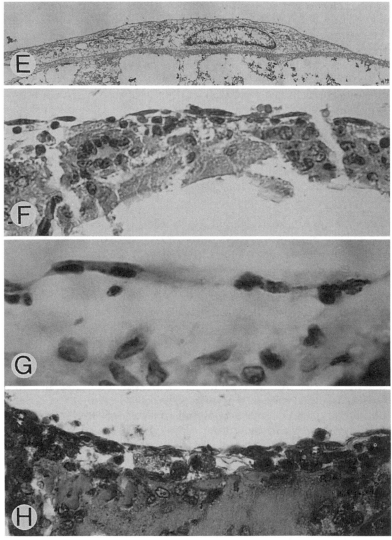

FIGURE 4.—E, transmission electron microscopy; original magnification ×3,050. F, confirmation of endothelium by positive factor VIII/von Willebrand's factor staining result; original magnification ×485. G, confirmation of endothelium by positive *Ulex europaeus* agglutinin staining result; original magnification ×1,210. H, confirmation of macrophages by HAM 56 immunocytochemistry staining; original magnification ×485. (Courtesy of Wu MH-D, Shi Q, Wechezak AR, et al: Definitive proof of endothelialization of a Dacron arterial prosthesis in a human being. *J Vasc Surg* 21:862–867, 1995.)

*Reference*

1. Sauvage LR: Presence of endothelium in an axillary-femoral graft of knitted Dacron with an external velour surface. *Ann Surg* 182:749–752, 1975.

**Differential Effect of the Retropleural and Retroperitoneal Environments on Healing of the Inner Wall of Porous Fabric Prostheses in the Thoracic and Abdominal Aorta of the Same Dog**
Hayashida N, Han M-T, Wu MH-D, et al (Univ of Washington, Seattle)
*Ann Vasc Surg* 9:369–377, 1995                                                            13–2

*Objective.*—The hypothesis that inner wall healing of preclotted knitted Dacron prostheses may be site specific was explored by comparing the healing around prostheses implanted in the descending thoracic aorta (DTA) and the abdominal aorta (AA) of the same dog.

*Methods.*—Prostheses were implanted in both the DTA and AA of 16 dogs, and healing was assessed after 4, 8, and 16 weeks. The degree of attachment of the tissue to the prosthesis was determined qualitatively. Light, scanning electron, and transmission electron microscopy, and immunofluorescent techniques were used to examine tissue samples to deter-

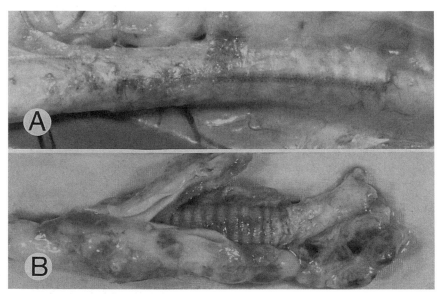

FIGURE 1.—Eight-week gross specimens of preclotted knitted Dacron grafts. **A,** mid–descending thoracic aorta graft showing thin tightly adherent outer capsule representative of all 16 grafts implanted in this location. **B,** abdominal aortic graft showing thick loosely attached outer capsule representative of 50% of the 16 grafts implanted in this location. (Courtesy of Hayashida N, Han M-T, Wu MH-D, et al: Differential effect of the retropleural and retroperitoneal environments on healing of the inner wall of porous fabric prostheses in the thoracic and abdominal aorta of the same dog. *Ann Vasc Surg* 9[4]:369–377, 1995.)

TABLE 1.—Thickness of Inner and Outer Capsules at the Midportion of the Graft

| | | Implant Time | | |
|---|---|---|---|---|
| | | 4 wk (n = 5) | 8 wk (n = 5) | 16 wk (n = 6) |
| DTA and AA grafts | | | | |
| Inner capsule (µm) | DTA | 112 ± 52 | 71 ± 21 | 82 ± 42 |
| | AA | 89 ± 50 | 193 ± 181 | 307 ± 154 |
| Outer capsule (µm) | DTA | 1,500 ± 300 | 1,100 ± 300 | 600 ± 200 |
| | AA | 3,500 ± 800 | 4,200 ± 2400 | 1,600 ± 800 |

| | Implant Time | | | | | |
|---|---|---|---|---|---|---|
| | 4 wk | | 8 wk | | 16 wk | |
| | T (n = 2) | L (n = 3) | T (n = 2) | L (n = 3) | T (n = 4) | L (n = 2) |
| AA Grafts with tight and loose perigraft tissue attachment | | | | | | |
| Inner capsule (µm) | 80 ± 15 | 76 ± 27 | 114 ± 85 | 245 ± 227 | 348 ± 118 | 227 ± 240 |
| Outer capsule (µm) | 2,800 ± 1000 | 3,800 ± 400 | 2,400 ± 600 | 5,500 ± 2300 | 1,300 ± 600 | 2,300 ± 900 |

*Abbreviations: T*, tight; *L*, loose.
(Courtesy of Hayashida N, Han M-T, Wu MH-D, et al: Differential effect of the retropleural and retroperitoneal environments on healing of the inner wall of porous fabric prostheses in the thoracic and abdominal aorta of the same dog. *Ann Vasc Surg* 9[4]:369–377, 1995.)

mine the thrombus-free surface (TFS) score, the thickness of the inner and outer capsules, and the distribution of microvascular ostia on the flow surface or the endothelial-like cell coverage (CC) score.

*Results.*—The DTA grafts had no surrounding seromas or hematomas (Fig 1), and all of the outer capsules were firmly attached to the grafts. In contrast, only 50% of the outer capsules were firmly adhered in the AA grafts, and seroma and hematoma involvement was noted in 3 of the 8 grafts to which the tissue was loosely attached. The outer capsules in the DTA grafts at 16 weeks were thin (600 μm), translucent, and compliant, whereas the 8 outer capsules that were not firmly adhered to the prostheses in the AA grafts were thick (1,600 μm), largely opaque, and semicompliant (Table 1). By 16 weeks, complete healing of the inner wall and endothe- lialization were noted in all of the DTA grafts and in the 50% of the AA grafts to which tissue was firmly bonded. No healing was observed in the 50% of the AA grafts to which tissue was loosely bonded. The graft surface was white and smooth in most of the DTA grafts but covered with red thrombotic areas in the AA grafts. The combined TFS and CC scores of the AA graft of each animal was lower than that of the DTA graft. The CC scores for grafts with loose attachments were significantly lower than those for grafts with tight attachments. The number of microvascular ostia on the flow surfaces was lower for DTA than AA grafts.

*Conclusion.*—The healing of the inner wall of Dacron arterial prosthe- ses is positively correlated with the tightness of the attachment of the outer capsule. In dogs, the healing is site specific, with faster and more complete healing in DTA than AA grafts.

▶ Dr. Sauvage's group in Seattle maintains an active interest in the healing of prosthetic vascular grafts (see Abstract 13–1). Perhaps the rate of healing of grafts in the thoracic aorta is different from that in the abdominal aorta in dogs. However, if there is 1 message we have learned over the past 40 years of graft study, it is that experimental animals and humans behave grossly differently in their ability to heal prosthetic grafts. As far as I can tell, pigs, goats, sheep, cows, and, I believe, elephants, all show very rapid and complete healing of prosthetic grafts. Unfortunately, humans do not. I al- ways thought it quaint that the initial design characteristics for grafts were directed toward early and complete healing in animals, a model almost totally unrelated to humans. This whole matter requires a fresh look.

## Graft Infection

**Infected Lower Extremity Extra-Anatomic Bypass Grafts: Management of a Serious Complication in High-Risk Patients**
de Virgilio C, Cherry KJ Jr, Gloviczki P, et al (Mayo Clinic, Rochester, Minn)
*Ann Vasc Surg* 9:459–466, 1995                                                                      13–3

*Introduction.*—Mortality rates from infections of arterial prosthetic grafts range from 13% to 58%, with amputation rates of 8% to 52%. Management of patients with infections of lower extremity extra-anatom-

TABLE 3.—Presenting Symptoms and Signs

| Symptom or sign | No. of patients (%) |
|---|---|
| Draining wound/sinus | 16 (57) |
| Tender mass | 11 (39) |
| Fever | 5 (18) |
| Hemorrhage | 1 (4) |
| Pseudoaneurysm | 1 (4) |
| Exposed graft | 1 (4) |

(Courtesy of de Virgilio C, Cherry KJ Jr, Gloviczki P, et al: Infected lower extremity extra-anatomic bypass grafts: Management of a serious complication in high-risk patients. *Ann Vasc Surg* 9:459–466, 1995.)

ical bypass grafts (EABGs) is particularly difficult, because these patients frequently have cardiac or pulmonary disease, limiting options for revascularization. The management of axillofemoral, axillopopliteal, and femorofemoral graft infections was described.

*Methods.*—The medical records of 28 patients with infected EABGs were retrospectively reviewed. Sixteen of the grafts were axillofemoral, 10 were femorofemoral, and 2 were axillopopliteal.

*Results.*—Indications for EABGs in the patients reviewed were severe lower extremity ischemia with high surgical risk (13 patients), aortic graft infection (9 patients), unilateral limb ischemia (5 patients), and mycotic aneurysm (1 patient). Previous groin dissection and prior graft infection were the 2 most common predisposing factors for EABG infection. The most frequent presenting signs of EABG infection were drainage from a wound (16 patients) or presence of a tender, palpable mass (11 patients) (Table 3). Fever was present in 5 patients; hemorrhage, pseudoaneurysm, or exposed graft were present in 1 patient. Coagulase negative *Staphylococcus* species were present in 36% of cases, anaerobes in 25%, and gram-negative rods in 18%.

Of the 10 patients with infected femorofemoral grafts, 9 were treated with complete graft resection and 1 with a partial resection. Methods of revascularization included prosthetic axillofemoral bypass, femorofemoral bypass with endarterectomy, and combined prosthetic axillopopliteal and saphenous vein femorofemoral bypass. No reconstruction was used in 3 patients. For infected axillofemoral and axillopopliteal grafts, drainage and débridement or muscle flap coverage were attempted as initial treatment in 6 patients and was successful in 2. Partial graft excision was used as initial management in 11 patients, with 4 failures. Complete graft excision was used in 6 patients. An average of 3.8 surgical procedures were performed. Femorofemoral grafts occluded in 4 patients; 3 of 10 prosthetic reconstructions performed for infected axillofemoral and axillopopliteal grafts became reinfected. Amputations were necessary in 10% of femorofemoral grafts, 25% of axillofemoral grafts, and in all axillopopliteal grafts. Overall operative mortality was 18%.

*Conclusion.*—Although EABG infections can be effectively treated, mortality and morbidity are high. Excision of the graft, débridement of infected tissue, and revascularization are primary steps in management of

EABG infections. Long-term follow-up is also necessary to monitor for graft patency and recurrence of infections.

▶ This is a classic Mayo Clinic retrospective review over 13 years of 28 patients with infected extra-anatomical grafts, doubtless treated by a multitude of surgeons with no standard protocol. It is difficult to make chicken soup out of chicken guano. Overall the authors experienced an 18% mortality and a 25% amputation rate, including 2 patients requiring hemipelvectomies and 1 patient with bilateral hip disarticulations. This is hardly the stuff dreams are made of. Nevertheless, it is important for us all to be reminded from time to time just how serious prosthetic graft infections are in our patient population. The surgical principles are clear: If a prosthetic graft is infected, excise it completely and replace it with a new graft through a clean field, or if you must use a contaminated field, use an autogenous conduit. I have little tolerance for those who recommend significant deviations from these established surgical principles.

---

**Differences in Early Versus Late Extracavitary Arterial Graft Infections**
Calligaro KD, Veith FJ, Schwartz ML, et al (Pennsylvania Hosp, Philadelphia; Albert Einstein College, New York)
*J Vasc Surg* 22:680–688, 1995                                                                13–4

---

*Introduction.*—Total graft excision is often recommended for the management of infected arterial grafts. However, graft preservation may have better outcomes in well-selected patients with infected extracavitary grafts. The characteristics of early and late graft infections and factors associated with successful complete graft preservation were investigated by comparing the manifestation, bacteriology, management, and outcomes of patients with early (EGIs) and late extracavitary graft infections (LGIs).

*Methods.*—A total of 141 patients were treated for infected extracavitary arterial grafts between 1979 and 1994. The infected grafts were prosthetic grafts in 112 patients (19 Dacron and 93 polytetrafluoroethylene grafts) and autologous vein grafts in 29 patients. The infected area involved an anastomosis in 123 patients and was only in the body of the graft in 18 patients. Graft infections were considered early if they occurred within 2 months of surgery. Systemic sepsis was an indication for total graft excision, whereas a disrupted anastomosis or occluded graft was treated with subtotal graft excision, as was an infected occluded graft with intact anastomoses. Complete graft preservation was attempted when the infection occurred only in a segment of a patent graft with intact anastomoses in the absence of systemic sepsis.

*Results.*—Of the 141 patients, 99 (70%) had EGIs and 42 (30%) had LGIs, which occurred 4 to 96 months after surgery. There were no significant differences between patients with EGIs and LGIs in the likelihood of a disrupted anastomosis of systemic sepsis or in the hospital mortality and amputation rates. Whereas LGIs were more likely to be associated with occluded grafts and be treated with subtotal graft excision, EGIs were more likely to be associated with patent intact grafts and be treated with complete graft preservation. Amputation was more likely in patients with occluded grafts, systemic sepsis, or graft hemorrhage and requiring subtotal or total graft excision than in patients with intact patent grafts treated with complete graft preservation. Successful wound healing and long-term intact grafts were almost twice as common in patients with EGIs treated with complete graft preservation than in patients with LGIs. There were no significant differences in the type of bacterial causing EGIs and LGIs.

*Conclusion.*—Complete graft preservation is likely to have a successful outcome in patients selected according to the following criteria: the presence of a patent graft and intact anastomoses, the absence of systemic sepsis and Pseudomonas infection, and the onset of the graft infection within 2 months of graft placement. If the first 4 criteria are satisfied, complete graft preservation may be successful in patients with graft infections occurring later than 2 months after graft placement but should be reserved for patients in whom secondary revascularization is contraindicated or to prevent major amputation secondary to total graft excision.

▶ If EGI is defined, as these authors suggest, as occurring less than 2 months after implantation and LGI occurs 4 to 96 months after implantation, one can only contemplate the terminology of a graft infection occurring precisely 3 months after implantation. On balance, there appears to be no substantial difference between the 2 time periods of graft infection. These authors continue to beat the drums for partial excision of infected grafts and preservation of infected grafts, but I regard this whole effort as silly. One must stick to one's principles and disregard things with which we disagree.

---

**Surgical Management of Infrainguinal Arterial Prosthetic Graft Infections: Review of a Thirty-Five–Year Experience**
Mertens RA, O'Hara PJ, Hertzer NR, et al (Cleveland Clinic Found, Ohio)
*J Vasc Surg* 21:782–791, 1995                                   13–5

---

*Background.*—Infrainguinal prosthetic graft infection (IAPGI) is an uncommon problem but has potentially devastating consequences. A series of 68 cases of IAPGI was reviewed to define the early and late morbidity and mortality and to clarify the optimal management.

*Methods.*—The infections occurred in 67 patients (53 men and 14 women, mean age 61) over a 34-year period. A femoropopliteal graft was involved in 85% of cases of IAPGI, a femorodistal graft in 9%, and other grafts or synthetic patches in 6%. The grafts were made of Dacron in 53% of cases, polytetrafluoroethylene in 41%, and human umbilical vein in 6%. In nearly one fourth of cases, the IAPGI was not recognized until the involved limb had to be amputated; the grafts were occluded in 14 of 16 amputated limbs. Overall 38% of grafts were thrombosed.

*Results.*—The results of culture were available in 59 IAPGIs, and staphylococcal organisms were involved in 58% of cases. The diagnosis of IAPGI was made a median of 3 months after graft implantation and 1 month after the last procedure involving the original graft. The initial treatment consisted of total graft excision in 59% of cases, partial removal or in situ graft replacement in 22%, and local treatment only in 19%. The total excision rate was 94% in patients with previous amputations vs. 48% in intact limbs. There were 12 early deaths for a postoperative mortality of 18%; 7 of these deaths resulted from sepsis, and all occurred in patients in whom limb salvage was still being attempted.

In the first year after diagnosis of IAPGI, the amputation rate in 52 intact limbs was 40%. Ongoing sepsis necessitated further operations in 82% of IAPGIs managed by incomplete graft removal, compared with 13% of those managed with complete excision. Among patients who survived the operation, cumulative 5-year survival was 77%, significantly lower than expected for the normal, age-matched population

*Conclusion.*—In patients who have undergone vascular reconstruction, IAPGI carries high early mortality and amputation rates. Recurrent sepsis is less frequent when the infected graft is completely excised. Incomplete graft excision should be used only with caution.

▶ If you did not use prosthetic grafts for leg bypass, you would not get prosthetic leg graft infections. However, these authors do, and they did. Overall mortality rate in these 67 patients was 18% and amputation was required in 21 of 52 limbs (40%) within 1 year. Eighty-two percent of infected grafts managed with incomplete graft removal required subsequent operations for continued sepsis compared with 13% of the 40 grafts treated with complete excision. The authors' conclusion that complete excision of infected graft material is the treatment of choice is precisely correct, as opposed to the conclusions reached in the previous abstract.

**Autogenous Reconstruction With the Lower Extremity Deep Veins: An Alternative Treatment of Prosthetic Infection After Reconstructive Surgery for Aortoiliac Disease**
Nevelsteen A, Lacroix H, Suy R (Univ Clinic Gasthuisberg, Leuven, Belgium)
*J Vasc Surg* 22:129–134, 1995                                                           13–6

*Introduction.*—Prosthetic infection after reconstructive vascular surgery is typically managed with prosthetic excision and ectopic bypass. However, the experience of autogenous reconstruction using the superficial femoropopliteal vein in 15 patients was reported.

*Methods.*—The records of 15 patients who underwent autograft repair with lower extremity deep veins for the management of prosthetic infection after reconstruction for aortoiliac disease between 1990 and 1994

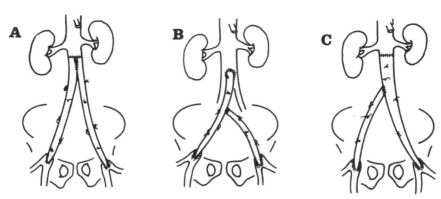

FIGURE 1.—Schematic drawing of operative techniques for aortobi(ilio)femoral reconstruction (A) "pantaloon" technique used in 9 cases, (B) end-to-side unilateral aortofemoral graft with side branch to the opposite groin, and (C) end-to-end unilateral aortofemoral graft with side branch to opposite groin. (Courtesy of Nevelsteen A, Lacroix H, Suy R: Autogenous reconstruction with the lower extremity deep veins: An alternative treatment of prosthetic infection after reconstructive surgery for aortoiliac disease. *J Vasc Surg* 22:129–134, 1995.)

were studied. The superficial femoropopliteal vein was harvested from either leg or both legs and was used either reversed or nonreversed or sewn together to replace the infected prosthesis after débridement of the periarterial tissues. Patients were followed for a mean of 17 months (range, 4–33 months).

*Results.*—The diagnosis of infection occurred 1 to 152 months after the initial surgery (median, 26 months). Of the 15 patients, 13 had primary graft infection and 2 had secondary graft-enteric erosion. Five patients had signs of sepsis; 4 had a groin abscess; and 5 had ischemic complications. A staphylococcal infection was found in 9 patients, and 4 had polymicrobial infections. Of the 15 patients, 11 had bilateral reconstruction. In all but 2 patients, the anastomoses were end to end using the bifurcation "pantaloon" graft technique in 9 patients. In the other 2 patients, anastomosis was accomplished with the nonreversed vein sutured to the aorta to form a unilateral aortofemoral graft, end to end in 1 and end to side in the other (Fig 1). One patient (7%) died perioperatively, and another patient had an occluded venous femorotibial homograft, requiring an above-knee amputation. There were 2 postoperative deaths, unrelated to the reconstruction. One of the graft reconstructions became occluded 16 months after surgery. None of the patients had recurrent infections. All but 1 patient was able to resume normal daily activities. Although limb swelling was common early in the postoperative period, it was controlled with routine use of bed rest, leg elevation, and elastic stockings. Only 1 patient had persistent limb swelling, with disability from venous hypertension lasting more than 2 years after reconstruction.

*Conclusion.*—Deep venous reconstruction is a viable management option in patients with prosthetic infection, offering the potential salvaging of life and limbs and preservation of function.

▶ The superb results reported herein include a mortality of 7%, with 1 patient sustaining limb loss. These results are dramatically superior to those reported in the previous articles in this section. As pointed out by both these authors and the Southwestern group,[1] the preferred conduit for this use is the superficial femoral vein (now officially known as the femoral vein). The saphenous vein does not appear to give as durable or satisfactory results. We have obtained excellent results with abdominal graft infections with axillary-femoral grafting in a clean field, followed by graft excision and aortic oversewing. To date we have not recognized aortic stump blowout, perhaps associated with our rather excessive method of aortic stump closure. Nonetheless, we regard revascularization in a contaminated field using superficial femoral veins as an acceptable alternative to the more conventional remote grafting with prosthetic excision. This is perhaps bending the principle slightly, but certainly it does not constitute the radical end run-around principles recommended in Abstract 13–4.

*Reference*

1. 1995 YEAR BOOK OF VASCULAR SURGERY, p 347.

---

**Avidin and ¹¹¹In-Labelled Biotin Scan: A New Radioisotopic Method for Localising Vascular Graft Infection**
Chiesa R, Melissano G, Castellano R, et al (Univ of Milano, Italy)
*Eur J Vasc Endovasc Surg* 10:405–414, 1995                                    13–7

---

*Background.*—Several imaging techniques are used to diagnose graft infection, but most have poor specificity, especially during the early phase. Although isotope scanning techniques have better sensitivity and specificity, their technical complexity precludes their routine use. However, a new avidin/biotin method is a simplified technique, which appears to have promising clinical utility. With this method, avidin, a protein that accumulates at sites of infection, is administered as a pretarget. After 24 hours, $^{111}$In–labeled biotin, which has a strong affinity for avidin, is injected, and scintigraphy is performed. The clinical utility of $^{111}$In-labeled avidin/biotin scintigraphy was assessed in the diagnosis of infected prosthetic vascular grafts.

*Methods.*—Over a 1-year period, 31 vascular grafts in 26 patients were studied, including 16 patients with suspected vascular graft infection and 10 control patients with no clinical evidence of graft infection. Whole-body scintigraphy was performed 2 hours after $^{111}$In-labeled biotin was injected, following pretargeting with avidin. The scans were evaluated for evidence of graft infection and compared with operative or clinical findings.

*Results.*—Two patients with suspected graft infection were excluded. Of the remaining 14 patients with suspected graft infection, the scanning findings yielded 6 true positives, 1 false positive, and 11 true negatives.

Scanning results in the control group yielded 10 true negatives. Therefore, avidin and [111]In-labeled biotin scanning had a sensitivity of 100%, specificity of 95%, accuracy of 96%, positive predictive value of 86%, and negative predictive value of 100%. The procedure was safe and well tolerated.

*Conclusion.*—Avidin and [111]In-labeled biotin scanning had good diagnostic accuracy in patients with vascular graft infections. Its further benefits include its noninvasiveness, simplicity, safety, and cost effectiveness.

▶ This is a 1-year study from 1 department, with 9 authors attesting to the 100% sensitivity of a technique that they have previously reported to show up inflammation, infection, and tumor. Besides the difficulties of any qualitative imaging technique, the high level of residual activity in the urinary tract may make this test of limited value in the very area where it is most necessary, namely, the diagnosis of deep intra-abdominal infection. Scans of the legs are not affected by this overlap, but in that site, infection is more easily assessed clinically. The principle is certainly elegant and the technique claimed to be simple. The question now is how well it will travel and whether it will reliably guide clinical management in those who might be harboring an infected intra-abdominal graft.

**A.E.B. Giddings, M.D.**

---

**Detection of Prosthetic Vascular Graft Infection Using Avidin/Indium-111-Biotin Scintigraphy**
Samuel A, Paganelli G, Chiesa R, et al (Univ of Milan, Italy)
*J Nucl Med* 37:55–61, 1996                                          13–8

---

*Objective.*—The use of nonspecific avidin/indium-111–biotin imaging in diagnosing prosthetic vascular graft infection was examined.

*Background.*—Prosthetic vascular graft infection is rare but causes high morbidity and mortality. Early diagnosis is key, but patients often have vague, nonspecific symptoms, and radiologic studies are often inconclusive. Patients sometimes undergo long periods of observation before prosthetic vascular graft infection is finally diagnosed.

*Methods.*—There were 25 patients with 29 grafts. The probability of disease was low in 18 patients, but surgical exploration was needed in the other 7. Avidin was administered intravenously, then [111]In-biotin was administered 24 hours later. Ten minutes and 2 hours after injection, whole-body images were obtained. One hour after injection, single-photon emission CT images were obtained.

*Results.*—Increased uptake along the length of the graft was considered evidence of infection. All infected grafts were correctly identified by avidin/[111]In-biotin scintigraphy. This was confirmed by culturing surgical specimens. Graft infection was correctly ruled out in all grafts but 1. In patients who did not have surgery, long-term follow-up was used to detect infection.

*Conclusion.*—For routine diagnosis of vascular graft infection, avidin/ [111]In-biotin scintigraphy is accurate, is simple compared with white blood cell imaging, and does not require special laboratory setup. This technique may be further simplified by the recent availability of a technetium-99m–labeled biotin molecule. Prognosis may be improved by early identification of this disease.

▶ A number of radionuclide scanning techniques have been developed for the detection and diagnosis of prosthetic graft infections, and here is yet another. None of its predecessors has withstood the test of time. So although this technique seems intuitively sound, with just a few patients, we'll have to wait and see. I'm skeptical.

**W. Abbott, M.D.**

▶ Dr. Abbott's typically understated skepticism is noted. See also Abstract 13–7.

**J.M. Porter, M.D.**

## Miscellaneous Topics

**Application of Computed Tomography for Surveillance of Aortic Grafts**
Berman SS, Hunter GC, Smyth SH, et al (Univ of Arizona, Tucson)
*Surgery* 118:8–15, 1995                                                    13–9

*Introduction.*—Because of their intra-abdominal location, it is difficult to detect subclinical aortic graft complications. Several imaging modalities have been used for surveillance. The clinical utility of CT for surveillance of aortic grafts was evaluated.

*Methods.*—Patients scheduled for abdominal CT scanning for aortic graft surveillance were followed prospectively. In addition, the medical records of patients with aortic grafts noted during diagnostic abdominal CT examinations were reviewed. Data were collected on patients identified either prospectively or retrospectively between 1987 and 1993. All scans were obtained after IV or oral contrast was administered and were reviewed by an investigator blinded to the graft type or placement indication. The degree of graft dilation, if present, was determined and correlated with graft type.

*Results.*—Of the 178 patients, 129 (72%) underwent CT surveillance and 49 (28%) underwent diagnostic CT scanning. There were bifurcated grafts in 128 patients (72%) and tube grafts in 50 patients (28%). The graft prostheses were woven Dacron (WD) in 74 patients (42%), knitted Dacron (KD) in 69 patients (38%), and polytetrafluoroethylene (PTFE) in 35 patients (20%). There were abnormal CT findings in 24 patients (13.5%). Aneurysmal dilation was the most common abnormality, including 7 supragraft aneurysms, 5 distal anastomotic aneurysms, and 3 proximal anastomotic aneurysms. Other abnormalities included 2 graft infections, 2 perigraft fluid collections, 2 graft aneurysms, and 3 neurovascular complications, including 1 ureteral obstruction and 2 pancreatic

TABLE 2.—Abnormalities Detected by Computed Tomography Scan

| Finding | No. (%) |
|---|---|
| Supragraft aneurysm | 7 (4) |
| Distal anastomotic aneurysm | 5 (3) |
| Proximal anastomotic aneurysm | 3 (1.7) |
| Graft infection | 2 (1.1) |
| Graft aneurysm with thrombus | 2 (1.1) |
| Pancreatic pseudocyst | 2 (1.1) |
| Perigraft fluid collection | 2 (1.1) |
| Ureteral obstruction | 1 (0.5) |

(Courtesy of Berman SS, Hunter GC, Smyth SH, et al: Application of computed tomography for surveillance of aortic grafts. *Surgery* 118:8–15, 1995.)

pseudocysts (Table 2). Multivariate analyses identified a significant correlation between graft dilation and the use of KD prostheses rather than WD or PTFE prostheses for both tube and bifurcated grafts. Graft dilation did not correlate significantly with recognized risk factors, the indication for graft placement, or the duration of graft placement. The incidence of anastomotic aneurysms was 10% with KD grafts, 4% with WD grafts, and 0% with PTFE grafts.

*Conclusion.*—Computed tomography is suitable for aortic graft surveillance. The KD aortic prosthesis was particularly associated with graft dilation. Surveillance should include a CT scan at 1 year and 5 years.

▶ As far as I can tell, 178 patients with aortic prosthetic grafts underwent a follow-up CT scan at a mean time of 43.3 months after implantation. Variations from expected CT appearance were noted in 13.5% of patients, including the expected spectrum of supragraft aneurysm, distal anastomotic aneurysm, proximal anastomotic aneurysm, and graft infection. The amount of dilatation noted in the grafts over preimplant size was significant but about in line with that reported by others. The propensity to dilate appeared especially prominent with KD, also a finding noted by others. Although I do not find the data in this article particularly persuasive, we do agree that CT scanning is indicated in the long-term follow-up of prosthetic grafts. I believe that a CT should routinely be obtained 4 to 5 years after graft implantation and probably 2 to 3 years thereafter.

---

**Boundary Layer Infusion of Heparin Prevents Thrombosis and Reduces Neointimal Hyperplasia in Venous Polytetrafluoroethylene Grafts Without Systemic Anticoagulation**

Chen C, Hanson SR, Lumsden AB (Emory Univ, Atlanta, Ga)
*J Vasc Surg* 22:237–247, 1995                                    13–10

---

*Background.*—Expanded polytetrafluoroethylene (e-PTFE) is currently the most widely accepted prosthetic graft material. Use of prosthetic graft materials in the venous system is limited by early graft thrombosis and frequent late suture line stenosis. Complications preclude use of long-term systemic heparin therapy for anticoagulation in vascular surgery. However, the authors have recently designed an e-PTFE–based local infusion device capable of delivering therapeutic agents directly through the wall of a synthetic graft to achieve high concentrations in the blood-fluid boundary layer along the graft wall and downstream at anastomotic sites (Fig 1). A rabbit model of inferior vena cava replacement was used to evaluate the feasibility of this approach and the effects of locally infused heparin on graft patency and anastomotic neointimal hyperplasia.

*Findings.*—Twelve rabbits were randomly assigned to undergo inferior vena cava replacement and local infusion with either saline solution or heparin for 14 days. Vascular cell proliferation was assessed via bromode-oxyuridine labeling. All grafts of heparin-treated animals remained patent 14 days after placement; all grafts in control animals were occluded at this time. However, measurements of systemic activated partial thromboplastin time before and during infusion of heparin did not differ significantly. Treated animals showed an 88% reduction in neointimal thickness, a 95%

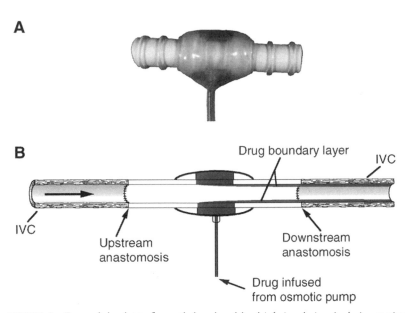

FIGURE 1.—Exapanded polytetrafluoroethylene–based local infusion device. **A,** device consists of silicone rubber cuff-reservoir glued in position between 2 rings of ringed 4-mm ID e-PTFE graft (30-µm internodal distance). Hub is attached to 1-mm ID silicone rubber catheter tubing, which is then attached to osmotic pump. **B,** soluble agent from osmotic pump will pass through graft wall, enter bloodstream in highest concentration at graft wall (boundary layer), and be transported downstream (axially) by blood flow (convection), with slower mixing in radial direction (i.e., toward centerstream blood flow), occurring primarily through diffusive mechanisms. *Long arrow* indicates direction of blood flow. *Abbreviations:* *e-PTFE,* expanded polytetrafluoroethylene; *ID,* inside diameter; *IVC,* inferior vena cava. (Courtesy of Chen C, Hanson SR, Lumsden AB: Boundary layer infusion of heparin prevents thrombosis and reduces neointimal hyperplasia in venous polytetrafluoroethylene grafts without systemic anticoagulation. *J Vasc Surg* 22:237–247, 1995.)

TABLE 1.—Effect of Heparin on Downstream Anastomotic Neointimal Hyperplasia and Cell Proliferation

| | Downstream | Upstream | p Value* | Reduction |
|---|---|---|---|---|
| Neointimal thickness | 0.144 ± 0.074 mm | 0.658 ± 0.192 mm | 0.006 | 88% |
| Neointimal area | 0.415 ± 0.209 mm² | 2.779 ± 0.239 mm² | 0.008 | 95% |
| Cell proliferation | 7% ± 2% | 25% ± 6% | 0.001 | 72% |

* A *P* value < 0.05 is considered significant.
(Courtesy of Chen C, Hanson SR, Lumsden AB: Boundary layer infusion of heparin prevents thrombosis and reduces neointimal hyperplasia in venous polytetrafluoroethylene grafts without systemic anticoagulation. *J Vasc Surg* 22:237–247, 1995.)

reduction in neointimal area, and a 72% reduction in bromodeoxyuridine labeling index at the locally treated downstream anastomosis as opposed to the untreated upstream anastomosis (Table 1).

*Conclusion.*—Overall inferior vena cava graft patency is increased, and downstream anastomotic neointimal hyperplasia and cell proliferation are greatly decreased by local boundary layer infusion of heparin. This technique appears promising as a method of antithrombolytic therapy for use in venous replacement with synthetic graft materials.

▶ The group in Atlanta has designed a Rube Goldberg apparatus for infusing heparin into a prosthetic graft. I am a little bit intrigued, but not much.

## Inguinal Wound Fluid Collections After Vascular Surgery: Management by Early Reoperation
Gordon IL, Pousti TJ, Stemmer EA, et al (Univ of California, Irvine)
*South Med J* 88:433–436, 1995                                                    13–11

*Background.*—Local wound complications may occur in one third of infrainguinal vascular grafting procedures. Seromas, hematomas, and other apparently minor complications may carry an increased risk of graft infection. Wound complications after vascular surgery have generally been managed conservatively by expectant observation or repeated aspiration. An experience with early surgical reexploration and drainage of inguinal fluid collections after vascular surgery was reported.

*Methods.*—Fourteen patients underwent early exploration for significant inguinal fluid collections after vascular grafting procedures. Reexploration was carried out within 24 hours after the complications were recognized. Management included evacuation and culture of the fluid collections, placement of closed suction drains, and reapproximation of the wound. The patients were given IV broad-spectrum antibiotics until 24 hours after the drains were removed. The results were analyzed in terms of such variables as spontaneous wound drainage, positive intraoperative wound cultures, graft exposure on reexploration, and graft type.

*Results.*—Follow-up averaged 14 months. There was just 1 case of graft infection, which occurred 6 months after reoperation. Reexploration did not cause any complications in wound healing.

*Conclusion.*—The use of early operative reexploration for patients with clinically significant inguinal fluid collections after vascular surgery was reported. This is a safe approach that results in primary healing and has a low rate of subsequent graft infection. It also avoids prolonged periods of drainage and dressing changes, though the wound must still be monitored closely.

▶ I certainly can't disagree with a recommendation to aggressively reexplore significant early groin wound fluid collection. The problem is: What is significant? As usual, clinical judgment is needed, which a paper such as this cannot address.

**W. Abbott, M.D.**

▶ I respectfully disagree slightly with Professor Abbott. When we identify any significant inguinal wound fluid collection after arterial surgery, especially if it is associated with prosthetic grafting, we reoperate within 7 days, evacuate the collection, and reclose. I do not use the closed-suction drains recommended by the authors. This aggressive approach has worked well in our hands. See also Abstract 16–13.

**J.M. Porter, M.D.**

---

**The Second Decade of Experience With the Umbilical Vein Graft for Lower-Limb Revascularization**
Dardik H (Englewood Hosp, NJ)
*Cardiovasc Surg* 3:265–269, 1995                                  13–12

---

*Background.*—The first clinical trials of umbilical vein grafting for revascularization of the lower limb were reported in 1974. Since then, reports of the effectiveness of these grafts have varied widely. A long experience with umbilical vein grafting for lower limb revascularization is updated.

*Methods.*—The authors reported a 10-year experience with umbilical vein grafting ending in 1985, describing the results of 907 bypass procedures in 799 limbs of 715 patients. Since that report, the authors have been using the umbilical vein less frequently because of a decision to use autologous saphenous vein whenever possible. The previous report was updated to include 167 additional umbilical vein bypass procedures performed from 1985 to 1993.

*Results.*—Five-year secondary patency rates of popliteal and crural reconstruction improved continuously during the experience. Five-year secondary patency rate was 61% for femoropopliteal grafts and 36% for femorotibial grafts. Five-year limb salvage rate was 73% for femoropopliteal grafts and 56% for femorotibial grafts. With increasing experience, infection, stenosis, and pseudoaneurysm became less frequent. Only 2 aneurysms developed during the latter part of the experience.

*Conclusion.*—When autologous vein is absent or inadequate, umbilical vein grafting offers an acceptable alternative for lower limb revascularization. The patency rates offered by umbilical vein grafts are exceeded only by those achieved with autologous vein. The risk of umbilical vein graft failure as a result of aneurysm appears to have been exaggerated.

▶ I suppose the umbilical vein graft still has a small role in lower extremity grafting, although it is not our choice. The results reported here appear similar to prosthetic grafting in general and considerably less than that obtained with autogenous grafting.

## The Upper Arm Basilic-Cephalic Loop for Distal Bypass Grafting: Technical Considerations and Follow-Up

Hölzenbein TJ, Pomposelli FB Jr, Miller A, et al (Harvard Med School, Boston)
*J Vasc Surg* 21:586–594, 1995                                                            13–13

*Background.*—Autogenous distal arterial revascularization in patients without adequate saphenous vein is difficult, because alternative sources of autologous vein are limited. A graft consisting of the upper arm basilic and cephalic veins in continuity was evaluated in patients undergoing distal bypass grafting.

*Methods.*—Fifty patients underwent 54 distal reconstructions using an upper arm vein loop graft over a 4-year period. Seventeen primary and 37 repeat procedures were included in the review. The patients consisted of 30 men and 20 women (mean age 69); three fourths were diabetic. A near-continuous incision, with a skin bridge left in the antecubital area, was made to harvest the vein grafts. During the operation, angioscopy was performed to make sure there was no endoluminal disease and to directly visualize the valvulotomy of the nonreversed portion of the graft.

TABLE 3.—Vein Graft Configuration and Quality of the Conduit as Judged With Angioscopy at the Final Inspection in 54 Upper Arm and Vein Loop Grafts

|  | No. | Good | Conduit quality Upgraded | Inferior |
|---|---|---|---|---|
| Upper arm loop | 38 | 22 | 14 | 2 |
| Upper arm loop with splicing* | 11 | 2 | 8 | 1 |
| Upper arm loop + other arm vein | 3 | 1 | 1 | 1 |
| Upper arm loop + leg vein | 2 | 2 | — | — |
| Total | 54 | 27 | 23 | 4 |

* Upper arm loop graft alone with onlay patch plasty, excision, and reanastomosis.
(Courtesy of Hölzenbein TJ, Pomposelli FB Jr, Miller A, et al: The upper arm basilic-cephalic loop for distal bypass grafting: Technical considerations and follow-up. *J Vasc Surg* 21:586–594, 1995.)

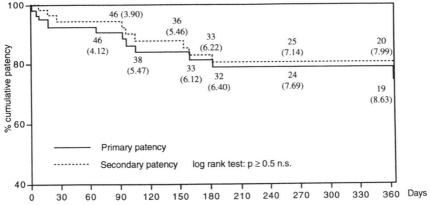

**FIGURE 1.**—Primary and secondary (corrected) patency rates of 54 upper arm loop grafts in 50 patients. Numbers give grafts at risk, and numbers in parentheses give standard error of the mean. *Abbreviation: n.s.,* not significant. (Courtesy of Hölzenbein TJ, Pomposelli FB Jr, Miller A, et al: The upper arm basilic-cephalic loop for distal bypass grating: Technical considerations and follow-up. *J Vasc Surg* 21:586–594, 1995.)

*Results.*—The objective of surgery was limb salvage in 98% of cases. A total of 33 femorotibial-pedal, 11 femoropopliteal, 7 popliteal-distal, and 2 outflow jump grafts were performed. The reason that the ipsilateral saphenous vein could not be used was previous infrainguinal bypass in 35 cases, previous coronary artery bypass grafting in 14, and poor saphenous vein quality in 5. Thirty-eight upper arm loop grafts were placed in continuity, whereas repair or splicing with additional vein segments was required in 16 cases (Table 3).

The primary 30-day patency rate was 93%, with 4 grafts becoming occluded. There were no operative deaths. At 1 year, cumulative patency rate was 74% and limb salvage rate was 91% (Fig 1).

*Conclusion.*—The upper arm vein loop graft for distal bypass grafting yields excellent patency rates in the short term and midterm. The graft can be made long enough to reach below the knee to the midtibial level. Intraoperative angioscopy helps to exclude endoluminal disease, which occurs most frequently in the median cubital vein. Patency is unaffected by straightening the curve of the median cubital vein and by valvulotomy. The upper arm vein loop graft may permit limb salvage in difficult vascular surgery cases.

▶ Bright people devise clever solutions to difficult problems. We are requiring the use of some combination of arm veins in 20% to 30% of all of our leg bypass patients. The Deaconess group[1] described the use of the basilic-cephalic vein in continuity in 1987. This experience has now been expanded to 54 patients and angioscopy is used to evaluate the graft. Standard Mill's valvulotome was used for value disruption. Patency rate and limb salvage with these grafts is excellent, and this is an occasionally useful technique for the vascular surgeon to keep in mind. However, I am unconvinced as to the value of the addition of angioscopy.

*Reference*

1. LoGerfo FW, Paniszyn CW, Menzoian J, et al: A new arm vein graft for distal bypass. *J Vasc Surg* 5:889–891, 1987.

# 14 Vascular Trauma

## Diagnosis

**Penetrating Injuries of the Neck in Patients in Stable Condition: Physical Examination, Angiography, or Color Flow Doppler Imaging**
Demetriades D, Theodorou D, Cornwell E III, et al (Univ of Southern California, Los Angeles)
*Arch Surg* 130:971–975, 1995                                                    14–1

---

*Background.*—Angiography is the current gold standard for the evaluation of vascular trauma in patients with penetrating neck injuries. However, its expense and invasiveness can limit its use. The accuracy of clinical examination in this setting is controversial. Color flow Doppler (CFD) has been shown to be accurate in evaluating vascular trauma in patients with penetrating extremity injuries, but its value in the evaluation of penetrating neck injuries is not known. Therefore, the accuracy of clinical examination and CFD was assessed in comparison with angiographic findings in the evaluation of penetrating neck trauma.

*Methods.*—Over an 18-month period, all stable patients with penetrating injuries of the neck were assessed first clinically, then with 4-vessel angiography, and finally with CFD imaging by independent assessors. The sensitivity, specificity, and positive and negative predictive values were determined for clinical examination and for CFD imaging, with angiographic findings used as the standard for comparison.

*Results.*—A total of 82 patients underwent the complete study protocol. A vascular lesion was detected by angiography in 11 patients (13.4%), with the lesions in 2 patients (2.4%) requiring treatment. Color-flow Doppler imaging correctly identified 10 of these 11 lesions and missed the small intimal tears in the common carotid and vertebral arteries in 1 patient who was managed nonoperatively. There were no false positive findings with CFD imaging. Color-flow Doppler imaging yielded a sensitivity of 91%, specificity of 98.6%, and accuracy of 98.8%. The sensitivity, specificity, and accuracy of CFD imaging all were 100% in the detection of lesions requiring treatment.

Clinical examination was able to detect small and large hematomas, minor and moderate bleeding, low systolic blood pressure, diminished peripheral pulse, and bruit as signs of vascular injury. Overall clinical examination had a sensitivity of 45.5%, specificity of 92.8%, and accuracy of 86.3%. In the detection of lesions requiring treatment, clinical examination had a sensitivity of 100%, specificity of 91%, and accuracy of 91.3%

*Conclusion.*—The combination of clinical examination and CFD imaging provided reliable accuracy, safety, and cost effectiveness in the evaluation of vascular trauma in patients with penetrating neck injuries and may therefore be a viable alternative to angiographic evaluation. Further prospective studies should be undertaken to validate these findings.

▶ I suspect these authors are correct that the combination of a careful physical examination and CFD provides a reliable method of assessing vascular injury. A worrisome consideration in the neck, of course, is the possibility of other injury, especially esophageal. Nonetheless, this and many previous articles have now established the usefulness of duplex in the diagnosis of arterial trauma. See also Abstract 14–2.

---

**Proximity Penetrating Extremity Trauma: The Role of Duplex Ultrasound in the Detection of Occult Venous Injuries**
Gagne PJ, Cone JB, McFarland D, et al (Univ of Arkansas, Little Rock)
*J Trauma* 39:1157–1163, 1995                                                    14–2

---

*Background.*—The management of penetrating proximity extremity trauma (PPET) has focused on diagnosing and repairing arterial injuries. The diagnosis of occult venous injuries has been given little attention. Therefore, the incidence and clinical significance of occult venous injuries in patients with PPET were investigated, and the diagnostic utility of color-flow duplex ultrasonography was explored.

*Methods.*—A total of 37 patients with gunshot wounds in proximity to a major vascular bundle in the lower extremity, but with no signs or symptoms of vascular injury, were studied. Each of the 48 injuries in 43 lower extremities was evaluated prospectively with an arteriogram, a venogram, and separate arterial and venous color-flow duplex ultrasonography. Clinical follow-up information was obtained from records and interviews.

*Results.*—Of the 40 extremities evaluated with arteriography, 37 had normal findings. The remaining 3 arteriograms showed evidence of external compression of a superficial femoral artery in 1, cutoff of a distal branch of a profunda femoris artery in 1, and occlusions of a small posterior tibial artery in 1. Color-flow duplex ultrasonography detected an intimal flap in the superficial femoral artery of 1 of 36 extremities; the remaining 35 arterial examinations were normal. The 3 arterial injuries not detected by color-flow duplex ultrasonography were not clinically significant.

Of the 36 extremities examined with venous color-flow duplex ultrasound, 14 revealed abnormalities, including 6 femoral-popliteal vein injuries, 1 peroneal vein injury, and extrinsic compression of venous segments in 7. Of the 17 extremities examined with venography, 7 had abnormalities, including 2 femoral-popliteal vein injuries, 1 anterior tibial/peroneal vein injury, 1 compressed superficial femoral vein, and 3 technically inadequate studies. The abnormalities detected by venography were also consistently found with venous color-flow duplex ultrasonography. Of the 6 patients with femoral-popliteal vein injuries, 3 (50%) had significant complications. Neither the patients with calf vein injuries nor the patients with extrinsic venous compression had complications during the follow-up (median, 11.75 months).

*Conclusion.*—Occult venous injuries occurred without concomitant arterial injuries in 22% of the study patients. Significant thromboembolic complications occurred in half of the patients with femoral-popliteal vein injuries. Color-flow duplex ultrasonography had greater diagnostic utility than venography in the detection of occult venous injuries of the lower extremities, although it did not contribute significantly to the diagnosis of arterial injuries.

▶ It appears that color-flow duplex is also useful in detecting extremity venous traumatic injuries.

---

## A Reassessment of Doppler Pressure Indices in the Detection of Arterial Lesions in Proximity Penetrating Injuries of Extremities: A Prospective Study

Nassoura ZE, Ivatury RR, Simon RJ, et al (Lincoln Med and Mental Health Ctr, Bronx, NY)
*Am J Emerg Med* 14:151–156, 1996                                    14–3

---

*Background.*—Though many investigators have studied the management of penetrating extremity injuries in proximity to major vascular structures, the best management has not been clearly established. The accuracy and reliability of noninvasive Doppler pressure measures for detecting occult arterial injury were assessed prospectively.

*Methods.*—Two hundred ninety-eight patients with 323 proximity extremity traumatic (PET) injuries underwent physical examination and Doppler pressure assessment. An ankle-brachial index (ABI)/brachial-brachial index (BBI) of less than 0.9 was considered abnormal. Arteriographic findings were used for comparison.

*Findings.*—Arteriography demonstrated 11 injuries (3.4%) associated with normal indices. Four injuries were repaired surgically, and 1 was treated by angiographic embolization of a bleeding vessel. All 5 of these injuries were proximal to the knee or elbow. The remaining 6 injuries were observed only. All 29 injuries associated with abnormal indices were associated with positive arteriographic results. Four lesions treated surgically were proximal, and 25 managed by observation only were distal. Compared with angiography, Doppler indices yielded 283 true negative findings, 11 false negative, 29 true positive, and no false positive results.

TABLE 4.—Results of Doppler Ratios According to the Site of Injury

| Doppler Ratio <.9 | Angiography | | Total |
| --- | --- | --- | --- |
| | Positive* | Negative | |
| Proximal Penetrating Injuries (proximal to the knee or elbow) | | | |
| Yes | 4 (4) | 0 | 4 |
| No | 10 (5) | 220 | 230 |
| Total | 14 (9) | 220 | 234 |
| Distal Penetrating Injuries (distal to the knee or elbow) | | | |
| Yes | 25 (0) | 0 | 25 |
| No | 1 (0) | 63 | 64 |
| Total | 26 (0) | 63 | 89 |

*Lesions that required treatment in parentheses.
(Courtesy of Nassoura ZE, Ivatury RR, Simon RJ, et al: A reassessment of Doppler pressure indices in the detection of arterial lesions in proximity penetrating injuries of extremities: A prospective study. *Am J Emerg Med* 14:151–156, 1996.)

The sensitivity of the Doppler indices was 72.5%; the specificity, 100%; positive predictive value, 100%; and negative predictive value, 96% (Table 4).

*Conclusion.*—Doppler indices should be part of the physical assessment of proximity penetrating injuries in the extremities. These indices can be used to screen patients with proximal injuries to determine the need for further studies, such as duplex sonography and arteriography.

▶ These authors belatedly conclude that simple Doppler indices are an important test in the evaluation of extremity arterial trauma. Using 0.9 or higher as normal, they found that an ABI less than 0.9 had a sensitivity of 72%, a specificity of 100%, a positive predictive value of 100%, and a negative predictive value of 96% in the detection of arterial injury. The worrisome thing here, of course, is a sensitivity of only 72%. Johansen and Lynch[1] of Seattle reached almost identical conclusions in an article published in 1991, although they found a sensitivity of 87%. I conclude from the current article, as well as the prior publication,[1] that false positives are rare, but there is definitely a moderate and worrisome incidence of false negatives using this method. I believe that the Doppler pressure indices should be obtained but should be combined with color duplex imaging of the site of suspected injury.

*Reference*

1. Lynch K, Johansen K: Can Doppler pressure measurement replace "exclusion" arteriography in the diagnosis of occult extremity arterial trauma? *Ann Surg* 214:737–741, 1991.

### Role of Transesophageal Echocardiography in the Diagnosis and Management of Traumatic Aortic Disruption

Vignon P, Guéret P, Vedrinne J-M, et al (Depuytren Hosp, Limoges, France; Henri Mondor Hosp, Créteil, France; Edouard Herriot Hosp, Lyon, France; et al)
*Circulation* 92:2959–2968, 1995                    14–4

*Background.*—Because patients with traumatic disruption of the aorta (TDA), usually caused by high-speed deceleration accidents, typically die quickly of massive hemorrhage, early diagnosis and immediate surgical repair is crucial. Aortography is currently considered the best diagnostic technique, but it is difficult to perform in patients with hemodynamic instability and multiple injuries. The diagnostic accuracy and clinical impact of transesophageal echocardiography (TEE) was evaluated prospectively in patients with suspected TDA.

*Methods.*—Over a 2-year period, patients with multisystem trauma or severe blunt chest trauma as a result of a high-speed deceleration accident and with a mediastinum widened to more than 8 cm on chest x-ray film underwent TEE examination. The findings of the TEE studies were compared against the findings at aortography, surgery, or necropsy. Complications of TEE and of aortography were noted.

*Results.*—Of the 32 study patients, 14 had TEE evidence of TDA. These findings were confirmed in all 14 patients by angiography, surgery, or necropsy findings. Transesophageal echocardiography detected 2 patterns of TDA. In 11 patients, subadventitial TDA appeared as an abnormal intraluminal thick flap, usually in association with a localized pseudoaneurysm. In 3 patients, intimal tears appeared as thin, moving intraluminal flaps in an area with unchanged diameter and contour. Transesophageal echocardiography failed to detect only 1 2-mm medial tear, which was confirmed by necropsy. Therefore, TEE had a sensitivity of 91% and specificity of 100% in the diagnosis of TDA. The patients who had subadventitial TDA underwent immediate surgical treatment. Patients with intimal aortic tears were successfully managed with conservative treatment. There were no complications with either TEE or aortography.

*Conclusion.*—Transesophageal echocardiography has good accuracy in the diagnosis of acute TDA in patients with multiple trauma or severe blunt chest trauma, which can direct the immediate and appropriate management of these patients. In addition, TEE is safe and portable. Therefore, it is recommended as the first-line imaging modality in this clinical setting.

▶ Clearly TEE is a highly accurate method of detecting traumatic aortic disruption, a finding repeatedly reported by others.[1, 2] The articles to-date have compared TEE to aortography. I wonder if we have now come to the point where TEE can stand alone? Be warned, the next publication reporting TEE is good for the diagnosis of traumatic aortic disruption will earn a CDA.

*References*

1. 1996 Year Book of Vascular Surgery, p 208.
2. 1996 Year Book of Vascular Surgery, p 210.

## Clinical Series

### Dislocation of the Elbow Complicated by Arterial Injury: Reconstructive Strategy and Functional Outcome

Kharrazi FD, Rodgers WB, Waters PM, et al (Boston; Massachusetts Gen Hosp, Boston; Brigham and Women's Hosp, Boston)

*Am J Orthop* May:11–15, 1995                                      14–5

*Objective.*—Twenty percent of elbow dislocations are complicated by arterial dislocations requiring revascularization. One approach to revascularization, reconstruction of the elbow, rehabilitation of the extremity, and functional outcome were reviewed.

*Methods.*—Four of 16 patients treated for elbow dislocations from January 1991 to December 1993 had complicating arterial injury. Functional outcome was assessed on the basis of patients' responses to a questionnaire. Cases of 4 patients (2 men and 2 women aged 24 to 68) were reviewed.

*Results.*—The dislocation was closed in 3 patients and open in 1. All patients had brachial transection as the arterial injury. Two patients had fractures of the lateral epicondyle, and 1 had multiple hand and wrist fractures. Three patients had neurologic deficits that varied from partial median nerve palsy to complete anterior interosseous palsy or complete palsies of the musculocutaneous, median, radial, and ulnar nerves. Three elbows redislocated before revascularization. Three patients began occupational therapy immediately. The fourth patient with multiple fractures was casted for 8 weeks. At follow-up, all elbows showed some restriction of motion. None of the nerve injuries had resolved completely. All patients complained of pain and weakness, 3 believed they were minimally disabled, and 1 was dissatisfied with the results.

*Conclusion.*—Even with aggressive treatment of elbow dislocation complicated by arterial injury using emergent revascularization and vigorous occupational therapy, some functional limitation will probably remain.

▶ These patients were not difficult to diagnose. They all were adults, and they all had brachial transection. Diagnosis was straightforward, as was repair. The real problem in elbow dislocation for me is when this injury occurs in an infant or very small child. These patients have notorious vasospasm and will frequently have no detectable distal pulses. Arteriography is difficult and potentially dangerous in these small children. We typically use the presence of a definite Doppler signal at the wrist as an indication for observation only. This is carefully followed over the next several days. If pulses return, fine; if pulses do not return, a decision is made for arteriography 1 or 2 days later after stabilization of the orthopedic injury. To date, I do not believe we have ever had to perform a delayed diagnostic arteriogram, because the pulses have invariably returned. I am sure, however, one day we are going to encounter a real arterial injury, and then we will be faced with the difficult problem of arterial repair in an extremely small artery.

## Exercise-Related Dissection of Craniocervical Arteries: CT, MR, and Angiographic Findings

Provenzale JM, Barboriak DP, Taveras JM (Duke Univ, Durham, NC; Shields Health Care, Brockton, Mass; Massachusetts Gen Hosp, Boston)
*J Comput Assist Tomogr* 19:268–276, 1995                14–6

*Introduction.*—Craniocervical arterial dissection (CAD) typically occurs after severe head or neck trauma but can occur with minor trauma, as may occur in exercise or sporting activities. In these cases diagnosis may be delayed. However, because of the risk of stroke, it is important to detect CAD as soon as possible. The neuroradiologic findings in 11 patients with exercise-related CAD were reviewed to identify the spectrum of findings and to compare the diagnostic value of different imaging modalities.

*Methods.*—Eleven patients with exercise-related dissection of the internal carotid artery (ICA) or vertebral artery (VA) were studied, with review of their medical records and neuroradiologic examinations. Of the 11 patients, 10 underwent CT, 9 underwent MRI, 4 underwent MRA, and 10 underwent contrast angiography.

*Results.*—Of the 11 patients, 7 had solitary dissections of the ICA, and 4 had solitary dissections of the VA. These injuries occurred while the patients were involved in running, paddleball, basketball, volleyball, wrestling, surfing, or trampoline jumping (Table 1). The symptoms began within minutes or up to 1 day after injury. Headache was the most common symptom of ICA dissection, and neckache was the most common symptom of VA dissection. Of the 10 patients who underwent CT examination, 4 had demonstrated infarction and 2 had a hyperdense artery, all of which were confirmed as dissections with either MRI or contrast angiography. Of the 5 patients with normal CT studies, 1 had abnormal MRI findings, 2 had normal MRI examinations, and 2 did not undergo MRI. Of the 9 patients examined with MRI, 7 had positive findings, including infarction and arterial signal abnormality in 3, infarction alone in 2, and arterial signal abnormality alone in 2. The 2 patients with false negative MRI findings had dissections located between the nonoverlapping cervical and intracranial examinations. Of the 4 patients who underwent MRA, 3 had abnormalities, and the remaining had an injury in an arterial segment not seen in nonoverlapping imaging volumes. All 10 patients who underwent contrast angiography had evidence of stenosis, including luminal irregularity in 5 patients, a pseudoaneurysm in 2, an intimal flap in 3, and occlusion of the distal branches in 2.

TABLE 1.—Clinical Course

| Case no./age/sex | Activity | Symptom onset | Symptoms and signs | Involved vessel | Residuum |
|---|---|---|---|---|---|
| 1/53/M | Running | Hours | Headache, Horner syndrome | L. ICA | Horner syndrome |
| 2/44/M | Paddleball | 1 day | Confusion, neckache | L. VA | Normal |
| 3/28/M | Basketball | 1 day | Hemianesthesia, hemiparesis | L. ICA | Mild hemiparesis |
| 4/24/M | Volleyball | Minutes | Hemiparesis, aphasia | L. ICA | Recurrent episodes of hemiparesis |
| 5/18/M | Wrestling | Minutes | Neckache, hemianesthesia, hemianopsia | R. VA | Quandrantanopsia |
| 6/40/M | Basketball | Minutes | Neckache, facial numbness, ataxia | R. VA | Normal |
| 7/44/M | Basketball | Hours | Headache, dysarthria, blurred vision | R. ICA | Normal |
| 8/35/M | Basketball | Minutes | Dizziness, dysarthria, coma | R. VA | Quadriparesis |
| 9/45/M | Surfing | Minutes | Headaches, Horner syndrome | R. ICA | None |
| 10/17/F | Trampoline jumping | Hours | Hemiparesis | R. ICA | Hemiparesis |
| 11/40/F | Basketball | Hours | Blurred vision, pulsatile tinnitus | L. ICA | None |

*Abbreviations: M,* male; *L.,* left; *R.,* right; *ICA,* internal carotid artery; *VA,* vertebral artery; *F,* female.
(Courtesy of Provenzale JM, Barboriak DP, Taveras JM: Exercise-related dissection of craniocervical arteries: CT, MR, and angiographic findings. *J Comput Assist Tomogr* 19:268–276, 1995.)

*Conclusion.*—Neuroradiologic findings indicating CAD include infarction and a hyperdense artery on CT, infarction and abnormal periarterial signal on MRI, and a narrowed arterial signal column on MRA. Computed tomography is not sensitive enough to be used as a screening examination. Either MRI or MRA (or both) of the head and neck may be a sensitive screening examination, but care must be taken to obtain overlapping images.

▶ Although I am interested in the CT findings reported herein, I am more concerned with the big picture raised by this article. These authors naively assume that these 11 patients with 7 ICA and 4 VA dissections had the dissections in every case caused by a sporting activity. I have been asked to give opinions on patients who had the symptoms come on while turning their head to look in an extreme direction. I have had occasional patients with some industrial injury such as a seemingly minor injury to the neck by a blow from a small piece of wood that did not break the skin and did not cause the patient to lose consciousness or to lose any time from work. A dissection occurring 4 days later was ascribed to the incident. Of course, there are much quoted examples of chiropractic manipulation putatively causing such injuries, usually diagnosed on a delayed basis. The problem is that once the event is recognized and the individual thinks back over his or her preceding 1 to 7 days' activities, he or she can almost always identify something that may have been causative. In many workman's compensation and insurance situations, the possible cause has great financial importance. I do not regard the cause and effect relationship to trauma as persuasive unless the effect appears almost immediately.

## Major Vascular Injuries During Laparoscopic Procedures

Nordestgaard AG, Bodily KC, Osborne RW Jr, et al (Cascade Vascular Associates, Tacoma, Wash)
*Am J Surg* 169:543–545, 1995                                                      14–7

*Background.*—Although laparoscopy has proved to be a safe, effective, and well-tolerated procedure, complications and failures can occur. Major vascular complications, although uncommon, carry a risk of serious morbidity or mortality when they do occur. Experience with 5 major vascular injuries occurring during laparoscopic procedures is reported, as are the findings of previously described major vascular injuries.

*Patients and Findings.*—Five major vascular injuries occurred in 3 women (aged 31–39 years) and 1 man (aged 76 years) over an 3-year period. All injuries were sustained during pelvic laparoscopy, which was performed for diagnostic reasons in 2 patients and for tubal ligation and hernia repair in 1 patient each. Vascular injuries were detected during laparoscopy in 3 patients, with immediate vascular surgery consultation required in 1 patient. Injuries to the iliac artery were noted in 3 patients. The iliac vein and the inferior epigastric artery also were injured in 1 patient each. In 2 patients, the mechanism of injury was the trocar. In the remaining 2 patients, vascular injuries were caused by sharp dissection for lysis of adhesions. Polytetrafluoroethylene (PTFE) interposition, PTFE patch angioplasty, resection and primary anastomosis, and ligation were used to repair arterial injuries in 1 patient each, and lateral venorrhaphy was used for venous repair. Three patients recovered without complications. The fourth patient had an ischemic cerebral accident, necessitating an extended stay in the rehabilitation unit.

Twenty previous major vascular injuries have been reported in the literature, all of which occurred as a result of the pneumoperitoneum needle or trocar insertion. The terminal aorta, vena cava, and iliac arteries and veins were most commonly injured, and most injures were managed by direct suture repair. Prompt identification of injuries was associated with patient recovery, whereas 3 of 8 patients with delayed recognition died.

*Conclusion.*—Although rare, major laparoscopic-related vascular injuries are serious and can be fatal. When such injures occur, prompt conversion to an open procedure and use of proper vascular surgical methods are needed to reestablish arterial and venous continuity and reduce complications and fatal outcomes.

▶ Four additional patients sustaining vascular injuries during laparoscopic procedures are reported. The injuries seemed to most frequently involve the iliac artery or vein, although other arteries are occasionally injured. We all have heard of patients with tragic or near-tragic outcomes as a result of unrecognized arterial injury during laparoscopy. This is another example of a form of treatment whose utilization far exceeds any proof of superiority.

---

**Prophylactic Greenfield Filter Placement in Selected High-Risk Trauma Patients**
Khansarinia S, Dennis JW, Veldenz HC, et al (Univ of Florida, Jacksonville)
*J Vasc Surg* 22:231–236, 1995                                                                14–8

---

*Background.*—Although prophylactic low-dose subcutaneous heparin (LDH) and sequential compression devices (SCDs) have been shown to reduce the incidence of deep venous thrombosis (DVT) and pulmonary embolus (PE) in severely injured patients, this management approach is contraindicated in a large number of patients and is not effective in all patients. The placement of prophylactic Greenfield filters (PGFs) in patients considered to be at high risk for thromboembolism has therefore been suggested. The safety and efficacy of PGF placement in patients with high-risk injuries were evaluated in comparison with a management strategy utilizing LDH or SCDs and venous surveillance.

*Methods.*—Over an 18-month period, PGF placement was considered in all patients who had an injury severity score (ISS) greater than 9 and 1 of the following injuries: severe head injury with lengthy ventilator depen-

TABLE 2.—Results

|  | No. | PE | PE deaths | Overall mortality rate |
|---|---|---|---|---|
| PGF | 108 | 0 | 0 | 18 (16%) |
| Control | 216 | 13 | 9 | 47 (22%) |
| p Value | — | < 0.009 | < 0.03 | NS |

*Abbreviations: PE, pulmonary embolus; PGF, prophylactic Greenfield filter.*
(Courtesy of Khansarinia S, Dennis JW, Veldenz HC, et al: Prophylactic Greenfield filter placement in selected high-risk trauma patients. *J Vasc Surg* 22:231–236, 1995.)

dence, severe head injury with multiple lower extremity fractures, spinal cord injury, major penetrating venous injury to the abdomen or pelvis, or pelvic fracture with lower extremity fractures. All patients in whom the PGFs were surgically placed also received LDH or SCDs. The outcomes of these patients were compared with those of trauma patients admitted earlier who were matched for age, ISS, mechanism of injury, and ICU length of stay.

*Results.*—Prophylactic Greenfield filter insertions were performed in 108 patients during the study period. There were 2 major complications among these patients: an internal jugular vein thrombosis that resolved spontaneously in 1 patient and a fluoroscopy C-arm malfunction leading to improper placement and filter migration into the right ventricle, which required retrieval with a thoracotomy, in another patient. There were no PEs in the 108 patients with a PGF compared with 13 (6%) in control patients (Table 2). Of the 13 control patients with PE, 9 (4.2%) died. The overall mortality rate was 16% in the PGF group and 22% in the control group, representing a reduction that was not statistically significant.

*Conclusion.*—The use of PGFs is safe and can be effective in preventing fatal and nonfatal PE in moderately or severely injured patients at high-risk for thromboembolism. The prevention of fatal PE may improve the survival rate of these patients.

▶ I remain confused by the incidence of DVT with trauma. One can find reports at all points of the compass. I agree that low-dose heparin and sequential compression devices remain the mainstay of prophylaxis in the trauma population, but clearly a significant number of patients are unable to have either of these modalities due to the nature of their injuries. In addition, the actual effectiveness of prophylaxis in the trauma setting is not clear, and certain articles have shown a disappointing incidence of both DVT and PE despite apparently adequate prophylaxis.[1, 2] In extremely high-risk patients reported herein, these authors placed a PGF in the vena cava. Significant benefits were shown for the PGF group, although this most assuredly was not a prospectively randomized study. An extremely important omission is that we are not told whether the historic control patients received any prophylaxis. Although I have inherent bias against the placement of inferior vena cava (IVC) filters in general and prophylactic IVC filters in particular, perhaps even I will have to conclude that highly selected high-risk trauma patients may be reasonable recipients of this extreme form of prophylaxis. I shall reserve judgment at present.

*References*

1. Dennis JW, Menant SS, Von Thron J, et al: Efficacy of deep venous thrombosis prophylaxis in trauma patients and identification of high-risk groups. *J Trauma* 35:132–139, 1993.
2. Knudson MM: Prevention of venous thromboembolism in trauma patients. *J Trauma* 37:480–487, 1994.

# 15 Venous Thrombosis and Pulmonary Embolism

## Prophylaxis

---

**Blood-Flow Augmentation of Intermittent Pneumatic Compression Systems Used for the Prevention of Deep Vein Thrombosis Prior to Surgery**
Flam E, Berry S, Coyle A, et al (UMDNJ-Robert Wood Johnson Med School, Piscataway; Englewood Hosp, NJ; et al)
*Am J Surg* 171:312–315, 1996                                    15–1

---

*Background.*—In patients undergoing surgery or periods of immobility, intermittent pneumatic compression (IPC) may be used to prevent deep vein thrombosis (DVT). Though several studies have compared the effectiveness of IPC with other treatments, none has compared different IPC systems. Two different types of IPC systems were compared using duplex ultrasonography.

*Methods.*—The randomized crossover study included 26 healthy young adults with no history of DVT, hypertension, diabetes, stroke, or vascular or cardiac disease. They were studied while wearing a knee-high, foam, single-pulse IPC device and a thigh-high, vinyl, sequential-pulse pneumatic compression system. Calf and thigh girth and leg length were measured before the start of the study. Flow measurements were made using duplex ultrasonography; average flow augmentation was used as a direct measure of the increase in femoral vein blood flow velocity over baseline.

*Results.*—Average flow augmentation was 107% ± 49% with the knee-high IPC device compared with 77% ± 35% with the thigh-high system. Sixty-two percent of patients showed a greater degree of augmentation with the knee-high system and 23% with the thigh-high system. Blood flow through the vein was documented during the decompression phase of IPC. However, with both systems, the blood flow velocity would sometimes fall to zero for short periods during the decompression phase, reflecting complete emptying. With the knee-high system, blood flow augmentation was not significantly affected by variations in limb anatomy.

This was not the case with the thigh-high system, with which augmentation decreased as thigh girth increased.

*Conclusion.*—Different levels of venous blood flow augmentation may be observed with different types of IPCs. Augmentation is significantly greater with a knee-high, foam, single-pulse IPC than with a thigh-high, vinyl, sequential pulse system.

▶ Surprise, surprise. I strongly suspected the thigh-high sequential-pulse IPC device would produce a significantly increased femoral vein flow velocity compared with the knee-high, single-pulse device. This study, however, indicates that the single-pulse, knee high-device produces significantly greater femoral vein velocity and, by implication, may be a more successful prophylactic device. On balance, I do believe that considerable evidence indicates the efficacy of the leg compressive system. If the single-chamber, below-knee device is equally or more effective than the more cumbersome thigh-high device with multiple chambers, it may indeed become the compressive device of choice.

## Venous Hemodynamics During Impulse Foot Pumping

Killewich LA, Sandager GP, Nguyen AH, et al (Univ of Maryland, Baltimore)
*J Vasc Surg* 22:598–605, 1995                                             15–2

*Background.*—Deep venous thrombosis (DVT) prophylaxis involves either antithrombotic medication or mechanical leg compression. However, antithrombotic medication has been associated with an increased risk of bleeding complications, and mechanical leg compression may be contraindicated in patients with lower limb trauma or may be considered cumbersome or uncomfortable by some patients. An alternative mechanical device that compresses the plantar venous plexus and simulates the normal physiologic pumping mechanism of ambulation has been developed. The effectiveness of impulse foot pumping with the device on lower limb venous outflow was evaluated with duplex ultrasound scanning.

*Methods.*—The venous velocities in the popliteal vein (PV) and common femoral vein (CFV) were measured with venous duplex scanning in 30 legs of 15 volunteers without venous dysfunction. Both resting venous velocities (RVVs) and maximum venous velocities (MVVs) were measured in both limbs with the subjects in the supine position and the 15-degree reverse Trendelenburg position at 2 pump impulse durations (1 second or 3 seconds) and 2 pressure settings (100 and 200 mm Hg).

*Results.*—The RVV in both veins did not change significantly with the change in position, although it was significantly higher in the CFV than in the PV. The mean MVV increased significantly in both veins during impulse foot pumping at both pressure settings, impulse cycles, and positions, with no statistically significant differences associated with any of these variables, except that in the supine position at the 100 mm Hg pressure setting, the PV MVV was higher with the shorter than with the longer impulse duration. In relation to the RVV, the increase in MVV was significantly greater in the PV than in the CFV. The impulse foot pumps caused no discomfort.

*Conclusion.*—The impulse foot pumping device caused increases in the venous velocities in the PV and CFV that were comparable or better than increases seen with other devices with proven efficacy for DVT prophylaxis. Therefore, the prospective evaluation of the device in patients requiring DVT prophylaxis is warranted.

▶ This investigation deals with 1 of the available mechanical methods for prophylaxis against postoperative venous thromboembolism—cyclic compression of the venous plexus in planta pedis. One interesting observation is the similar effect on venous velocity in the supine and the reversed Trendelenburg position, and it would therefore be interesting to investigate the method in patients undergoing laparoscopic surgical procedures.

**D. Bergqvist, M.D., Ph.D.**

▶ Before this article I did not realize that simple compression of the foot would result in such impressive increases in both PV and CFV duplex-determined velocities. Although the authors cautiously note that this study does not establish the efficacy of this therapy for DVT prophylaxis, the method appears to hold great promise. See also Abstract 15–3.

**J.M. Porter, M.D.**

## Prophylaxis of Deep Venous Thrombosis After Total Hip Arthroplasty by Using Intermittent Compression of the Plantar Venous Plexus

Stannard JP, Harris RM, Bucknell AL, et al (Brooke Army Med Ctr, San Antonio, Tex)
*Am J Orthop* 25:127–134, 1996                                                       15–3

*Background.*—Deep venous thrombosis is a common complication of total hip arthroplasty, and numerous methods of prophylaxis have been reported. Despite prophylaxis, however, the incidence of deep venous thrombosis in this situation remains substantial. Pulsatile intermittent compression of the plantar venous plexus was evaluated for its clinical effectiveness in prevention of deep venous thrombosis after total arthroplasty.

*Methods.*—A randomized, prospective, blind study compared outcome for 75 patients undergoing total hip replacement arthroplasty and receiving either heparin-aspirin therapy (group 1), intermittent pulsatile pneumatic-pump compression of the plantar venous plexus (group 2), or both (group 3). Compression was achieved using the PlexiPulse foot pump (NuTech, San Antonio, Texas) (Fig 2). The veins of the plantar plexus are emptied when the pump inflates the bladder for 3 to 5 sec. The pulsatile ejection of blood achieved resembles that occurring during ambulation. All patients underwent duplex ultrasonography before surgery and 1 and 2

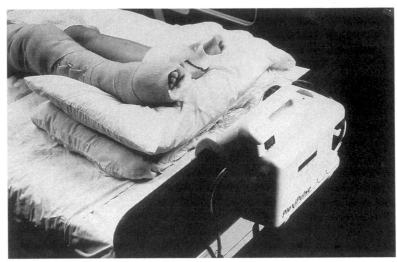

**FIGURE 2.**—The right lower extremity has a bladder placed under the postoperative dressing and the left lower extremity has a bladder over a single layer of cast padding. (Reprinted by permission of the publisher from Stannard JP, Harris RM, Bucknell AL, et al: Prophylaxis of deep venous thrombosis after total hip arthroplasty by using intermittent compression of the plantar venous plexus. *Am J Orthop* 25:127–134, Copyright 1996 by Quadrant Healthcom Inc.)

weeks after surgery; positive indications of deep venous thrombosis were confirmed with venography.

*Results.*—Deep vein thrombosis developed in 5 of the 25 patients in group 1, and pulmonary embolism also developed in 1 of these patients. Among patients in groups 2 and 3, no deep venous thrombi were detected. Use of intermittent compression of the plantar venous plexus provided a significant reduction in detectable deep venous thrombosis. Patients in group 2 also experienced a significant decrease in wound drainage by 2 to 3 days.

*Conclusion.*—Intermittent plantar compression provided outstanding prophylaxis against proximal deep vein thrombosis relative to prophylaxis with heparin and aspirin. However, limited sample size and the fact that only deep vein thromboses proximal to the calf were measured must be considered. Combination therapy with heparin-aspirin (group 3) appeared to confer no additional benefit over use of intermittent plantar compression alone.

▶ See also Abstract 15–2. This article presents, as far as I know, the first clinical study on the foot pump as venous thrombosis prophylaxis. The foot pump appeared superior to heparin-aspirin prophylaxis in a prospective randomized study. On balance, I am impressed with the potential of intermittent foot compression to be as effective as other types of lower extremity pneumatic compression. Certainly this would appear easier to use than the other types.

## Comparing Subcutaneous Danaparoid With Intravenous Unfractionated Heparin for the Treatment of Venous Thromboembolism: A Randomized Controlled Trial

de Valk HW, Banga JD, Wester JWJ, et al (Academic Hosp Utrecht, The Netherlands; St Anthonius Hosp, Nieuwegein, The Netherlands; Eemland Hosp, Amersfoort, The Netherlands)

*Ann Intern Med* 123:1–9, 1995                                                  15–4

*Objective.*—Danaparoid, a low–molecular weight sulfated glycosaminoglycan, has little effect on platelet function and low cross-reactivity with heparin-induced antibodies. Its safety and efficacy in the treatment of deep vein thrombosis or pulmonary embolism have not been assessed. The results of a randomized, open, multicenter, parallel group study comparing the safety and efficacy of 2 subcutaneous doses of danaparoid with continuous IV administration of heparin in the treatment of deep venous thrombosis or pulmonary embolism were presented.

*Methods.*—Patients were given either a low-dose IV bolus of 1,250 anti–factor Xa units of danaparoid, followed by subcutaneous injections of 1,250 anti-factor Xa units every 12 hours (n = 65) or a high-dose IV bolus of 2,000 anti–factor Xa units, followed by 2,000 anti–factor Xa units every 12 hours (n = 63). A loading dose of 2,500 units of heparin was given intravenously, followed by an adjusted maintenance dose of approximately 30,000 units/24 hr (n = 60). Patients were treated for at least 5 days until satisfactory anticoagulation was achieved. Bleeding times were determined daily. Ultrasonography, contrast venography, ventilation-perfusion scanning, or combination thereof was performed at 24 hours, 5 to 8 days after treatment, and when otherwise clinically indicated. Blinded investigators evaluated the findings.

*Results.*—Venous thromboembolism was diagnosed in 188 of 209, 30 of whom had pulmonary embolism. Two lung tests were performed in each of 179 patients, 2 leg tests were performed in each of 179 patients, and both tests were repeated in 166 patients. Recurrence or extension of venous thromboembolism was significantly reduced in patients treated with high dose danaparoid compared with patients treated with heparin (13% vs. 28%). Pulmonary embolism recurred in 7% of high-dose danaparoid-treated patients and in 24% of heparin-treated patients. Deep vein thrombosis recurred in 5% of high-dose danaparoid-treated patients and in 11% of heparin-treated patients. One low-dose and 1 high-dose danaparoid-treated patient and 2 heparin-treated patients had major bleeding. One heparin-treated patient died of intracranial hemorrhage on day 6.

*Conclusion.*—High-dose danaparoid is at least as safe and effective as heparin for treatment of venous thromboembolism.

▶ Yet another study appears to show superiority of a low–molecular weight heparinoid over unfractionated heparin in the treatment of established deep vein thrombosis.[1] The superiority of low–molecular weight heparin in many clinical settings is being increasingly recognized. I do believe that this represents a major therapeutic advance in treatment, as well as prophylaxis of deep vein thrombosis.

*Reference*

1. 1993 YEAR BOOK OF VASCULAR SURGERY, pp 359–360.

## Routine Prophylactic Vena Cava Filter Insertion in Severely Injured Trauma Patients Decreases the Incidence of Pulmonary Embolism

Rogers FB, Shackford SR, Ricci MA, et al (Med Ctr Hosp of Vermont, Burlington)
*J Am Coll Surg* 180:641–647, 1995                                          15–5

*Background.*—Standard prophylactic measures designed to prevent pulmonary embolism are often ineffective or contraindicated in the trauma patient. Patients with head injuries, spinal cord injuries, complex pelvic fractures, and hip fractures appear to be at particularly high risk for pulmonary embolism. In an attempt to decrease the incidence of this complication, physicians at the study institution have employed prophylactic vena cava filters. Results were reported for 63 patients.

*Methods.*—Starting in July 1991, prophylactic vena cava filters were inserted percutaneously in the radiology suite in all high-risk trauma patients (Table 2). Excluded were elderly patients with isolated hip fractures who could safely undergo anticoagulation if venous thromboembolism were to occur. The filters were normally inserted through the right femoral vein. Patients were followed for development of deep vein thrombosis (DVT) by weekly impedance plethysmography. Filter position and patency were checked by abdominal duplex ultrasonography 1 month after discharge, at 6 months, and then yearly.

*Results.*—The trauma service admitted 3,151 patients between July 1991 and July 1994. Of the 71 patients considered to be at high risk for pulmonary embolism, 63 had a prophylactic vena cava filter inserted as soon as their condition was stabilized. The mean time between admission and insertion of the filter was 4.3 days. Two cases of DVT developed within 48 hours of insertion, and 3 cases occurred after hospital discharge. Overall, deep vein thrombosis developed in 30% of patients (19/63) with prophylactic vena cava filters, a significant reduction compared with historical controls. There was 1 case of pulmonary embolism; an obese, 19-year-old man with a severe pelvic fracture died 10 days after fracture fixation with a sudden, massive pulmonary embolism. Five of 6 patients who did not receive the vena cava filter and in whom pulmonary embolism developed were elderly individuals with isolated hip fractures. Patency rates for the filters were 100% at 30 days and 96.1% at 1 and 2 years.

*Conclusion.*—Standard prophylactic regimens do not prevent venous thromboembolism in trauma patients. The use of vena cava filters was effective in decreasing the risk of pulmonary embolism in patients at high

TABLE 2.—Demographics of Patients Receiving a Prophylactic
Vena Cava Filter

|  | PVCF | All trauma patients |
| --- | --- | --- |
| Number of patients | 63 | 3,088 |
| Age, y | 38.9 ± 19.3 | 38.8 ± 25.9 |
| Male:female, percent | 73:27 | 60:40 |
| Injury Severity Score | 31.5 ± 9.4 | 9.2 ± 7.3 |
| Mortality, percent | 4.8 | 2.9 |

Note: Patients receiving a prophylactic vena cava filter were compared with all trauma patients admitted to the Medical Center Hospital of Vermont during July 1991 to July 1994 (mean ± standard deviation).
Abbreviations: PVCF, patients in whom a prophylactic vena cava filter was inserted; y, year.
(Rogers FB, Shackford SR, Ricci MA, et al: Routine prophylactic vena cava filter insertion in severely injured trauma patients decreases the incidence of pulmonary embolism. *J Am Coll Surg* 180:641–647, 1995. By permission of the *Journal of the American College of Surgeons*.)

risk for this complication, although at a high cost (approximately $5,000). A serum marker that would predict which patients require a filter would allow the prophylactic device to be inserted selectively.

▶ High-risk patients (including those with head injuries, spinal cord injuries, and complex pelvic fractures) underwent prophylactic vena caval filter placement. Thirty percent of these patients suffered DVT, but pulmonary embolism was diagnosed in only 1 patient. Unfortunately, this proved fatal. The authors state this experience was superior to historic controls, but, unfortunately, they provide few details of the prior experience. A significant weakness in this paper is the detection of DVT by venous impedance methodology, a testing method that I thought went out of date with the widespread use of the wedge. On balance, just as in Abstract 14–8, these results are suggestive. Before I accept this radical recommendation, however, I do insist on a prospective, randomized trial. Only then will the data be sufficiently persuasive to justify adoption of this radical policy.

## Phlegmasia Complicating Prophylactic Percutaneous Inferior Vena Caval Interruption: A Word of Caution
Harris EJ Jr, Kinney EV, Harris EJ Sr, et al (Stanford Univ, Calif)
*J Vasc Surg* 22:606–611, 1995                                                                 15–6

*Background.*—In patients with deep vein thrombosis (DVT), anticoagulation permits natural thrombolysis to occur and prevents the development of the 2 major complications of DVT: phlegmasia cerulea dolens and pulmonary embolism. Some authors are recommending placement of an inferior vena cava (IVC) filter instead of anticoagulation for patients with venous thromboembolic disease. Thrombotic complications after percutaneous IVC interruption in patients with DVT were evaluated.
*Methods.*—The retrospective study included 32 patients who underwent placement of 33 percutaneous IVC filters. Fifty-three percent had DVT and

47% had pulmonary embolism; all patients with pulmonary embolism who were evaluated for DVT proved to have DVT. The patients were 18 women and 14 men (mean age 64). The most common indication for IVC filter insertion was DVT with a relative contraindication to anticoagulation, 31%, followed by prophylactic filter insertion in a patient with pulmonary embolism and therapeutic anticoagulation, 25%; pulmonary embolism and absolute contraindication to anticoagulation, 16%; prophylactic insertion in a patient with DVT and therapeutic anticoagulation, 16%; prophylactic insertion in a patient with pulmonary embolism and therapeutic coagulation, 8%; and DVT and absolute contraindication to anticoagulation, 6%. Overall, 17 patients did not receive anticoagulation, 10 because of relative contraindications and 7 because of absolute contraindications. The remaining 15 patients did receive anticoagulation.

*Results.*—Phlegmasia cerulea developed in about one fourth of patients who received a percutaneously inserted IVC filter without anticoagulant therapy. In contrast, none of the patients who received an IVC filter in addition to anticoagulation had phlegmasia.

*Conclusion.*—In patients with DVT, percutaneous IVC filter insertion can prevent pulmonary embolism. However, it has no effect on the patient's underlying thrombotic process and may even contribute to progressive thrombosis if the patient is not receiving anticoagulation as well. Percutaneous IVC filter insertion should not replace anticoagulation therapy for patients with routine proximal DVT. When IVC filter placement is required because of failed anticoagulation, heparin treatment of the underlying thrombotic process should continue. The decision to perform IVC interruption in place of anticoagulation for patients with relative contraindications for the latter form of therapy should be carefully considered.

▶ As previously stated, I have a deep-seated, although perhaps mildly irrational, aversion to IVC filters. Clearly, one of the indications for IVC filter placement is a patient with a DVT or pulmonary embolism who has an absolute contraindication to therapeutic anticoagulation. In 17 such patients reported herein, 4 (24%) developed phlegmasia cerulea dolens. Three patients recovered; 1 died. The authors appropriately recommend that when a patient receives a vena caval filter for contraindication to anticoagulation, one should very carefully review these contraindications and decide if perhaps an exception could be made. The risk of phlegmasia in patients without anticoagulation with a new IVC filter appears significant indeed. The authors appropriately recommend anticoagulation be maintained along with IVC filtration if at all possible. I agree.

### Low Molecular Weight Heparin Started Before Surgery as Prophylaxis Against Deep Vein Thrombosis: 2500 Versus 5000 Xal Units in 2070 Patients

Bergqvist D, Burmark US, Flordal PA, et al (Univ Hosp, Uppsala, Sweden; Danderyds Hosp, Södersjukhuset Stockholm; Kärnsjukhuset, Skövde; et al)
*Br J Surg* 82:496–501, 1995                                             15–7

*Background.*—Low–molecular weight heparins (LMWHs) are of proven effectiveness for the prevention of postoperative venous thromboembolism. However, the optimal dose of LMWHs remains to be established. Two doses of LMWH (2,500 and 5,000 Xal units) were compared for safety and efficacy in the prevention of deep vein thrombosis (DVT).

*Methods.*—The prospective, randomized, double-blind, multicenter trial included 2,070 patients undergoing elective general abdominal surgery. Two thirds of patients had malignant disease. They were randomized to receive 2,500 or 5,000 Xal units of the LMWH dalteparin beginning the evening before surgery and once daily every evening thereafter. The fibrinogen uptake test was performed to detect DVT, and bleeding complications were assessed. The results were analyzed by both intention to treat and in patients receiving the correct prophylaxis, as 86% did.

*Results.*—A total of 1,957 patients had a technically correct fibrinogen uptake test. Deep vein thrombosis occurred in 7% of patients receiving the 5,000 Xal units of dalteparin vs. 13% of those receiving 2,500 Xal units. The higher dose also produced better results on intention-to-treat analysis (7% vs. 13%) and in patients with malignant disease (9% vs. 15%) (Table 3). Thirty-day mortality was about 3% in both dose groups; 2 patients died of pulmonary embolism. Bleeding complications occurred in 5% of patients receiving the higher dose of LMWH vs. 3% in those receiving the

TABLE 3.—Frequency of Deep Vein Thrombosis

| | Dose of dalteparin | | | |
| | 2500 units | 5000 units | 95% c.i. of difference | *P* |
|---|---|---|---|---|
| Total study group | | | | |
| Intention to treat (*n* = 1957) | 12·7 | 6·6 | 2·8–7·8 | < 0·001 |
| Correct prophylaxis (*n* = 1732) | 13·1 | 6·8 | 3·0–8·5 | < 0·001 |
| Patients with malignancy | | | | |
| Intention to treat (*n* = 1303) | 14·9 | 8·5 | 2·1–8·9 | < 0·001 |
| Correct prophylaxis (*n* = 1154) | 15·1 | 8·8 | 2·1–9·4 | 0·001 |

*Note:* Values are percentages.
*Abbreviation: c.i.,* confidence interval.
(Courtesy of Bergqvist D, Burmark US, Flordal PA, et al: Low molecular weight heparin started before surgery as prophylaxis against deep vein thrombosis: 2500 versus 5000 Xal units in 2070 patients. *Br J Surg* 82:496–501, 1995; Blackwell Science Ltd.)

lower dose. This difference was not significant in the patients with malignant disease.

*Conclusion.*—In patients undergoing high-risk general surgery, 5,000 XaI units of the LMWH dalteparin offers effective prophylaxis against DVT. There is a small associated risk of bleeding complications. Even in the high-risk group studied, fatal pulmonary embolism appears to be a very infrequent complication with dalteparin treatment.

▶ The authors herein compare 2 dosing regimens of LMWH (2,500 vs. 5,000 XaI units daily) in the prophylaxis of DVT, concluding the higher dose of LMWH was twice as effective for prophylaxis as the lower dose but also resulted in twice the incidence of bleeding. A potential weakness of this paper is the use of the fibrinogen uptake test for the diagnosis of DVT, a test that has been severely questioned.[1] On balance, I believe this to be an important dose ranging study, which helps us establish the optimal dose for this particular LMWH in DVT and pulmonary embolism prophylaxis.

*Reference*

1. Lensing AWA, Hirsh H: $^{125}$I-fibrinogen leg scanning: Reassessment of its role for the diagnosis of venous thrombosis in postoperative patients. *Thromb Haemost* 69:2–7, 1993.

---

**A Trial of a Low Molecular Weight Heparin (Enoxaparin) Versus Standard Heparin for the Prophylaxis of Postoperative Deep Vein Thrombosis in General Surgery**
Nurmohamed MT, Verhaeghe R, Haas S, et al (Academic Med Ctr, Amsterdam; Univ Hosp Leuven, Belgium; Technischen Univ München, Germany; et al)
*Am J Surg* 169:567–571, 1995                                   15–8

---

*Introduction.*—Results have been conflicting in investigations comparing low–molecular weight heparin (LMWH) with standard heparin (SH) for preventing deep vein thrombosis (DVT) in general surgery patients. The efficacy and safety of LMWH and SH were compared in a prospective, randomized, double-blind international multicenter trial.

*Methods.*—Patients were randomized to receive either 20 mg of LMWH (enoxaparin) once daily or 5,000 IU of SH 3 times daily starting preoperatively and continuing daily for 10 days or until discharge. Patients were observed daily for venous thromboembolism, bleeding complications, and other clinical problems. Fibrinogen iodine-125 uptake leg scanning was used daily for up to 10 days postoperatively to detect DVT.

*Results.*—In all, 718 patients received LMWH and 709 patients received SH. A total of 103 patients had abnormal leg scans or were symptomatic for venous thromboembolism. Of these, 45 patients received SH and 58 received LMWH. The incidence of patients with abnormal leg scans or symptomatic venous thromboembolism was 3.7% in patients treated with

TABLE 4.—Confirmation of Thromboembolic Complications in the Two Study Groups

| Outcome | Standard Heparin (n = 709) | LMWH (n = 718) |
|---|---|---|
| Deep vein thrombosis | | |
| Abnormal fibrinogen uptake test | | |
| Confirmed by venogram | 8 | 25* |
| No or inadequate venogram | 15 | 17 |
| Confirmed clinical suspicion† | 2 | — |
| Pulmonary embolism | | |
| Confirmed clinical suspicion† | 1 | — |
| Confirmed by autopsy | 0 | 1 |
| Total | 26 (3.7) | 43 (6.0) |

*Note:* Data reported as number of patients (%). Unless otherwise indicated, comparisons were not statistically significant.
*$P < 0.05$; the other comparisons were not statistically significant.
†Without abnormal fibrinogen uptake test.
*Abbreviation:* LMWH, low–molecular weight heparin.
(Reprinted by permission of the publisher from Nurmohamed MT, Verhaeghe R, Haas S, et al: A comparative trial of a low molecular weight heparin (enoxaparin) versus standard heparin for the prophylaxis of postoperative deep vein thrombosis in general surgery. *American Journal of Surgery* 169:567–571, Copyright 1995 by Excerpa Medica Inc.)

SH and 6.0% in those treated with LMWH (Table 4). Eleven (1.5%) patients treated with LMWH and 18 (2.5%) patients receiving SH experienced major bleeding complications. Reoperation was needed by 13 patients (1.8%) in the SH group and 4 patients (0.6%) in the LMWH group. Six patients treated with SH and 4 patients treated with LMWH died. One patient treated with LMWH died of pulmonary embolism. Two patients treated with SH and 1 patient treated with LMWH had major bleeding–associated deaths. All other deaths were not related to bleeding or embolism.

*Conclusion.*—There were no between-group differences in the prevention of postoperative venous thromboembolism for patients treated with SH or LMWH. The major advantage of using LMWH over SH is its convenience of administration; thus, it may be the preferred approach in thromboprophylaxis.

▶ The conclusions are predictable; LMWH appears as effective and safe as unfractionated heparin and much more convenient to give. The problems with this admirable multicenter trial is that [125]I fibrinogen was used to diagnose DVT and that the dose of enoxaparin is reported in milligrams. I believe the patients reported herein received only about 2,000 Xa inhibitory units of drug daily. According to Dr. Bergqvist, this would not be an optimal amount. I suspect we will have to hash out for some time the optimal dose of the LMWHs.

## Is DVT Prophylaxis Overemphasized? A Randomized Prospective Study

Kosir MA, Kozol RA, Perales A, et al (Wayne State Univ, Detroit)
*J Surg Res* 60:289–292, 1996                                    15–9

*Objective.*—Mechanisms of determining risk factors for deep vein thrombosis (DVT) in general surgical patients have improved in the last decade. The use of conventional prophylaxis has decreased the incidence of DVT. The incidence of DVT in surgery patients receiving conventional prophylactic therapies was evaluated in a prospective study.

*Methods.*—A total of 139 patients undergoing emergency abdominal, thoracic, head, or neck surgery were randomized to receive pneumatic compression (group 1, n = 25), subcutaneous heparin (group 2, n = 38), or no prophylactic therapy (group 3, n = 45) 1 hour before and for 7 days after surgery. Duplex venous studies of both lower extremities were performed using a color-flow duplex scanner with a 7.5-MHz probe and a 8.1-MHz pencil probe Doppler preoperatively and 1, 3, and 30 days postoperatively. A prognostic index was calculated for each patient, and incidences of DVT were recorded.

*Results.*—Prognostic indices (PIs) were calculated for each patient and included as risk factors: age, obesity, hemoglobin level, colorectal procedures, diabetes, chronic obstructive pulmonary disease, peripheral vascular disease, immobilization, and cancer. Prognostic indices were similar among groups and predicted a 20% incidence of DVT. Twenty-nine patients were discontinued from the study. No DVTs were detected in any group, but DVTs were detected in 8 patients not in the study during the study period.

*Conclusion.*—No DVTs occurred within 30 days of surgery in any group. There were no predictors of DVT that accurately predicted the incidence of DVT in this study.

▶ There are several problems with this paper, making the conclusions invalid. The mean age is much lower than usually encountered in thrombo-prophylactic studies. One must remember age is 1 of the most important risk factors for postoperative thromboembolism. Several studies have documented the poor sensitivity of duplex in surveillance of postoperative thrombosis. The sample size of the study is much too small; moreover, it is armed. The results of this 1 small study do not invalidate the overwhelming documentation of the beneficial effect of thromboprophylaxis in surgical risk groups.

**D. Bergqvist, M.D., Ph.D.**

▶ For reaching grandiose conclusions wholly unsupported by the presented data, these authors are awarded the prestigious CDA.

**J.M. Porter, M.D.**

## Treatment

### Prospective Study of Safety of Lower Extremity Phlebography With Nonionic Contrast Medium

AbuRahma AF, Powell M, Robinson PA (West Virginia Univ, Charleston, WVA; Pfizer Central Research, Groton, Conn)
*Am J Surg* 171:255–257, 1996                                                                 15–10

---

*Objective.*—The incidence of lower extremity deep venous thrombosis (DVT) after high osmolar ionic contrast phlebography varies between 9% and 31%. The incidence of minor and major adverse reactions and post-phlebographic DVT when nonionic contrast medium iopamidol was used was determined in a prospective study.

*Methods.*—Between 1991 and 1992, 157 patients with clinically suspected DVT underwent phlebography using iopamidol (mean amount 102 mL). Of these, 111 patients had prephlebography venous color duplex ultrasound of the lower extremities and 102 were examined for delayed side effects 1 week after phlebography. The presence of phlebography-induced DVT was assessed using color duplex ultrasound.

*Results.*—The prephlebography duplex findings revealed 81 negative studies and 30 positive studies that included 17 cases of acute DVT of the lower extremity and 13 cases of chronic DVT. Phlebography revealed 91 normal studies and 38 cases of acute DVT, 16 cases of chronic DVT, and 12 cases of DVT of undetermined age. There were no major complications or cases of postphlebography DVT. Minor adverse reactions occurred in 7% of patients and included nausea, local pain, and dizziness. The maximum hypothetical true rate of major complications, given that no patients in the study were observed to have any major adverse effects, was 2.9.

*Conclusion.*—Lower extremity phlebography using nonionic contrast medium is safe, with no incidence of postphlebography DVT in this series of patients. Phlebography with nonionic contrast material should be used if duplex ultrasound is not available or inconclusive.

▶ The lack of complications associated with the use of nonionic contrast media for lower extremity phlebography is gratifying. The complete absence of phlebography-induced DVT is noteworthy and quite different from the 10% to 30% incidence of contrast agent–induced DVT associated with high osmolar ionic contrast media. This would have been much more persuasive had it been a prospective randomized study comparing the 2 types of contrast media. Even so, I take this as valuable information concerning the relative safety of the nonionic media.

### Preliminary Results of a Nonoperative Approach to Saphenofemoral Junction Thrombophlebitis

Ascer E, Lorensen E, Pollina RM, et al (Maimonides Med Ctr, Brooklyn, NY)
*J Vasc Surg* 22:616–621, 1995                                                                                                15–11

*Background.*—Surgical ligation of the greater saphenous vein (GSV) has long been the recommended treatment for saphenofemoral junction thrombophlebitis (SFJT). A nonoperative approach to the management of SFJT was studied.

*Methods.*—The nonrandomized study included 20 consecutive patients with SFJT, all of whom were admitted to the hospital and placed on a full course of heparin. The diagnosis was confirmed and the deep venous system assessed by a preadmission duplex ultrasound study. A follow-up scan was performed on hospital day 2 to 4. Warfarin therapy continued for 6 weeks in patients who had SFJT alone and in those whose SFJT had resolved on the follow-up duplex scan. Warfarin therapy continued for 6 months in patients who had deep venous thrombosis (DVT) in addition to SFJT. The results of treatment were assessed in terms of SFJT resolution, recurrent SFJT, and occurrence of pulmonary embolism.

*Results.*—Forty percent of patients had concurrent DVT: unilateral in 4 cases, bilateral in 2 cases, and developing during anticoagulation in 2 cases (Fig 1). Five patients had DVT contiguous with SFJT, and 3 had noncontiguous DVT. Follow-up duplex scans were performed in 13 patients at 2 to 8 months. These scans showed partial resolution of SFJT in 7 cases, complete resolution in 5, and nonresolution in 1. At up to 14 months'

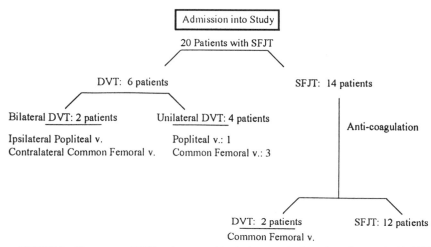

FIGURE 1.—Occurrence of DVT as documented by duplex scanning in patients diagnosed with SFJT. Of 20 patients with SFJT admitted into the study, 6 had associated DVT at the time of admission, 2 had bilateral DVT, and 4 had unilateral DVT. All patients were treated with hospitalization and anticoagulation. Of 14 patients with SFJT alone on admission, 2 developed DVT. *Abbreviations: DVT,* deep venous thrombosis; *SFJT,* saphenofemoral junction thrombophlebitis; *v.,* vein. (Courtesy of Ascer E, Lorensen E, Pollina RM, et al: Preliminary results of a nonoperative approach to saphenofemoral junction thrombophlebitis. *J Vasc Surg* 22:616–621, 1995.)

follow-up, none of the patients experienced pulmonary embolism, recurrent SFJT, or complications of anticoagulation.

*Conclusion.*—In patients with SFJT, anticoagulation therapy is effective in achieving resolution and preventing recurrence of SFJT, as well as in preventing pulmonary embolism. Many patients with SFJT will have concurrent DVT. Thus, the deep venous system must be closely monitored during treatment for SFJT.

▶ From this small flawed study comes a useful message for anyone whose thinking about SFJT remains stuck in the intuitive approach of the 1930s. It is not the superficial phlebitis that is really dangerous but the 40% chance of an associated DVT. This can extend and embolize despite conventional anticoagulation in hospital, and SFJ ligation may actually increase the risk. A fatal postligation embolism was the stimulus for the authors' prospective study, which may actually underestimate the associated DVT because the gap between diagnosis and initial follow-up scans was only 2 to 4 days. In addition, although it was a prospective study, only 13 of the 20 patients had follow-up scans at 2 months or more. Saphenofemoral junction ligation is outdated and anticoagulation the best management, but it is certainly no panacea. The next question for the authors is why they admitted all these patients to hospital and put them on strict bed rest. Diagnosis and anticoagulation can be achieved on an outpatient basis, and maintaining mobility is a significant advantage.

**A.E.B. Giddings, M.D.**

▶ Especially with once-daily low–molecular weight heparin!

**J.M. Porter, M.D.**

---

**Low Molecular Weight Heparins (LMWH) in the Treatment of Patients With Acute Venous Thromboembolism**
Hirsh J, Siragusa S, Cosmi B, et al (Hamilton Civic Hosp Research Ctr, Ont, Canada)
*Thromb Haemost* 74:360–363, 1995                                    15–12

---

*Introduction.*—Randomized trials to compare the relative efficacy and safety of low–molecular weight heparins (LMWHs) and unfractionated heparin (UFH) in the treatment of deep venous thrombosis (DVT) have shown trends for better efficacy and safety with the use of LMWH. A meta-analysis was carried out to further investigate the relative efficacy and safety of LMWH and UFH for the treatment of DVT and recurrent venous thromboembolism (VTE).

*Methods.*—The study material consisted of 13 randomized clinical trials that compared LMWH and UFH when used to treat patients with a first episode of acute DVT or pulmonary embolism. Only patients with objectively confirmed symptomatic recurrent VTE and major bleeding were included in the analysis. Studies were classified as level 1 if they were double blind or if the assessment of outcomes was blinded and as level 2 if they were not double blind or if the assessment of outcomes was not blinded.

*Results.*—The incidence of recurrent VTE during the first 15 days of anticoagulant therapy was 0.8% in the LMWH-treated group and 3.2% in the UFH-treated group. The incidence of recurrent VTE during subsequent treatment with oral anticoagulants from days 16 to 90 was 1.9% in the LMWH group and 3.2% in the UFH group. During the 3-month period of anticoagulant therapy, 10 of 365 LMWH-treated patients (2.9%) and 24 of 371 UFH-treated patients (6.4%) had recurrent VTE. The differences were statistically significant. The overall mortality rate was 3.2% in the LMWH group and 5.9% in the UFH group in favor of LMWH. The incidence of fatal pulmonary embolism for the entire treatment period was 0.4% among LMWH-treated patients and 0.7% among UFH-treated patients. The relative risk of recurrent VTE when only level 1 studies were considered was 0.24 for the first 15 days of anticoagulant therapy and 0.39 for the entire treatment period in favor of LMWH. The overall relative risk for major bleeding was 0.42 in favor of LMWH. For the level 2 studies, there were no significant differences in VTE recurrence or major bleeding between the 2 treatment groups.

*Conclusion.*—In the treatment of patients with VTE, LMWHs are at least as safe and effective as UFH and are probably more effective and safer than UFH in the treatment of DVT. The beneficial effects of LMWHs become apparent within the first 15 days of treatment and are maintained during the 3 months of oral anticoagulant therapy.

▶ A meta-analysis comparing LMWH to unfractionated heparin in the treatment of venous thrombosis is reported herein. Overall, in the best clinical studies, classified as level 1, significant benefits in favor of LMWH were recognized. See also Abstracts 15–4, 15–7, and 15–8. The general superiority of LMWH in both prophylaxis and treatment of DVT is becoming more firmly established every day.

---

**A Comparison of Six Weeks With Six Months of Oral Anticoagulant Therapy After a First Episode of Venous Thromboembolism**
Schulman S, and the Duration of Anticoagulation Trial Study Group (Karolinska Hosp, Stockholm; Huddinge Hosp, Stockholm; Danderyd Hosp, Södersjukhuset, Stockholm; et al)
N Engl J Med 332:1661–1665, 1995                                    15–13

---

*Background.*—Prophylactic oral anticoagulants are given routinely to patients with deep vein thrombosis (DVT) or pulmonary embolism to prevent recurrence. However, the optimal duration of anticoagulant therapy has been debated. The efficacy of 6 weeks of therapy was compared with that of 6 months of therapy in preventing recurrence, hemorrhagic complications, and death in patients after a first episode of DVT or pulmonary embolism.

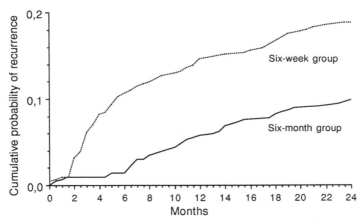

**FIGURE 1.**—Cumulative probability of recurrent venous thromboembolism after a first episode according to the duration of anticoagulation. (Reprinted by permission of *The New England Journal of Medicine*. Schulman S, and the Duration of Anticoagulation Trial Study Group: A comparison of six weeks with six months of oral anticoagulant therapy after a first episode of venous thromboembolism. *N Engl J Med* 332:1661–1665, Copyright 1995, Massachusetts Medical Society.)

*Methods.*—Consecutive patients at least 15 years old diagnosed with a first episode of either pulmonary embolism or DVT were randomly assigned to receive oral anticoagulation therapy for either 6 weeks or 6 months after prothrombin times were stable within the target range (international normalized ratio 2.0–2.85). The patients were followed for 2 years to determine the incidence of recurrent venous thromboembolism, major hemorrhage, and death in each treatment group.

*Results.*—Of 897 patients enrolled, 443 were assigned to receive 6 weeks of therapy and 454 were assigned to receive 6 months of therapy. There were major hemorrhages in 1 patient in the 6-week group and in 5 patients in the 6-month group; none was fatal. Three of these patients were receiving anticoagulant doses exceeding the target range. Twenty-two patients in the 6-week group and 17 patients in the 6-month group died during the 2-year study period. There were 123 episodes of recurrent venous thromboembolism, with a significantly higher incidence in the 6-week than in the 6-month group (18.1% vs. 9.5%) (Fig 1). The incidence of recurrence increased sharply immediately after anticoagulant therapy was discontinued in the 6-week group.

*Conclusions.*—The risk of recurrent thromboembolism was reduced significantly by increasing the duration of oral anticoagulant therapy from 6 weeks to 6 months, which supports the use of at least 6 months of anticoagulant therapy after an initial thromboembolic episode. However, the monthly incidence of recurrent thromboembolism was comparable in the 2 groups after 6 months, suggesting that venous thromboembolism is an ongoing condition with a persistent risk of recurrence.

▶ A controversy has raged for years as to the optimal duration of anticoagulant therapy after an episode of DVT. In the carefully conducted study reported herein, 6 months of prophylactic oral anticoagulation after the first episode of DVT led to a markedly lower recurrence rate than did anticoagulant treatment for only 6 weeks. The entire difference occurred between 2 months and 6 months, and after 6 months the recurrence in both groups paralleled each other at about 5% to 6%. It seems important that we recognize DVT as part of a continuous ongoing disease process and most assuredly not as a 1-hit event with low likelihood of recurrence. Six months of warfarin treatment after DVT appears minimal.

---

**Treatment of Venous Thrombosis With Intravenous Unfractionated Heparin Administered in the Hospital as Compared With Subcutaneous Low-Molecular-Weight Heparin Administered at Home**
Koopman MMW, for the Tasman Study Group (Academic Med Ctr, Amsterdam; Slotervaart Hosp, Amsterdam; Istituto di Semeiotica Medica, Padua, Italy; et al)
*N Engl J Med* 334:682–687, 1996                          15–14

---

*Background.*—The standard in-hospital treatment for patients with deep vein thrombosis (DVT) consists of an IV course of unfractionated heparin, with dose adjustments to prolong the activated partial-thromboplastin time to the length desired. However, fixed-dose subcutaneous low–molecular weight heparin (LMWH), which can be given on an outpatient basis, appears to be as safe and effective. The 2 treatments were compared in symptomatic outpatients with proximal vein thrombosis but no signs of pulmonary embolism.

*Methods and Findings.*—By random assignment, 198 patients were given adjusted-dose IV standard heparin in the hospital, and 202 received fixed-dose subcutaneous LMWH at home. Thromboembolism recurred in 8.6% of the patients receiving standard heparin and 6.9% of those receiving LMWH. Major bleeding occurred in 2% of the former and 0.5% of the latter. Both groups showed improvement in quality of life. Patients given LMWH had better physical activity and social functioning. Thirty-six percent of those receiving LMWH were never hospitalized. Forty percent were discharged early. The number of days spent in the hospital was reduced by 67%.

*Conclusion.*—Outpatient treatment with fixed-dose subcutaneous LMWH in the treatment of proximal vein thrombosis is effective and safe. Such treatment does not adversely affect physical or mental well-being and decreases costs.

▶ It was inevitable. First, LMWH was proved equal or superior to unfractionated heparin (UF) in DVT prophylaxis. Next it was proved to be as good or probably superior in treatment. The logical conclusion is reported in this article; treat DVT patients as an outpatient with once-daily LMWH injection without the need for coagulation studies. I suspect in the very near future it will be the rare patient admitted to the hospital for the treatment of DVT with

IV heparin. I believe we are witnessing the passing of an era and the appearance of a new therapeutic principal.

## Clinical Series

**The Superficial Femoral Vein: A Potentially Lethal Misnomer**
Bundens WP, Bergan JJ, Halasz NA, et al (Univ of California, San Diego; US Naval Med Ctr, San Diego, Calif)
*JAMA* 274:1296–1298, 1995                                    15–15

*Background.*—Duplex scanning has represented a major advance in the early diagnosis of deep venous thrombosis of the lower extremity. However, the term "superficial femoral vein" in duplex sonography reports refers to a vein that is actually part of the deep venous system. This reporting practice is potentially misleading. The potential for error related to this term was examined in a mail survey study.

*Methods.*—Three separate mail surveys were performed: 1 targeted to multispecialty medical groups, 1 to the anatomy departments of U.S. medical schools, and 1 to vascular laboratories. Response rates were around 75%. Responses were received from 46 family practitioners and general internists, who were asked what treatment they would suggest for a patient with leg pain and an acute thrombosis of the superficial femoral vein; from 95 anatomy department heads, who were asked about the "correct," "acceptable," "preferred," and "taught" terms for the deep thigh veins; and from 85 laboratory directors, who were asked what terms they use in reports of lower limb venous duplex scanning.

*Results.*—In the clinical scenario described, just one fourth of respondents said they would prescribe anticoagulation. Only 3% of the anatomists considered the term "superficial femoral vein" to be correct. Though 22% judged it an acceptable alternative, just 9% taught it to medical students, and only 7% reported it was the preferred term for everyday use. Nevertheless, 93% of vascular laboratories responding used this term for lower limb venous duplex reports.

*Conclusion.*—Most vascular laboratories use the misleading term "superficial femoral vein"in reporting venous duplex scan results. This practice is potentially dangerous for patients. Primary care physicians are generally unaware that this term actually refers to a deep vein and that acute thrombosis of the "superficial femoral vein" is potentially life threatening.

▶ I wonder how many people have died of a fatal pulmonary embolism because internists and general practitioners receiving a report from the vascular laboratory that the patient had "superficial femoral vein thrombosis" mistakenly thought this meant superficial venous thrombosis? The authors of this paper have done us all a service. We must henceforth stop referring to the portion of the artery and vein between the profunda femoris and the popliteal as the "superficial femoral anything." Both the nomina anatomica, as well as the edition 38 of *Gray's Anatomy*[1] (1995) speak to the vascular structures between the external iliac and the popliteal as the femoral artery and the femoral vein, without any subdivision into common or superficial. We must learn to live with this nomenclature and let us once and for all abandon the term superficial femoral artery and vein, because the confusion caused by this terminology has finally become unacceptable.

*Reference*

1. *Gray's Anatomy*, ed 38. 1995.

---

**Venous Thromboembolic Disease and Combined Oral Contraceptives: Results of International Multicentre Case-Control Study**
World Health Organization Collaborative Study of Cardiovascular Disease and Steroid Hormone Contraception (Univ College London Med School)
*Lancet* 346:1575–1582, 1995                                    15–16

---

*Introduction.*—The formulation and use of oral contraceptives (OCs) have changed since previous studies of the OC-associated risk of venous thromboembolism (VTE). Also, the results obtained in European and U.S. studies do not necessarily apply to populations with different rates of and risk factors for VTE. Data from a case-control study of stroke, acute myocardial infarction, and VTE in Africa, Asia, Europe, and Latin America were used to assess the association between current OC use and risk of a first VTE.

*Methods.*—The hospital-based study was conducted in 21 centers in 17 countries. The patients were women in their twenties through forties who had been admitted to the hospital with a discharge diagnosis of deep vein thrombosis (DVT), pulmonary embolism (PE), or both. Each case of DVT or PE was categorized as definite or probable based on the clinical and radiologic findings. The controls were women admitted to the same hospital with a diagnosis considered to be unrelated to OC use. Cases and controls were evaluated in a standardized interview.

*Results.*—One thousand eleven women with DVT and 206 with PE were recruited into the study. Forty-two percent of the DVT diagnoses and 25% of the PE diagnoses were confirmed by definitive investigations, and more than 80% of both case types were categorized as definite or probable. The analysis included a total of 1,143 DVT/PE patients and 2,998 matched controls. European patients with DVT or PE were better educated and more likely to have had hypertension during pregnancy than their controls. Patients with DVT or PE in the developing countries were more likely than their controls to have had 1 or more live births and to have a previous history of high blood pressure and rheumatic heart disease.

Crude odds ratios (ORs) of VTE were 2.32 in European women and 33.0 in women in developing countries, were 2.70 for European women and 33.0 for women in developing countries for a history of rheumatic heart disease, were 2.70 for European women and 4.61 for women in developing countries for body mass index (BMI) greater than 30 kg/m$^2$ vs. 20 kg/m$^2$ or less, 2.65 for European women and 3.81 for women in developing countries for a history of varicose veins, 2.59 for European women and 1.22 for women in developing countries for moderate smoking, 1.66 for European women and 1.16 for women in developing countries for hypertension during pregnancy, and 0.95 for European women and 1.82 for women in developing countries for a history of high blood pressure. Europe and all 3 regions of the developing world showed an increased overall OR for VTE associated with current OC users compared with nonusers and never-users. The risk estimates, about 4.2 in Europe and 3.3 in the developing world, were not significantly altered by duration of current and lifetime use.

Risk increased significantly with increasing BMI. The increased risk was apparent within 4 months of the start of OC use and resolved within 3 months of stopping. Though risk estimates were similar for OCs containing lower vs. higher estrogen doses, the risks associated with first- and second-generation progestagens were somewhat greater when used in combination with a higher dose of estrogen. Risks were higher for women whose OC contained third-generation progestagens, which are given only with low-dose estrogen, than for those receiving first- and second-generation progestagens. The odds ratio of VTE was greater for European women who used other progestagens combined with a low-dose estrogen.

*Conclusion.*—In the developing world, as in Europe, OC use is associated with an increased risk of VTE. The overall OC-related risk estimates are lower than in most previous studies of nonfatal idiopathic VTE. The only confounder is a history of hypertension during pregnancy among European women; the only other VTE risk factors are history of varicose veins, BMI greater than 25 kg/m$^2$, and history of rheumatic heart disease.

▶ I keep including articles on this topic, attempting to once and for all reach the definitive answer to the haunting question as to whether OCs cause VTE disease. This large study finds that the use of combined OCs is associated with a significantly increased risk of VTE, with odds ratios averaging 4.2 in Europe and 3.3 in developing countries. Of interest is the observation that the third-generation progestagens currently in use have a higher odds ratio of causing VTE than the progestagens of the first and second generation. I doubt this will be the last word on this subject. See also the references for additional information.

*References*

1. 1993 Year Book of Vascular Surgery, p 332.
2. 1993 Year Book of Vascular Surgery, p 364.

## Prospective 12-Year Follow-Up Study of Clinical and Hemodynamic Sequelae After Deep Vein Thrombosis in Low-Risk Patients (Zürich Study)

Franzeck UK, Schalch I, Jäger KA, et al (Univ Hosp, Zürich, Switzerland)
*Circulation* 93:74–79, 1996                                                      15–17

*Introduction.*—There are no prospective investigations in the literature for the long-term sequalae of more than 10 years after acute deep vein thrombosis (DVT). The natural history of postthrombolic syndrome was evaluated in 58 patients considered to be low risk for DVT.

*Methods.*—Patients underwent clinical and hemodynamic evaluations at time of admission; after 3, 6, and 12 months; after the second, third, fourth, and fifth years; and after the twelfth year. Each patient received heparin initially, then oral anticoagulants.

*Results.*—At 12-year follow-up, 64% of 39 available patients had normal clinical findings of the lower limbs. Other findings were 28% mild skin changes, 5% marked trophic changes, and 1 venous ulcer. Fifty-four percent of patients with multilevel thrombosis reported regular use of compression stockings. In highly compliant patients there were no relevant trophic skin lesions. These patients had no or mild postthrombotic symptoms at 12 years. The patient with a venous ulcer used compression stockings occasionally. The mean maximum outflow was significantly decreased in the affected leg compared with the contralateral leg throughout follow-up. However, 6 months after DVT, a significant improvement in venous outflow was observed in the affected leg. Also at 6 months after DVT, 50% of patients demonstrated recanalization, with 20% valvular incompetence of the posterior tibial veins and 17% with partial recanalization. At 12-year follow-up, 54% of patients had normal findings and 46% had valvular insufficiency. Eight of the initial 58 patients died (14% mortality rate). Of these deaths, 5 were related to vascular events.

*Conclusion.*—There was a low incidence of DVT at 12-year follow-up in patients treated with oral anticoagulants and regular compression therapy. However, with a mortality rate of 14% and a recurrence rate of 24%, the prognosis after DVT is not favorable, even in patients who are considered low risk.

▶ This is a small study with only 39 available patients at follow-up, but it is important in that it prospectively analyzes the development of a posthrombotic syndrome. The authors chose a group of patients with cryptogenetic DVT defined as a low-risk population. After 12 years this definition turned out to be true concerning both survival (86%) and the occurrence of venous ulcer (3%). One highly remarkable detail in the treatment protocol is the initial 5 days' bedrest, immobilization probably being 1 of the great risk factors for the development of thrombosis.

**D. Bergqvist, M.D., Ph.D.**

### Propagation, Rethrombosis and New Thrombus Formation After Acute Deep Venous Thrombosis

Meissner MH, Caps MT, Bergelin RO, et al (Univ of Washington, Seattle)
*J Vasc Surg* 22:558–567, 1995                    15–18

*Background.*—Though recanalization frequently occurs after an episode of deep venous thrombosis (DVT), further thrombotic events are also possible. Patients with first episodes of acute DVT were studied to determine the incidence, timing, and outcome of further thrombotic events.

*Methods.*—The study included venous thrombi of 204 lower extremities in 177 patients. Each thrombus was followed with duplex sonography at 1 day, 1 week, and 1 month; then every 3 months for 1 year; then yearly.

*Results.*—Thrombi propagated to new segments in 30% of initially involved extremities and rethrombosis in 31%. Thirteen percent of segments had both propagation and rethrombosis in different segments, and 9 initially uninvolved limbs showed new thrombi. None of the clinical risk factors studied was significantly related to these events, though rethrombosis occurred in limbs that were initially more extensively involved. The median time to propagation in initially involved extremities was 40 days in all segments; new thromboses in initially uninvolved extremities and rethromboses were later events. Reflux was more likely to occur in initially uninvolved segments to which the thrombus extended. Reflux was also common in rethrombosed middle and distal superficial femoral and popliteal artery segments.

*Conclusion.*—Many patients with acute DVT will go on to have recurrent thrombotic events. Ultimately these events have a negative impact on valvular competence. No known clinical risk factors can predict recurrent thrombotic events, which occur even in patients receiving standard anticoagulation therapy.

▶ Our suspicions have been confirmed by this careful study. The authors have not included events in the iliac veins in their report, but the evidence needs to be taken very seriously; DVT is not usually a discrete threat but a dynamic, continued menace. See also Abstract 15–13. Despite the availability of specific diagnosis and conventional anticoagulation (often poorly administered and monitored), the management of DVT is frequently inadequate because it is poorly understood. We must prevent extension, rethrombosis, contralateral thrombosis, and late venous incompetence, but improvement is unlikely to be achieved until there is new knowledge. At best, anticoagulation influences only 1 of the major causes. Effective anticoagulation, early mobility, and vigilant, perhaps lifelong, follow-up is mandatory, particularly for patients who have developed thrombosis without a discrete and reversible cause being identified. Further research is likely to uncover greater prevalence and greater complexity.

**A.E.B. Giddings, M.D.**

## Distribution and Occlusiveness of Thrombi in Patients With Surveillance Detected Deep Vein Thrombosis After Hip Surgery

Ascani A, Radicchia S, Parise P, et al (Univ di Perugia, Italy)
*Thromb Haemost* 75:239–241, 1996                                                                 15–19

*Background.*—Most postoperative deep vein thromboses (DVTs) are asymptomatic, and the existing noninvasive imaging methods are inaccurate in screening for asymptomatic DVTs. The characteristics of postoperative thrombi may account for the inability of noninvasive imaging techniques to detect them. A large series of venograms performed in hip surgery patients was analyzed to determine the distribution and occlusiveness of postoperative DVT.

*Methods and Results.*—Patients underwent venography a mean of 10 days after surgery for hip fracture or elective implantation of a hip prosthesis. Twenty-eight percent of limbs studied were found to have DVT. Isolated calf thrombi accounted for 55% of the DVTs detected, proximal and distal thrombi for 31%, and isolated proximal thrombi for 14%. Of the proximal DVTs, 46% involved the common femoral vein, 48% involved the superficial femoral vein, and 54% involved the popliteal vein. Sixty-eight percent of the common femoral vein DVTs, 56% of the superficial femoral vein DVTs, and 59% of the popliteal vein DVTs were nonocclusive.

*Conclusion.*—Most asymptomatic DVTs in hip surgery patients are nonocclusive. Thus, noninvasive techniques to detect DVTs by measurement of venous flow are unlikely to improve the detection rate of asymptomatic thromboses. Isolated thromboses of the superficial femoral vein are common, suggesting the need to perform real-time B-mode ultrasound examination of the entire proximal venous system.

▶ In a study using phlebography to detect postoperative DVT in 321 asymptomatic hip surgery patients, these authors found DVT in 28% of patients, with about half involving the proximal veins of the leg and half involving the calf veins. A majority of the affected veins were subtotally occluded, meaning that impedance plethysmography would be a poor diagnostic test. I believe that our duplex is sufficiently sensitive to detect subtotally occlusive calf vein thrombi with a high degree of accuracy, although we have never subjected this to simultaneous phlebography. On balance, the pattern of disease reported in this study is about as predicted.

## Prevalence of Deep Venous Thrombosis Among Patients in Medical Intensive Care

Hirsch DR, Ingenito EP, Goldhaber SZ (Harvard Med School, Boston)
*JAMA* 274:335–337, 1995                                                                 15–20

*Introduction.*—The rate of deep vein thrombosis (DVT) is well documented in surgical patients, but few studies have examined the frequency of this complication in medical patients. The prevalence of DVT was determined in a prospective study conducted in the medical ICU (MICU) of a large tertiary care hospital.

*Patients and Methods.*—Eligible patients were 18 years or older and expected to have a stay of at least 48 hours in the MICU. Excluded were those with an admitting diagnosis of DVT or pulmonary embolism and patients unable to have ultrasound (US) examination. Serial venous US examinations of the upper and lower extremities of 100 patients were performed with color Doppler imaging twice weekly during their MICU stay and 1 week after discharge from the unit. The diagnosis of DVT in lower extremities was confirmed by absent or diminished Doppler flow, lack of respiratory variation, and failure to augment flow with calf compression. About half of the enrolled patients had pulmonary diagnoses. Prophylaxis against venous thromboembolism was administered to 61 patients.

*Results.*—Deep venous thrombosis was detected by US examination in 33 of the 100 patients studied. Sixteen patients had proximal lower extremity DVT, and 5 had upper extremity DVT associated with central venous catheters. Both upper extremity DVT and proximal lower extremity DVT were present in 1 patient. The first US examination in the MICU yielded positive results in 23 of 33 patients. Therapeutic interventions were performed in 21 patients on the basis of US findings. Ten patients received low-dose subcutaneous heparin, 4 had full-dose anticoagulation, 3 received an inferior vena cava filter, 3 had follow-up US, and 1 had a central line removed. Overall in-hospital mortality for the 100 MICU patients was 27%, and the mortality rate was higher for patients with DVT (36%) than for those without DVT (24%). Patients with and without DVT had similar characteristics and similar causes of death.

*Conclusion.*—Despite prophylaxis against venous thromboembolism in more than half of these MICU patients, DVT was detected in one third of the group using US with color Doppler imaging. Patients who developed DVT did not differ from those without DVT in traditionally recognized risk factors for this complication. Patients admitted to MICUs may benefit from more intensive prophylaxis regimens or routine US surveillance.

▶ A large number of long-term stay patients in medical ICUs develop DVT, estimated in this study at 33%. About half of these will have proximal lower extremity DVT, one third will have isolated calf DVT, and 15% will have upper extremity DVT usually associated with catheters. Although the quantitation of this population is interesting, I find little of surprise here.

### The Incidence of Occult Cancer in Patients With Deep Venous Thrombosis: A Prospective Study

Bastounis EA, Karayiannakis AJ, Makri GG, et al (Univ of Athens, Greece)
J Intern Med 239:153–156, 1996                                        15–21

*Objective.*—The association between diagnosed cancer and deep vein thrombosis (DVT) is well known. The potential relationship between DVT and occult cancer in apparently healthy patients was studied prospectively.

*Methods.*—Between 1987 and 1992 venography or Doppler examinations were performed on 487 patients with suspected DVT. Patients with known malignancies, thrombophlebitis, or recurrent venous thrombosis were excluded. Others were followed for 2 years.

*Results.*—First-episode DVT was diagnosed in 293 patients, 86 (29%) of whom had idiopathic DVT. Cancer was diagnosed on admission in 22 patients (7.5%), 16 (18.6%) of whom had idiopathic DVT and 6 of whom had secondary DVT (known risk factors for DVT). Ten patients had other signs of malignancy, but 12 appeared to be healthy. These 22 patients were excluded from follow-up. During the follow-up period, cancer was diagnosed in 5 (7.35%) of patients with idiopathic DVT and in 2 (1%) patients with secondary DVT. Significantly more patients with idiopathic DVT (25%) than secondary DVT (4%) developed cancer. There were no other significant differences between groups. Cancer was detected by CT in 7 asymptomatic patients, colonoscopy in 4, chest radiograph in 1, and blood testing in 1. Cancers were detected early and curative treatment was possible.

*Conclusion.*—Although the appearance of DVT made early detection of cancer possible in this study, additional prospective studies need to be conducted to validate these findings.

▶ Numerous studies have consistently shown that a distressing percentage of patients with idiopathic DVT will subsequently be proven to have cancer. The numbers seem to range between 5% and 25%. The 25% reported in this study does appear a bit high. Nonetheless, the occurrence of apparently idiopathic DVT should alert the clinician to a significant likelihood of undiagnosed cancer.[1]

*Reference*

1. Prandoni P, Lensing AWA, Buller HR, et al: Deep vein thrombosis and the incidence of subsequent symptomatic cancer. N Engl J Med 327:1128–1133, 1992.

## Calf Vein Thrombi Are Not a Benign Finding

Lohr JM, James KV, Deshmukh RM, et al (Good Samaritan Hosp, Cincinnati, Ohio)

*Am J Surg* 170:86–90, 1995                                                    15–22

*Introduction.*—The literature disagrees regarding which patients with calf vein thrombi are at increased risk for proximal propagation. A total of 288 patients with isolated calf vein thrombi were prospectively evaluated. Serial scans were performed at 3-day intervals to determine propagation of thrombi. Late scans were taken at 3 and 4 weeks.

*Results.*—Sequential follow-up scans were available for 192 patients. Of these, 53 (28%) had propagation of the initial thrombi. The most proximal level of the propagation in these patients was popliteal vein, 11; superficial femoral vein, 5; common femoral vein, 5; adjacent tibial or soleal veins, 24; adjacent soleal veins alone, 7; and lesser saphenous vein, 1. Free-floating thrombus tips were observed in the large veins of the thighs of 3 patients with thrombus propagation. There were no significant differences in results of deep venous thrombosis prophylaxis in patients with and without propagation (Table 2). Three (13%) of 23 patients treated with systemic heparin developed thrombus propagation; none reached the popliteal vein or any other venous segment above the knee.

*Conclusion.*—No significant risk factors for propagation of calf vein thrombi were determined despite a 28% overall rate of propagation. No patients treated with heparin propagated a thrombus above the knee. It seems that calf vein thrombi are as not as benign as previously believed. The role of subcutaneous low–molecular weight heparin needs to be explored in the treatment of calf vein thrombosis.

▶ This paper deals with a debated and controversial topic, the danger of isolated calf vein thrombosis. It clearly shows that, left untreated, some propagate proximally. It seems certain that symptomatic calf vein thrombosis has the potential to cause pulmonary embolism. Symptomatic calf vein thrombi treated with anticoagulation for only 1 week recurs significantly more frequently than those anticoagulated for 3 months.[1] Asymptomatic calf

TABLE 2.—Deep Vein Thrombosis Prophylaxis in Patients With and Without Propagation

|  | With Propagation (n = 53) | Without Propagation (n = 139) |
|---|---|---|
| Compression stockings | 9 (17%) | 20 (14%) |
| Subcutaneous heparin | 7 (13%) | 8 (6%) |
| Coumadin | 2 (4%) | 7 (5%) |
| Aspirin | 7 (13%) | 10 (7%) |
| Persantine | 0 | 3 (2%) |
| Pneumatic compression | 4 (8%) | 3 (2%) |

(Courtesy of Lohr JM, James KV, Deshmukh RM, et al: Calf vein thrombi are not a benign finding. *Am J Surg* 170:86–90, 1995.)

vein thrombosis does not, however, seem to be a danger, not even for postthrombotic venous insufficiency.[2] To conclude, symptomatic calf vein thrombi are not benign.

*References*

1. Lagerstedt C, Fagher BO, Olsson CG, et al: Need for long-term anticoagulant treatment in symptomatic calf vein thrombosis. *Lancet* 2:515–518, 1985.
2. Lindhagen A, et al: Deep venous insufficiency after postoperative thrombosis diagnosed with [125]I-labelled fibrinogen uptake test. *Br J Surg* 71:511–515, 1984.

### Surgical Treatment of Septic Deep Venous Thrombosis
Kniemeyer HW, Grabitz K, Buhl R, et al (Heinrich-Heine-Univ Düsseldorf, Germany)
*Surgery* 118:49–53, 1995                                                      15–23

*Background.*—Septic deep vein thrombosis (SDVT) may cause death. Most reported cases of SDVT are related to IV drug abuse or percutaneously inserted central venous catheters. Most cases of SDVT respond to catheter removal, antibiotics, and anticoagulation. On occasion, however, the condition can progress to thrombosis and septic embolism. The role of surgery in the treatment of SDVT was examined in a retrospective study.

*Methods.*—The review included 5 patients with SDVT who underwent venous thrombectomy with arteriovenous fistula over a 7-year period. There were 3 males and 2 females (mean age 21). None was an IV drug abuser; 2 had osteomyelitis, 1 had SDVT after delivery, and 2 had no recognized cause of SDVT. Severe systemic complications of SDVT were present in 3 patients. Three patients had iliofemoral plus vena caval SDVT, and 1 each had femoropopliteal and iliofemoral involvement. All patients received IV antibiotics and anticoagulation in addition to venous thrombectomy. Two patients underwent simultaneous transabdominal caval thrombectomy.

*Results.*—Respiratory failure from previous septic embolism occurred in 2 patients. Multiorgan failure occurred before thrombectomy in another patient. The patients required intensive care for a mean of 28 days; however, all survived. All were alive, with no recurrent septic or embolic complications, at a mean 50 months' follow-up.

*Conclusion.*—Venous thrombectomy may be indicated for patients with complicated SDVT whose condition does not improve with conservative therapy. In this situation, thrombectomy can be lifesaving. Conservative and surgical management are supplemental rather than competitive treatment approaches.

▶ Short of draining an abscess, I do not believe there is any established role for surgery for a presumed SDVT. The cases presented in this article are not convincing. I have little use for attempted venous thrombectomy in this setting. I believe the authors should significantly rethink their position.

# 16 Chronic Venous and Lymphatic Disease

## Biology

**Role of Leukocyte Activation in Patients With Venous Stasis Ulcers**
Pappas PJ, Fallek SR, Garcia A, et al (UMDNJ-New Jersey Med School, Newark)
*J Surg Res* 59:553–559, 1995                                          16–1

*Introduction.*—Leukocyte activation has been implicated in the pathogenesis of chronic venous stasis ulcers (CVSUs). Differences in the levels of activated circulating leukocytes and cytokines were compared in patients with CVSUs and healthy controls.

*Methods.*—Blood samples were obtained from 11 men with class III venous insufficiency and CVSUs and from 12 age-matched healthy controls. Serum measurements of soluble interleukin-1β (IL-1β), IL-2, IL-6, tumor necrosis factor–α (TNF-α), and TNF-β microglobulin levels were obtained. The percentage of lymphocytes (CD3), monocytes (CD14), and granulocytes (CD15) expressing cell surface activation markers was determined with fluorescence flow cytometry. Ulcer samples from the patients were cultured, and the bacteria were identified.

*Results.*—Compared with the controls, patients had significant decreases in the expression of the CD3+/DR+ and CD3+/CD38+ markers on T lymphocytes and significant increases in the expression of CD14+/CD38+ markers on monocytes. The ratio of T-helper cells to T-suppressor cells was significantly increased in the patients, indicating good immune function. There were increased systemic levels of IL-6 but normal systemic levels of TNF-α, IL-1β, IL-2, and β2-microglobulin. Of the 9 patients with wound cultures, 8 had *Streptococcus aureus* infections.

*Conclusion.*—The elevated systemic IL-6 levels, downregulated T-lymphocyte levels, and upregulated monocyte activation present in patients with CVSUs may be mediated by bacterial staphyloccal enterotoxins in the wound itself. No systemic neutrophil activation was found in these patients, suggesting that their involvement may be a local microcirculatory phenomenon.

▶ These authors purport to have found a variety of differences in monocytes and lymphocytes from patients with CVSUs compared with normal controls. A broad interpretation of these results is that there is increased monocyte activity in CVSU patients but no evidence of systemic neutrophil activation. The general theory seems to be that venous hypertension or its sequelae cause activation of certain white blood cells, which, in turn, cause local tissue damage. I wonder. Biologic phenomenon are almost never that neat. See also Abstract 16–3.

## Expression of the Adhesion Molecules ICAM-1, VCAM-1, and E-Selectin and Their Ligands VLA-4 and LFA-1 in Chronic Venous Leg Ulcers

Weyl A, Vanscheidt W, Weiss JM, et al (Univ of Freiburg, Germany)
*J Am Acad Dermatol* 34:418–423, 1996                                    16–2

*Background.*—In certain systems, leukocyte binding to endothelial cells (ECs) is regulated by the interaction of adhesion molecules, including intracellular adhesion molecule–1 (ICAM-1), vascular cell adhesion molecule–1 (VCAM-1), and E-selectin on ECs and leukocyte function-associated antigen-1 (LFA-1) and very late activated antigen–4 (VLA-4) on leukocytes. Increased expression of these adhesion molecules may play a role in the pathogenesis of chronic venous insufficiency. This hypothesis was investigated in the present study.

*Methods.*—Monoclonal antibodies against ICAM-1, VCAM-1, LFA-1, VLA-4, and E-selectin were used to stain 27 biopsy specimens of inflamed dermatoliposclerotic skin that was proximal to venous leg ulcers. Normal skin specimens also were subjected to immunohistochemical analysis, and staining intensity was compared between healthy and affected skin.

*Results.*—No epidermal expression of ICAM-1, VCAM-1, LFA-1, VLA-4, and E-selectin was found in healthy skin. In comparison, increased expression of ICAM-1 and VCAM-1, but not E-selectin was noted on ECs in the specimens of leg ulcers caused by chronic venous insufficiency. An increased perivascular accumulation of leukocytes, strongly expressing LFA-1 and VLA-4 on their surfaces, was observed in specimens from patients with chronic venous insufficiency. Analysis revealed that 61% of capillary loops were surrounded by LFA-1–positive leukocytes in specimens from patients vs. 20% from healthy individuals and that 68% of capillary loops were surrounded by VLA-4–positive leukocytes in specimens from patients vs. 21% from healthy controls.

*Conclusion.*—In patients with chronic venous insufficiency, increased adherence and extravasation of LFA-1 and VLA-4-positive leukocytes may occur in response to upregulation of ICAM-1 and VCAM-1 on ECs. In a recent study, pentoxifylline was found to inhibit T-cell adhesion to activated ECs in vitro. Thus, downregulation of adhesion molecules on ECs and leukocytes also may be achieved with pharmacologic intervention in patients with chronic venous insufficiency.

▶ Tissue from skin biopsy specimens taken adjacent to venous leg ulcers showed increased expression of various adhesion molecules and leukocyte function–associated antigens, as well as VLA-4. The authors take this as indirect evidence that there may be an upregulation of adhesion molecules on endothelial cells in areas of venous hypertension, which may contribute to the increased adherence and extravasation of selected leukocytes in chronic venous insufficiency. Increasing but not yet convincing evidence suggests abnormal leukocyte function in patients with venous ulceration.

**Diminished Mononuclear Cell Function Is Associated With Chronic Venous Insufficiency**
Pappas PJ, Teehan EP, Fallek SR, et al (UMDNJ-New Jersey Med School, Newark)
*J Vasc Surg* 22:580–586, 1995                                    16–3

*Background.*—The association between venous hypertension and chronic venous insufficiency (CVI) is clearly established. However, the mechanisms involved in clinical disease progression are not understood. Recent studies have implicated lymphocytes and monocytes in the pathophysiology of CVI. The possibility of functional alteration of lymphocytes and monocytes was explored by measuring their proliferative response to mitogenic stimuli.

*Methods.*—Fifty patients were assigned to 4 groups: the control group of 14 patients with no history of CVI, group 2 with 10 patients with class 2 CVI, group 3 with 15 patients with active venous ulcers and class 3 CVI, and group 4 with 11 patients with a history of multiple venous ulcers and current lipodermatosclerosis (LDS). Blood was obtained from all patients. The lymphocytes and monocytes were isolated and cultured with staphylococcal enterotoxins A, B, $C_1$, D, and E at 1, 8, 31, and 125 µg/well and with phytohemagglutinin (PHA) as the control mitogen at 5 µg/well. After culturing for 96 hours, the cells were pulsed with tritiated thymidine for 6 hours, and thymidine incorporation was measured.

*Results.*—All of the cells responded to PHA, although there was less proliferation in group 2 cells compared with the other 3 groups. The proliferative responses of cells in the CVI groups to all of the staphylococcal enterotoxins were significantly lower than in the control group, with a consistently diminishing responsiveness in association with clinical disease progression.

*Conclusion.*—The consistency of the relationship between reduced proliferative responsiveness and clinical disease progression strongly suggests biological significance. Because cytokine production, which regulates epidermal regeneration, extracellular matrix production, and tissue repair, is dependent on cellular proliferation, alterations in mononuclear cell responsiveness to challenges may result in delayed wound healing.

▶ This study shows that mononuclear white blood cell function diminishes with increasing degree of venous insufficiency. Although an interesting observation, nothing can be said of the importance of this finding in pathogenesis of deep vein insufficiency and venous ulceration.

**D. Bergqvist, M.D., Ph.D.**

▶ This study appears to conflict with Abstract 16–1. Does monocyte activity increase or decrease in these patients?

**J.M. Porter, M.D.**

## Diagnosis

### Comparison of Venous Reflux in the Affected and Non-Affected Leg in Patients With Unilateral Venous Ulceration
Bradbury AW, Brittenden J, Allan PL, et al (Royal Infirmary, Edinburgh, Scotland)
*Br J Surg* 83:513–515, 1996                                              16–4

*Background.*—Venous disease is the most common cause of lower limb ulcerations, and most venous ulcers appear to result from venous reflux. However, there are few data on the contributions of reflux at varying sites in the deep and superficial venous system. Venous reflux was assessed in the affected and unaffected legs of patients with unilateral venous ulcers.

*Methods.*—The 54 patients studied had unilateral ulcers with characteristics strongly suggesting a purely venous origin. Each patient underwent color-flow duplex ultrasonography of the deep and superficial venous systems of both the affected and unaffected legs. Pathologic reflux was considered to be present if there was reverse flow exceeding 0.5 sec.

*Results.*—Proximal popliteal vein reflux was present in 42 affected legs vs. 31 unaffected legs and distal popliteal vein reflux in 39 vs. 26 legs. Venous reflux of the posterior tibial and anterior tibial veins was also significantly more frequent in the ulcerated legs. There were no differences between legs in the pattern of venous reflux in the common femoral, proximal and distal superficial femoral, peroneal, long saphenous, and short saphenous veins.

*Conclusion.*—Many lower extremities may have deep and superficial venous reflux without the characteristic skin changes of chronic venous insufficiency. The findings suggest that information on the unaffected, contralateral leg is needed to determine the significance of venous reflux in a leg with venous ulceration. The goal of surgery should be to correct reflux in the affected but not the unaffected limb. In most patients, this would be best achieved by correction of deep venous incompetence.

▶ This study emphasizes that many patients with unilateral venous leg ulceration have distinctly abnormal venous function in the opposite leg. In fact, the incidence of venous reflux in the opposite leg appeared as frequent as that in the symptomatic leg. The authors' suggestion that one should not attempt to ascribe significance to reflux in the symptomatic leg until determining its presence in the asymptomatic leg appears to be well taken. This again emphasizes the theory put forward earlier that we must regard venous thrombosis as an ongoing disease process in which almost no patient suffers a single hit. The episodes of deep venous thrombosis appear repetitious, continuous, and unpredictable and probably involve both legs in most patients. See also Abstract 15–13.

**Duplex-Derived Valve Closure Times Fail to Correlate With Reflux Flow Volumes in Patients With Chronic Venous Insufficiency**
Rodriguez AA, Whitehead CM, McLaughlin RL, et al (Tufts Univ, Boston)
*J Vasc Surg* 23:606–610, 1996                                    16–5

*Introduction.*—The most common cause of chronic venous insufficiency is valvular reflux. There is still debate for methods of quantifying reflux, although a number of noninvasive methods effectively screen for the presence of reflux. One method more commonly used because of its ability to be easily measured is studying the duplex-derived valve closure times. However, the abnormal valve closure times have wide variances. The relationship between valve closure times and other duplex-derived measurements of reflux volumes was explored in patients who have chronic venous insufficiency.

*Methods.*—Duplex scan and air plethysmography were used to examine 69 legs in 45 patients with varying degrees of chronic venous insufficiency. It was determined whether a correlation exists between total volume refluxed and air plethysmography–derived residual volume fraction and between total valve closure times and venous filling index obtained from air plethysmography.

*Results.*—A history of deep venous thrombosis was found in 20% of patients, with 29% having undergone venous surgery. There was no correlation between flow volume and valve closure time or between flow at peak reflux and valve closure time at any of the anatomical locations, including the greater saphenous vein, the saphenofemoral junction, superficial femoral vein, saphenous vein, popliteal vein, and profunda femoris vein. There was no correlation between total flow volumes and air plethysmography–derived residual volume fraction or between total valve closure time and air plethysmography–derived venous filling index. A moderate correlation was found between total flow volumes and total valve closure times.

*Conclusion.*—Although duplex-derived valve closure times are extremely useful in determining the presence of reflux, they should not be used to quantitate the degree of reflux because they do not correlate with the magnitude of reflux. Patients about to have surgery should have ascending and descending phlebography. Further studies are necessary because currently no test is available to identify who will progress in degree of reflux.

▶ There are only several things we can measure about venous reflux. We can measure the time required for venous valve closure using duplex; we can approximate the volume of venous reflux, as well as the velocity of venous reflux using the duplex, although certain assumptions are required concerning diameter, which may not be valid; and we can use the air plethysmograph to determine venous filling index and such other variables as residual volume fraction. In fact, almost no correlation was found between the valve closing time and the flow volume, the peak flow velocity, the venous filling index, or residual volume fraction. I wonder how the reflux volume and velocity correlated with the air plethysmography data. I do not find this given. It is interesting to note that in previous studies neither valve closure time nor air plethysmography appeared capable of discriminating between class II and class III patients. Clearly we have a way to go in quantitating venous reflux. Presently not only do the varying tests have little internal agreement, but they also seem to have very poor agreement with the clinical categorization of the severity of venous reflux disease. We currently have chaos. We need order.

## Duplex Ultrasonography Scanning for Chronic Venous Disease: Patterns of Venous Reflux

Myers KA, Ziegenbein RW, Zeng GH, et al (Monash Univ, Melbourne, Australia)
*J Vasc Surg* 21:605–612, 1995                                          16–6

*Background.*—It is generally believed that lipodermatosclerosis or venous ulceration associated with chronic venous disease is caused by reduced valve function in the deep and perforating veins, leading to chronic congestion in the calf muscle venous plexuses, causing blood ejection from muscle contraction through perforators to damage overlying tissues. However, this belief has been challenged by recent findings suggesting that deep venous reflux is uncommon and outward flow in perforators occurs commonly in healthy patients. Patterns of venous flow were studied in patients with both uncomplicated and complicated varicose veins with duplex ultrasonography.

*Methods.*—Duplex ultrasonography scanning was performed on 776 lower limbs with primary uncomplicated varicose veins, 70 limbs with lipodermatosclerosis, and 96 limbs with past venous ulceration. Venous flow was studied in the long and short saphenous veins, the common and superficial femoral veins, popliteal veins, 3 sets of crural veins, and medial calf perforators. Differences between the findings in the different patient groups were analyzed.

*Results.*—Deep venous obstruction was found in only 2 limbs, including 1 with lipodermatosclerosis and 1 with past venous ulceration. Superficial venous reflux alone was substantially more common in all limbs than deep venous reflux. Both superficial and deep venous reflux was more common in patients with complications than in patients with uncomplicated varicose veins. Superficial reflux was most common in limbs with ulceration. Overall, there was a greater frequency of long saphenous reflux than of

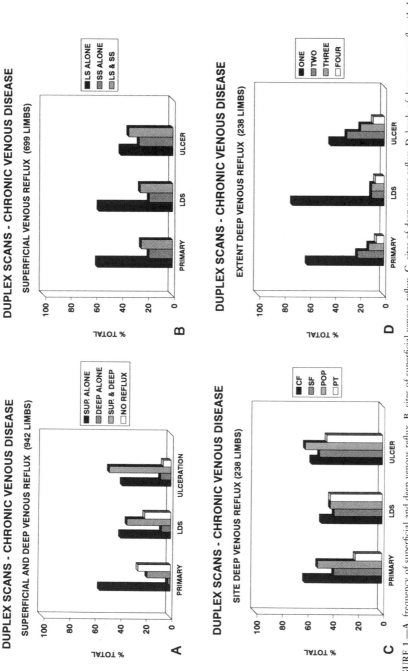

FIGURE 1.—A, frequency of superficial and deep venous reflux. B, sites of superficial venous reflux. C, sites of deep venous reflux. D, levels of deep venous reflux (1–4 contiguous levels) according to clinical manifestation. *Abbreviations: sup.,* superficial; *LS,* long saphenous; *SS,* short saphenous; *CF,* common femoral; *SF,* superficial femoral; *POP,* popliteal; *PT,* posterior tibial. (Courtesy of Myers KA, Ziegenbein RW, Zeng GH, et al: Duplex ultrasonography scanning for chronic venous disease: Patterns of venous reflux. *J Vasc Surg* 21:605–612, 1995.)

short saphenous reflux. Short saphenous reflux was seen more frequently in limbs with complicated than in limbs with uncomplicated varicose veins (Fig 1). There was outward flow in the medial calf perforators in 57% of the uncomplicated limbs, 67% of the limbs with lipodermatosclerosis, and 66% of the limbs with past ulceration, usually with deep or superficial reflux. Isolated outward flow in medial calf perforators was seen in only 10% of the uncomplicated limbs, 10% of the limbs with lipodermatosclerosis, and 2% of the limbs with past ulceration.

Conclusion.—Deep venous reflux in the lower limb and incompetent deep vein valves were rare in patients with and without complications of varicose veins. Outward flow in medial calf perforators was seen frequently in limbs without complications. These findings contradict the common belief that deep and perforator venous disease typically cause complications and indicate the greater significance of superficial reflux. The relative efficacy of treating the superficial veins alone should be investigated prospectively.

▶ Most patients with symptomatic lower extremity venous valvular insufficiency have saphenous reflux, either alone or combined with deep reflux. After mulling over considerable information, these authors conclude that treatment directed to the superficial veins alone may be sufficient for most patients with symptomatic valvular reflux. This seems to be the same opinion put forward by St. Mary's group. I suspect that they are correct. In the majority of cases, the application of gradient compressive elastic stockings seems sufficient for the task. Even in patients with the advanced symptoms of venous ulceration, we have never yet identified a patient in whom we believed deep vein valvular repair was warranted.

## Venous Valvular Reflux in Veins Not Involved at the Time of Acute Deep Vein Thrombosis

Caps MT, Manzo RA, Bergelin RO, et al (Univ of Washington, Seattle)
J Vasc Surg 22:524–531, 1995                                      16–7

Introduction.—What happens at the histologic level after deep vein thrombosis (DVT) has not been well documented. Patients with a history of acute DVT episodes were evaluated to determine if incompetence develops in veins that were not the site of thrombosis.

Methods.—After detection of DVT, patients were monitored at 1 day, 1 week, and 1, 3, 6, 9, and 12 months with serial duplex ultrasonography at the common femoral, greater saphenous, proximal superficial femoral, deep femoral, popliteal, and posterior tibial venous segments. The incidence of reflux development in thrombosed and uninvolved venous segments was observed. Venous segments which developed reflux were classified as transient or permanent (Table 1).

Results.—Serial duplex ultrasonography was used to evaluate 227 limbs in 188 patients. Of 1,423 segments, 403 developed reflux, 118 of which

TABLE 1.—Classification of the Venous Segments That Developed Reflux Into "Transient," "Permanent," and "Unknown" Categories

| Segment | No. | No. reflux | History of thrombosis | | | No history of thrombosis | | |
|---|---|---|---|---|---|---|---|---|
| | | | Transient | Permanent | Unknown | Transient | Permanent | Unknown |
| CFV | 221 | 80 | 7 | 35 | 6 | 13 | 17 | 2 |
| GSV | 197 | 49 | 6 | 12 | 5 | 9 | 12 | 5 |
| DFV | 190 | 34 | 4 | 19 | 4 | 2 | 4 | 1 |
| SFP | 201 | 67 | 6 | 36 | 9 | 6 | 8 | 2 |
| PV | 208 | 79 | 13 | 46 | 13 | 2 | 5 | 0 |
| PTV | 406 | 94 | 17 | 33 | 14 | 9 | 15 | 6 |
| Pooled | 1423 | 403 | 53 | 181 | 51 | 41 | 61 | 16 |

*The segments are further stratified according to prior or concurrent history of involvement with thrombosis.
*Abbreviations: CFV,* common femoral vein; *GSV,* greater saphenous vein; *DFV,* deep femoral vein; *SFP,* superficial femoral vein; *PV,* popliteal vein; *PTV,* posterior tibial vein.
(Courtesy of Caps MT, Manzo RA, Bergelin RO, et al: Venous valvular reflux in veins not involved at the time of acute deep vein thrombosis. *J Vasc Surg* 22:524–531, 1995.)

had no prior or concurrent history of thrombosis. In the segments that developed incompetence, the percent at each level with no prior or concurrent history of thrombosis was 40.0% common femoral vein, 53.1% greater saphenous vein, 20.6% deep femoral vein, 23.9% proximal superficial femoral vein, 8.9% popliteal vein, and 31.9% posterior tibial vein. The incidence of transient incompetence was significantly higher for uninvolved segments (40.2%) compared with segments with prior or concurrent thrombosis (22.6%).

*Conclusion.*—It is possible for permanent venous valvular damage to occur in the absence of thrombosis after DVT. In uninvolved segments, reflux has a different anatomical distribution and is more likely to be transient compared with the incompetence associated with thrombosis.

▶ This study reminds us that venous segments uninvolved in deep vein thrombosis may develop venous reflux and that reflux after thrombosis may be transient. The frequency of reflux increases with time, also in nonthrombosed legs. The information in this article is important when studies on pathology of postthrombotic syndrome and deep vein insufficiency are designed. See also Abstract 16–4.

**D. Bergqvist, M.D., Ph.D.**

## Treatment

### Surgical Technique and Preliminary Results of Endoscopic Subfascial Division of Perforating Veins

Gloviczki P, Cambria RA, Rhee RY, et al (Mayo Clinic and Found, Rochester, Minn)
*J Vasc Surg* 23:517–523, 1996                                                    16–8

*Background.*—Although direct surgical ligation of incompetent perforating veins is effective in the treatment of severe chronic venous insuffi-

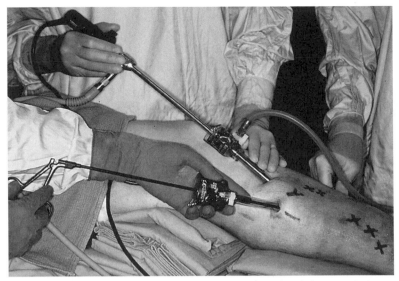

FIGURE 3.—Clipping and division of perforators are performed with laparoscopic instruments through second port; first port is used for video control. (Courtesy of Gloviczki P, Cambria RA, Rhee RY, et al: Surgical technique and preliminary results of endoscopic subfascial division of perforating veins. *J Vasc Surg* 23:517–523, 1996.)

ciency, significant wound complications can occur. One experience with endoscopic subfascial division of the perforating veins was reported.

*Methods.*—Nine patients underwent endoscopic subfascial division of perforating veins in 11 legs between August 1993 and December 1994. Venous ulcers were active or recently healed in 9 legs. Ulcers had been present for a mean 5.6 years. Using laparoscopic equipment with 2 10-mm ports, surgeons clipped and divided medial perforating veins through 2 small incisions just below the knee. The area of ulcer and lipodermatosclerosis was avoided. Dissection was facilitated by insufflating carbon dioxide into the subfascial space at a pressure of 30 mm Hg. A bloodless operating field was obtained with a pneumatic thigh tourniquet. In 8 limbs, superficial veins were removed concomitantly. Patients were followed for 2 to 13 months.

*Outcomes.*—Overall, the mean number of perforating veins divided was 4.4. The mean tourniquet time was 58 minutes. Early complications included wound infection of a groin incision and superficial thrombophlebitis, occurring in 1 patient each. Ulceration healed or did not recur in 7 legs, was improved in 3, and was unchanged in 1 (Fig 3).

*Conclusion.*—These preliminary findings suggest that endoscopic subfascial division of perforating veins is safe and beneficial in the short term. Further studies of this technique are warranted.

▶ There seems little doubt that if you are willing to accept a certain surgical complication rate, you can put a modified laparoscope under the fascia of the lower leg and divide incompetent perforating veins. An expanded version of this same paper was presented at the Vascular Society Meetings in June 1996. The question remains, however, that although one obviously can do an endoscopic subfascial division of perforating veins, why would one want to? It is my emotionally maintained position that there is not 1 substantial piece of evidence that interruption of perforating veins accomplishes anything. Dr. Browse[1] and his associates at St. Thomas randomized patients with venous ulcers to maximum conservative therapy alone or maximum conservative therapy plus ligation of perforating veins. Guess what? Both groups behaved exactly the same.

*Reference*

1. Browse N: Personal communication, 1996.

---

**Subcutaneous Jugulofemoral Bypass: A Simple Surgical Option for Palliation of Superior Vena Cava Obstruction**
Graham A, Anikin V, Curry R, et al (Royal Victoria Hosp, Belfast, Northern Ireland; Belfast City Hosp, Northern Ireland)
*J Cardiovasc Surg* 36:615–617, 1995                                    16–9

---

*Background.*—Surgical bypass is usually not possible in patients with superior vena cava (SVC) obstruction, because it typically involves a median sternotomy, and most patients have incurable malignant disease. Subcutaneous jugulofemoral bypass does not necessitate thoracotomy. The results of this procedure in 3 patients with SVC obstruction were described.

*Methods.*—The patients were 2 men (aged 83 and 55) and 1 woman (aged 34). In 2 patients, SVC obstruction resulted from lung cancer. The third patient underwent surgery after radiochemotherapy for malignant mediastinal teratoma. Intraluminal stenting had been considered but proved unfeasible in all patients. Instead, a jugulofemoral bypass was done. The long saphenous vein, tunneled subcutaneously from the femoral to the jugular vein, was used (Fig 1). Wound exploration for bleeding was necessary in 1 patient.

*Findings.*—In all patients, the operation resulted in good palliation. One patient died of lung cancer 3 months after surgery. The other 2 patients were alive without symptoms 6 weeks and 13 months after the operation.

*Conclusion.*—When nonoperative methods for SVC obstruction are not feasible in patients with SVC obstruction, subcutaneous jugulofemoral bypass offers good palliation. This procedure is simple and allows surgeons to avoid thoracotomy.

▶ What a straightforward proposition! In patients with severely symptomatic SVC obstruction in whom intraluminal stenting appeared impossible, these authors passed a saphenous vein from the jugular to the femoral vein. They have only 3 patients, but all enjoyed excellent palliation. I shall keep this technique in mind.

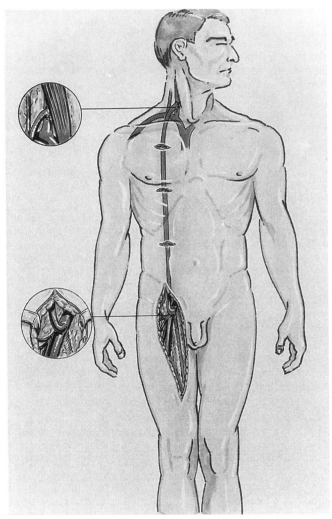

FIGURE 1.—The long saphenous vein is mobilized, swung around without being disconnected from the femoral vein, and fed through a subcutaneous tunnel to be anastomosed to the external or internal jugular vein. (By permission of Graham A, Anikin V, Curry R, et al: Subcutaneous jugulofemoral bypass: A simple surgical option for palliation of superior vena cava obstruction. *J Cardiovasc Surg* 36:615–617, 1995.)

## Healing of Venous Ulcers in an Ambulatory Care Program: The Roles of Chronic Venous Insufficiency and Patient Compliance

Erickson CA, Lanza DJ, Karp DL, et al (Med College of Wisconsin, Milwaukee)

*J Vasc Surg* 22:629–636, 1995                                        16–10

*Introduction.*—The development of venous ulceration is clearly associated with venous insufficiency, but the role of hemodynamic parameters and postthrombotic changes are not clear. Compliance with treatment has been shown to hasten venous ulcer healing and to delay recurrence. A nurse-managed/physician-supervised ambulatory ulcer clinic was set up, with a specialized protocol for management, education, and follow-up. The efficacy of the protocol was evaluated, and the influence of patient compliance and the degree of venous insufficiency on healing and recurrence were analyzed.

*Methods.*—A total of 71 patients with 99 venous ulcers were studied. All patients were evaluated initially by a surgeon, with clinical evaluation performed by a vascular nurse clinician. The evaluations included ankle-brachial indices, photoplethysmography, and venous duplex ultrasonography. Treatment was prescribed according to 1 of 2 protocols: a zinc oxide paste–impregnated bandage covered with a self-adhesive elastic wrap or an adhesive hydrocolloid patch covered with a graded elastic stocking. Patients were given comprehensive education regarding the pathophysiology and the importance of compression therapy and leg elevation. Initially follow-up was performed twice weekly, then less frequently during healing. After the ulcer was completely healed, patients were given graduated compression stockings with 30 to 40 mm Hg of compression and instructions for stocking replacement every 3 to 6 months.

*Results.*—The degree of venous insufficiency, based on venous refill times, was severe in 8%, moderate in 75%, and mild in 10% of the extremities, with 6 extremities having normal refill times. There was superficial-only venous insufficiency in 17% of the ulcerated extremities and deep or combined superficial and deep venous insufficiency in 83%. Healing occurred significantly more quickly in extremities with a median refill time of less than 10 sec, although the degree of venous insufficiency did not influence the time to first recurrence. Strict compliance was maintained for 32 of 99 extremities. At 5 months, complete healing had occurred in 73% of the compliant group and 59% in the noncompliant group. The median time of complete healing was 2.4 months in 97% of the compliant group and 4.3 months in 89.6% of the noncompliant group. At 2 years, recurrence occurred in 41% in the compliant group and 71% in the noncompliant group.

*Conclusion.*—Conservative treatment of venous ulcers is effective with extensive nurse/patient interaction that can increase treatment compliance, an essential element in speeding healing and delaying recurrence. Patients at risk for delayed healing can be identified by the presence of a venous refill time of more than 10 sec with photoplethysmography.

▶ Here is another study showing that venous ulcers healed when treated adequately by a dedicated team and that recurrence rate is much lower if the patients are compliant with the treatment. It was also interesting to note that between 20% and 25% of patients with venous ulcers had a history of deep vein thrombosis. We have found similar frequency in several studies, so it seems reasonable to conclude that around one fifth to one fourth of venous ulcer patients have a postthrombotic syndrome.

**D. Bergqvist, M.D., Ph.D.**

## Miscellaneous Topics

### Limited Range of Motion Is a Significant Factor in Venous Ulceration

Back TL, Padberg FT Jr, Araki CT, et al (Univ of Medicine and Dentistry of New Jersey, Newark)

*J Vasc Surg* 22:519–523, 1995                                    16–11

*Introduction.*—Calf muscle pump dysfunction is a known factor in chronic venous insufficiency (CVI). It is possible that reduced range of motion (ROM) of the ankle may contribute to the poor calf pump function associated with venous ulceration. Thirty-two limbs of 26 men were evaluated to determine if reduced ankle ROM in limbs of patients with CVI is a significant factor in venous ulceration.

*Methods.*—The 32 limbs were selected on the basis of clinical manifestation. Limbs were assigned CVI classifications: 6 normal, 9 class 1 or 2 CVI with no history of ulceration, 9 class 3 CVI with healed ulceration, and 8 class 3 CVI with active ulceration. A goniometer was used during maximal plantar flexion and dorsiflexion to determine ankle ROM. Air plethysmographic measurement of ejection fraction (EF) and residual volume fraction (RVF) were used to evaluate calf pump function.

*Results.*—Compared with age-matched controls, ankle ROM was significantly reduced in all CVI classification groups. Calf pump function, as determined by decreased EF and increased RVF, was significantly impaired in ulcerated limbs. There was a significant correlation between reduced ROM and abnormal EF and RVF findings. There was an association between impaired ROM and calf pump function and deterioration in the clinical classification of venous disease.

*Conclusion.*—Findings indicate that limbs with CVI have a limited ankle ROM. This limited ROM increases with increasing severity of clinical symptoms. The decreased ROM is also associated with and may contribute to poor calf function in patients with CVI.

▶ Here we have a classic chicken-egg problem. Patients who have severe venous disease up to and including ankle ulcerations appear to have significantly restricted ROM at the ankle. The restricted ROM leads to significant abnormality of calf muscle pump function as assessed by air plethysmography. The question is, does the impaired ankle motion result in bad calf muscle pump, which results in ambulatory venous hypertension, which results in ulceration? Alternately, a patient develops ulceration, and over a period chronic pain and inflammation associated with the ulcer impairs ankle motion, leading to the famous vicious circle. The authors wisely observe that the data from this study do not permit a clear differentiation between cause and effect. On balance, I find their observations interesting but interpretation difficult.

## Persistent Sciatic Vein: Diagnosis and Treatment of a Rare Condition

Cherry KJ Jr, Gloviczki P, Stanson AW (Mayo Clinic and Found, Rochester, Minn)

*J Vasc Surg* 23:490–497, 1996

16–12

*Background.*—Persistent sciatic vein (PSV), a rare anomaly, is usually associated with Klippel-Trenaunay syndrome (KTS). This entity is being diagnosed more often now because of the availability of MRI and the extended use of phlebography. One experience with PSV was reviewed.

*Methods and Findings.*—The MR studies and phlebograms of all patients with KTS seen since 1985 were reviewed. Of 186 patients with KTS, 41 underwent MRI. Twenty (48.8%) were diagnosed as having PSV. Another patient without KTS but with PSV was also identified. Altogether, the patients with PSV ranged in age from 5 to 71. Sixty-two percent were female. Thirty-eight percent of the patients had PSVs in the entire thigh and buttock; 28.6% in the upper half of the thigh and the buttock, and 33.3% in the lower half of the thigh. Anorectal arteriovenous malformations with heavy bleeding were present in 28.6% of patients. Pulmonary embolization was documented in 23.8%. Mortality was 9.5%. One patient (4.8%) underwent amputation. No specific surgery for PSV was done in 90.5% of the patients. Successful excision of PSVs was performed in 9.5%.

*Conclusion.*—Excision of PSV may be indicated for localized symptoms in patients with acceptable conditions and anatomies. In general, PSV excision is rarely indicated. The presence of PSV may be a marker for more extensive arteriovenous malformations and for increased risk for rectal bleeding and pulmonary embolization. The vascular malformations associated with PSV affect prognosis.

▶ This paper contains a great deal of important information. Despite the prior publication from the Mayo Clinic, I personally had not focused on the PSV in KTS.[1] I have known that patients with KTS seem to have unpredictable segmental interruption of the deep venous system, and I now suspect that in many of these patients this was associated with a PSV. The authors' observation that patients with a PSV have an increased incidence of deep venous thrombosis and pulmonary embolism is interesting and does bring up the potential role of prophylactic vena caval filter placement. On balance, I do not believe that the information contained in this paper is going to lead to any different future treatment for patients with KTS, but I do believe it does help explain some of the pathophysiologic features.

*Reference*

1. Gloviczki P, Stanson A, Strickler G, et al: Klippel-Trenaunay syndrome: The risks and benefits of vascular interventions. *Surgery* 110:469–479, 1991.

## A Comparison of Conservative Therapy and Early Selective Ligation in the Treatment of Lymphatic Complications Following Vascular Procedures

Schwartz MA, Schanzer H, Skladany M, et al (Mount Sinai School of Medicine, New York)
*Am J Surg* 170:206–208, 1995                                                    16–13

*Introduction.*—Lymphatic leakage, particularly at the groin level, is a somewhat uncommon, yet serious complication of vascular procedures. Conservative treatment includes bed rest, bed elevation, prophylactic antibiotics, compressive dressings, and intermittent aspiration. This condition takes a long time to heal, and infection is an ongoing concern. A more aggressive approach of wound exploration and ligation of the leaking lymphatic has been proposed. The results of conservative and aggressive treatment approaches were reported.

*Methods.*—Ten of 17 patients (59%) with groin complications were treated by selective ligation assisted with isosulfan blue dye injection. The remaining patients (41%) received conservative treatment.

*Results.*—The mean hospital stay for patients in the surgical group was 2.4 days and was 19 days for patients in the conservative group. One patient (10%) in the surgical group had an immediate recurrence that was successfully treated with reoperation. Four (57%) patients in the conservative groups developed groin infections.

*Conclusion.*—The use of surgical ligation assisted by isosulfan blue for patients with lymphatic leakage in the groin resulted in decreased hospital stay, lower complication rate, and fewer recurrences. This more aggressive approach may be the best form of treatment for these patients.

▶ A persistent lymph leak from the groin or the occurrence of a lymphocele leads us to very early reoperation with tight closure, usually without drainage. We have never used the selective dye injection or made any attempt for selective ligation of the offending lymphatic. Rather, we close the entire cavity very tightly, hoping to encompass the offending lymphatic in our deep sutures. If not, we try to give the lymph nowhere to go by obliterating all the space. This approach has generally been quite successful. I agree totally with the thrust of the position taken by these authors, namely, that early and aggressive reoperation is indicated in patients with persistent lymphatic leak or seroma of the groin after vascular surgery. I am convinced our patients are doing much better than they did in the earlier days when we treated these nonoperatively. See also Abstract 13–11.

# 17 Portal Hypertension

**The Transjugular Intrahepatic Portosystemic Stent-Shunt Procedure for Refractory Ascites**
Ochs A, Rössle M, Haag K, et al (Albert Ludwig Univ, Freiburg, Germany)
*N Engl J Med* 332:1192–1197, 1995                                          17–1

*Objective.*—The transjugular intrahepatic portosystemic stent shunt, a nonoperative side-to-side shunt between a main portal vein branch and a hepatic vein, has been used effectively to treat uncomplicated ascites in patients with variceal bleeding. It is an expandable metallic mesh device. This type of shunt was used in 50 of 62 consecutive patients having hepatic cirrhosis and treatment-resistant ascites. All patients had, besides ascites, other liver-related complications such as recent variceal bleeding or severe comorbidity.

*Results.*—The average follow-up was 426 days. A shunt was successfully established in all 50 patients, and the portal venous pressure gradient

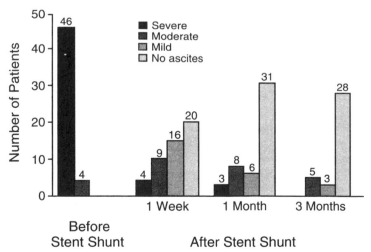

FIGURE 1.—Severity of ascites before and after the stent-shunt procedures. Ascites was graded by ultrasound as severe or tense ascites, moderate ascites with fluid in the flanks, or mild ascites with fluid around the liver and in Douglas's and Morison's pouches. (Reprinted by permission of *The New England Journal of Medicine.* Ochs A, Rössle M, Haag K, et al: The transjugular intrahepatic portosystemic stent-shunt procedure for refractory ascites. *N Engl J Med* 332:1192–1197, Copyright 1995, Massachusetts Medical Society.)

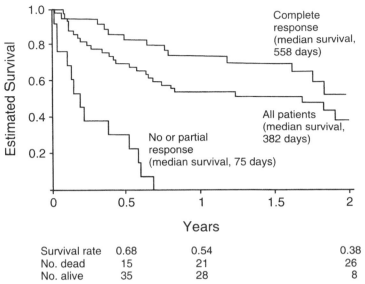

FIGURE 2.—Kaplan-Meier survival analysis of all patients and of patients according to their responses to treatment. (Reprinted by permission of *The New England Journal of Medicine*. Ochs A, Rössle M, Haag K, et al: The transjugular intrahepatic portosystemic stent-shunt procedure for refractory ascites. *N Engl J Med* 332:1192–1197, Copyright 1995; Massachusetts Medical Society.)

declined by 63% on average. Sixteen patients had 20 complications. Ascites lessened in 92% of patients and disappeared in 74%. Significant improvement took place within 1 week of stent placement (Fig 1). The serum creatinine level and creatinine clearance both improved significantly at 6 months. Serum bilirubin levels increased initially but subsequently improved. Hepatic encephalopathy improved in 3 patients after stent placement but developed for the first time in 8 patients. Median survival was enhanced for patients whose ascites resolved (Fig 2).

*Conclusion.*—The transjugular intrahepatic portosystemic stent-shunt procedure is an effective treatment of refractory ascites in many patients with cirrhosis.

▶ Although the transjugular intrahepatic portosystemic TIPS stent-shunt procedure has been shown to be effective in the treatment of ascites in patients with variceal bleeding, no prior study directed toward refractory ascites has been reported. This study indicates that the transjugular intraheptic portosystemic stent shunt overall was quite effective in controlling refractory ascites in cirrhotics. As the authors note, mortality in these patients was quite substantial from underlying disease, but the refractory ascites was markedly improved in most. This is a valuable treatment modality in selected patients.

### Splenic Venous Hypertension Presenting as Variceal Hemorrhage Caused by Portal Hypertension

Rozenblit G, Del Guercio LRM, Savino J, et al (New York Med College, Valhalla)

*J Am Coll Surg* 182:63–68, 1996

17–2

*Introduction.*—Bleeding caused by portal hypertension (PH) may be clinically indistinguishable from variceal hemorrhage resulting from splenic venous hypertension (SVH). Identification of the cause of bleeding is more difficult when SVH and PH coexist, and the potential for incorrect treatment is considerable. Patients with variceal hemorrhage referred for transvenous intrahepatic portosystemic shunt (TIPS) placement for PH were reviewed retrospectively to examine the diagnostic role of CT and angiography in this setting.

*Methods.*—Over an 18-month period, 7 of 58 consecutive cases of gastroesophageal variceal bleeding referred for interventional treatment were attributed to SVH. Diagnosis of SVH as the cause of bleeding was obtained by the use of contrast-enhanced nonhelical CT, duplex ultrasound (US), and angiography. Demonstration of an absent or disproportionally narrowed splenic vein at CT was considered diagnostic of SVH. Obstruction of the splenic vein was the basis for duplex US diagnosis of SVH. Findings of splenoportography and arterial portography were considered diagnostic when these methods failed to visualize a normal splenic vein showing splenic venous drainage through gastric or gastroesophageal varices.

*Results.*—The 7 patients with SVH required blood transfusion before admission and during the first 24 hours of hospitalization. All were known to have chronic alcoholic liver disease. Although endoscopy confirmed the presence of gastric and esophageal varices and blood in the stomach, the precise source of bleeding could not be determined. Because all patients had alcoholic liver disease, the source of variceal bleeding was assumed to be PH. Imaging studies performed when the patients were referred for TIPS placement or transmesenteric variceal sclerotherapy (or both) for control of hemorrhage yielded the correct diagnosis. Contrast-enhanced CT was diagnostic in 3 patients, duplex CT in 1, and arterial portography in 5; splenoportography unequivocally demonstrated SVH in the 2 patients unable to be diagnosed with certainty by arterial portography.

*Conclusion.*—Varices in SVH cause hemorrhage that is similar to that resulting from PH. The 2 conditions require completely different treatment approaches, but clinical data may not permit a differential diagnosis. Patients scheduled for TIPS placement for PH should undergo CT and angiography, if necessary, to exclude SVH.

▶ Our old friend SVH rears its head anew. These authors point out quite correctly that in these days of TIPS therapy for presumed portal hypertension, it is important to prevent inappropriate placement of a shunt in patients who have SVH due to splenic vein occlusion (frequently from pancreatic disease). These authors suggest that an imaging modality, preferably contrast-enhanced CT, be performed in every patient before placement of a TIPS. Their experience with this problem is emphasized by a recent experience with 58 patients with gastroesophageal variceal bleeding at their institution. Seven of the 58 had this condition as a result of SVH.

## Selective Distal Splenorenal Shunts for Intractable Variceal Bleeding in Pediatric Portal Hypertension

Evans S, Stovroff M, Heiss K, et al (Emory Univ, Atlanta, Ga)

*J Pediatr Surg* 30:1115–1118, 1995                                                                17–3

*Introduction.*—During the past decade, endoscopic sclerotherapy has emerged as the treatment of choice for children with hemorrhagic portal hypertension. Because of the efficacy of sclerotherapy, only children with refractory hemorrhage are managed with surgical shunting. A 10-year experience with surgical shunting used for the emergent care of such children was reported.

*Methods.*—The medical records of all children who underwent portosystemic shunting for intractable hemorrhagic portal hypertension despite extensive medical treatment between 1983 and 1994 were reviewed. Medical therapy had included restoration of blood volume, correction of the coagulopathy, use of splanchnic vasoconstrictors, and sclerotherapy. Either the distal splenorenal shunt (DSRS) or the mesocaval shunt was used.

*Results.*—Ten shunts were placed in 9 patients, including 8 selective DSRSs and 2 nonselective mesocaval shunts, which successfully relieved the acute hemorrhage. Six of the patients had intrahepatic disease, 2 had portal vein thrombosis, and 1 had splenic vein thrombosis. No intraoperative deaths occurred, but 2 patients with advanced disease died subsequently. Of the 9 patients, 3 underwent subsequent orthotopic liver transplantation, after which 1 died. One child with a mesocaval shunt developed fulminant hepatic failure and profound encephalopathy several weeks after the procedure. No patients with selective shunting developed encephalopathy.

*Discussion.*—The DSRS has a role in the management of children with emergent hemorrhagic portal hypertension. Its benefits include a low rate of hepatic encephalopathy and rebleeding and preservation of liver function. It can often be life sustaining in patients awaiting orthotopic liver transplantation, because it avoids the porta hepatitis, unlike the nonselective shunts.

▶ Portal hypertension in the pediatric population rarely requires shunting. Most of these are treated by endoscopic sclerotherapy. However, a few patients have such severe symptomatic portal hypertension that shunting is required. Over a 10-year period, 9 patients at the authors' institution underwent portosystemic shunting. This paper presents a general overview of the indications and outcome of shunting in these patients. Predictably, pediatric patients with sufficiently severe portal hypertension as to require shunting have a far more dismal outlook than those less severely afflicted.

**Mesocaval Shunt or Repeated Sclerotherapy: Effects on Rebleeding and Encephalopathy-Randomized Trial**
Isaksson B, Jeppsson B, Bengtsson F, et al (Lund Univ Hosp, Sweden)
*Surgery* 117:498–504, 1995                                          17–4

*Background.*—Sclerotherapy is most frequently used to treat acute esophageal variceal bleeding, but it has been associated with relatively high rebleeding rates. Surgical treatment with portal decompression has been effective in preventing rebleeding but has been associated with altered liver perfusion and encephalopathy. The relative effectiveness of interposition mesocaval shunt and sclerotherapy was evaluated in a prospective randomized study.

*Methods.*—Forty-five adult patients with endoscopically verified esophageal varices, portal hypertension, and histologically proven liver cirrhosis were stratified by Child's classification and randomly assigned to treatment with either mesocaval shunt surgery or transesophageal sclerotherapy. The patients were followed 4 months after surgery or sclerotherapeutic eradication of the varices with endoscopy, biochemical, and hematologic evaluation and clinical assessment of their mental status. Episodes of rebleeding and the need for additional sclerotherapies were recorded.

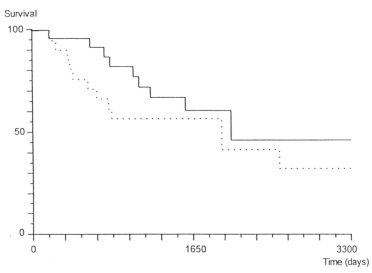

FIGURE 1.—Actuarial survival curves for mesocaval shunt and endoscopic sclerotherapy (all Child's groups). *Vertical axis* indicates survival time. No significant difference is noted. *Solid line*, shunt; *dotted line*, sclerotherapy. (Courtesy of Isaksson B, Jeppsson B, Bengtsson F, et al: Mesocaval shunt or repeated sclerotherapy: Effects on rebleeding and encephalopathy-randomized trial. *Surgery* 117:498–504, 1995.)

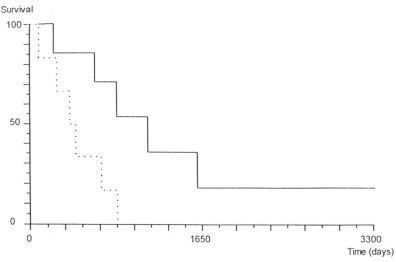

FIGURE 2.—Actuarial survival curves for mesocaval shunt and endoscopic sclerotherapy (patients in Child's class C). *Vertical axis* indicates survival time. Mesocaval shunt group has significantly longer survival compared with sclerotherapy group ($P < 0.05$). *Solid line*, shunt; *dotted line*, sclerotherapy. (Courtesy of Isaksson B, Jeppsson B, Bengtsson F, et al: Mesocaval shunt or repeated sclerotherapy: Effects on rebleeding and encephalopathy-randomized trial. *Surgery* 117:498–504, 1995.)

*Results.*—Of the 45 patients, 24 were treated with mesocaval shunt surgery and 21 with sclerotherapy. There were no differences between the stratified groups in baseline laboratory findings. The sclerotherapy group had significantly more rebleeding episodes after eradication of varices and required more additional sclerotherapies compared with the shunt group after surgery. There were no significant differences between the treatment groups in esophagitis. In the shunt group, there were no postoperative deaths and only 1 occluded shunt. No patients in this group still had a hepatopetal flow 1 year after surgery. Mental status deteriorated in 3 of 8 patients with baseline signs of encephalopathy and in 2 of 8 patients without such baseline signs in the shunt group and in just 1 patient in the sclerotherapy group. There were no statistically significant differences in the length of hospital stay or in the length of ICU stay. There was no difference in survival overall between the treatment groups (Fig 1). However, among patients with Child's class C disease, survival was significantly improved in the shunt group compared with the sclerotherapy group (Fig 2).

*Conclusion.*—Mesocaval shunting is significantly more effective in preventing rebleeding of esophageal varices than repeated sclerotherapy. In addition, mesocaval shunting prolongs the survival of patients with Child's 3 cirrhosis, suggesting that it may be the preferred treatment in these patients who have contraindications for transplantation.

▶ This curious study reports a prospective randomized assignment of variceal bleeding patients to repeat sclerotherapy or mesocaval shunt. The results appear to generally favor mesocaval shunting, especially in patients with Child's class C cirrhosis. We have little personal experience with this area, because vascular surgery seems to be less involved all the time with portal hypertension, a trend I incidentally heartily endorse and encourage.

**Prospective Randomised Study of Effect of Octreotide on Rebleeding From Oesophageal Varices After Endoscopic Ligation**
Sung JJY, Chung SCS, Yung MY, et al (Chinese Univ of Hong Kong, Shatin)
*Lancet* 346:1666–1669, 1995                                                    17–5

*Purpose.*—Endoscopic variceal ligation is safer than injection sclerotherapy for treating esophageal varices, but it is associated with early rebleeding rates of 20% to 40%. Octreotide, a synthetic analogue of somatostatin, has been used to treat variceal hemorrhage when endoscopic expertise is not available. The use of octreotide infusion as an adjunct to endoscopic variceal ligation was examined to determine whether it would lower the risk of early rebleeding.

*Patients.*—The study population consisted of 94 patients with endoscopically confirmed esophageal variceal bleeding, of whom 47 (mean age 56) were randomly allocated to endoscopic variceal ligation alone and 47 (mean age 58) were randomly allocated to octreotide infusion plus endoscopic variceal ligation. All patients underwent a second variceal ligation 5 days after the first treatment.

*Results.*—Bleeding was controlled in 44 patients treated with variceal ligation alone and in 45 patients who received the combination treatment. None of the patients treated with octreotide experienced drug-related side effects requiring discontinuation of the infusion. Early rebleeding occurred in 18 patients (38%) treated with ligation alone and in 4 patients (9%) who had the combination treatment. The difference was statistically significant. Ten patients in the ligation-alone group and 1 patient in the combination treatment group required balloon tamponade for massive hematemesis and hemodynamic instability. Nine patients (19%) in the ligation-alone group and 4 (9%) in the combination treatment died in the hospital, but this difference did not reach statistical significance. The 30-day mortality rates were 23% in the ligation-alone group and 11% in the combination treatment group.

*Conclusion.*—Octreotide infusion, when used as an adjunct to endoscopic variceal ligation in the management of variceal hemorrhage, significantly lowers early rebleeding rates and reduces the need for balloon tamponade.

▶ The ubiquitous octreotide again rears its readily recognized head. In a prospective randomized study, these investigators found that patients undergoing esophageal endoscopic variceal ligation who also received octreotide did better than those undergoing ligation alone. Octreotide indeed appears to be a magic bullet, but it frequently fails to reach statistical significance. See also Abstract 17–6.

---

**Sclerotherapy With or Without Octreotide for Acute Variceal Bleeding**
Besson I, Ingrand P, Person B, et al (Ctr Hosp Univ de Poitiers, France)
*N Engl J Med* 333:555–560, 1995                                                  17–6

---

*Introduction.*—Acute variceal bleeding is a major concern for patients with cirrhosis. Sclerotherapy is usually employed to stop this bleeding, but rebleeds are common. Octreotide, a synthetic somatostatin analogue, is also effective in controlling this type of bleeding. The effectiveness of sclerotherapy alone and in combination with octreotide therapy in controlling bleeding in patients with acute variceal bleeding was studied.

*Methods.*—One-hundred and ninety-nine patients with cirrhosis and either acute active bleeding or evidence of recent bleeding were enrolled in

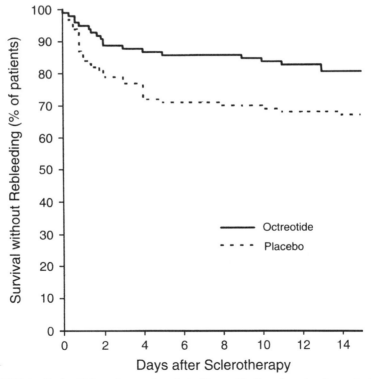

FIGURE 1.—Kaplan-Meier estimates of survival without rebleeding after sclerotherapy in the octreotide and placebo groups. The analysis was done on an intention-to-treat basis, and death was considered to be related to variceal bleeding regardless of the precise cause (*P* = 0.02 by the adjusted Mantel-Haenszel test). (Reprinted by permission of *The New England Journal of Medicine.* Besson I, Ingrand P, Person B, et al: Sclerotherapy with or without octreotide for acute variceal bleeding. *N Engl J Med* 333:555–560, Copyright 1995, Massachusetts Medical Society.)

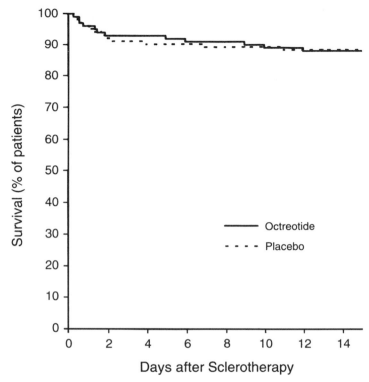

**FIGURE 2.**—Kaplan-Meier estimates of survival after sclerotherapy in the octreotide and placebo groups ($P = 0.95$ by the log-rank test). (Reprinted by permission of *The New England Journal of Medicine*. Besson I, Ingrand P, Person B, et al: Sclerotherapy with or without octreotide for acute variceal bleeding. *N Engl J Med* 333:555–560, Copyright 1995, Massachusetts Medical Society.)

this study. After emergency sclerotherapy, the patients were randomly assigned to receive by infusion either 500 µg of octreotide or a placebo. The principal measure was survival for 5 days after sclerotherapy without rebleeding, and a second measure was the amount of transfused blood required for these patients.

*Results.*—At 5 days a significantly higher percentage of patients who received octreotide survived without rebleeding (87% vs. 71%). The number of units of blood transfused during the first 24 hours was also less in the octreotide group (1.2 units vs. 2.0 units). Also, among those who were survivors at 5 days, less required blood transfusions after octreotide treatment. However, the mean overall survival between the 2 groups over a 15-day period was 88% in both groups (Fig 1). Side effects were minimal.

*Discussion.*—A higher survival at 5 days was found for patients who received octreotide in addition to sclerotherapy for bleeding, but the 15-day cumulative survival time was unaffected by mode of therapy (Fig 2). The rate of rebleeding documented in the placebo group was similar to the rate established in previous studies. Finally, 2 side effects (a decrease in glomerular filtration and encephalopathy) that may occur were not increased in those patients receiving octreotide.

▶ In a study similar to that of Abstract 17–5, a number of bleeding variceal patients were randomized to emergency sclerotherapy alone or sclerotherapy and octreotide. The proportion of patients surviving without rebleeding was statistically significantly higher in the octreotide group. This information, together with that in the preceding article, does suggest that octreotide has a role in the treatment of patients with acute variceal bleeding.

---

**Budd-Chiari Syndrome: Technical, Hemodynamic, and Clinical Results of Treatment With Transjugular Intrahepatic Portosytemic Shunt**
Blum U, Rössle M, Haag K, et al (Univ Hosp Freiburg, Germany)
*Radiology* 197:805–811, 1995                                            17–7

---

*Introduction.*—Patients with the Budd-Chiari syndrome (BCS) have been treated surgically by portosystemic shunt placement and liver transplantation. A recently reported nonsurgical strategy, use of a transjugular intrahepatic portosystemic shunt (TIPS), was evaluated in 12 patients with BCS.

*Patients and Methods.*—The patients, 6 men and 6 women aged 31 to 71, represented 2% of the 542 patients with portal hypertension referred to the study institution between December 1991 and January 1995 for TIPS placement. Duration of symptoms at the time of referral ranged from 2 days to 70 months. Budd-Chiari syndrome was subacute in 5 patients, chronic in 5, and fulminant in 2. Diagnosis was determined by demonstration of hepatic venous obstruction at CT and color duplex sonography and confirmed histologically in all cases. Patients were followed after TIPS placement for liver function, shunt function, ascites, and mortality.

*Results.*—Placement of a TIPS, with rapid inflow into the shunt tract, was successful in all patients. The 2 patients with fulminant BCS died 3 and 7 days after the procedure, 1 of septicemia and the other of progressive liver failure. Cancer was the underlying disease in both cases. Mean follow-up for the remaining 10 patients was 13 months. Treatment with a TIPS reduced the portal venous pressure gradient by 75% and brought about a mean shunt flow of 2,300 mL/min. Within 1 week these patients experienced clinical improvement and reduction of ascites. Four of 5 patients who had recurrent ascites required repeat intervention because of stenosis. One patient underwent successful liver transplantation 1 month after TIPS placement and was doing well; another died 11 months after the procedure of cardiac failure. The remaining 8 patients remained asymptomatic.

*Conclusion.*—Development of BCS is associated with a wide spectrum of disorders. The Western type of BCS is often caused by thrombosis within the small or large hepatic veins. Medical therapies have been ineffective, and most patients die of portal hypertension or cirrhosis.

Although liver function did not substantially improve in these patients, creation of a shunt led to clinical improvement and a favorable change in hemodynamics.

▶ I have always found BCS a mystical disease. It appears to be caused by portal hypertension resulting from occlusion of small or large hepatic veins, possibly by a prior thrombotic episode with subsequent fibrosis. If one can establish a TIPS into a nonaffected hepatic vein, the procedure has an excellent chance of being of significant benefit, as shown in this study. One must obviously be careful that the recipient vein is unobstructed in performance of this shunt.

# Subject Index*

## A

Abdomen
aortography, with digital subtraction
carotid and cerebral angiography,
97: 168
injury, exsanguinating penetrating,
damage control for improved
survival, 95: 377
insufflation for laparoscopic
cholecystectomy, venous stasis after,
95: 403
Acetazolamide
test, for risk identification of
post-carotid endarterectomy
hyperperfusion syndrome, 95: 323
Acetylcholine
sweat test, for lumbar sympathectomy
patient selection, 96: 294
Adenoma
aspirin use and risk for, in male health
professionals, 96: 177
Adenosine
in postischemic spinal cord injury
complete prevention, 95: 159
vasodilator effect of, endothelial release
of nitric oxide contributing to,
97: 39
Adhesion molecule
1, intercellular, shear stress upregulating
expression of in vascular
endothelial cells, 96: 62
ICAM-1, VCAM-1 and E-selectin, in leg
ulcer, chronic venous, 97: 430
Adrenal
hemorrhagic necrosis after aortic
surgery, 96: 251
Age
aortic diameter as function of, 95: 172
related differences in peripheral
atherosclerosis distribution,
97: 222
in venous physiologic parameters,
95: 408
Aged
80, survival after, 97: 64
aneurysm of, abdominal aortic, aortic
replacement for, 95: 188
healthy, low dose aspirin adverse effects
in, 95: 16
men, screening-detected abdominal
aortic aneurysm, prognosis,
97: 255

myocardial infarction, routine
non-invasive tests do not predict
outcome after, 95: 146
over 80, critical limb ischemia in, in
general hospital, 97: 301
women, ankle arm blood pressure index
decrease and mortality decrease in,
95: 1
AGM-1470
for murine hemangioendothelioma,
96: 60
Air
plethysmography, in chronic venous
insufficiency, 95: 419
Alcohol
consumption
and carotid atherosclerosis, Bruneck
Study results, 96: 1
and mortality of women, 97: 67
moderate intake, and myocardial
infarction risk decrease, 95: 8
Alcoholic
cirrhosis, portacaval shunt for, 95: 438
Allograft
saphenous vein
cryopreserved, as conduit for limb
salvage procedures, 95: 344
cryopreserved, for below-knee lower
extremity revascularization,
96: 360
vein, 95: 343
vein bypass, as alternative for
infrapopliteal revascularization,
95: 343
Alpha$_2$ adrenergic antagonists
blockade of vasospastic attacks by, in
idiopathic Raynaud's disease,
97: 176
Alpha-tocopherol
low level of, as risk factor in
myocardial infarction, 96: 3
Alteplase
for femoral artery thrombosis after
cardiac catheterization in children,
95: 83
Ambulatory
care program, venous ulcer healing in,
97: 440
Amputation, 95: 264, 96: 287
below-knee
for ischemia, and prostacyclin
analogue in healing of, 95: 264
medially based flap for, 96: 289

---

revascularization by, limb swelling
after, 97: 296
trends in vascular surgery since
introduction of, 96: 281
polytetrafluoroethylene patch, after
carotid endarterectomy, for
recurrent stenosis, 95: 307
renal artery, in ostial renal artery
atherosclerosis, 97: 113
results, dialysis access grafts, 97: 334
subintimal, of femoropopliteal artery
occlusion, 95: 63
Angioscopy
to assist saphenous vein graft, 96: 357
graft, 95: 357
intracoronary, in ischemia related lesion
in angina, 97: 164
saphenous vein, to detect unsuspected
venous disease, 95: 358
of thrombectomy, unilateral aortic graft
limb, 95: 359
of valvular disruption during in situ
saphenous vein bypass, 95: 357
Angiotensin
converting enzyme inhibition
with captopril, for Doppler
ultrasound of renal artery stenosis,
97: 167
stabilizing effect on creatinine and
proteinuria in type II diabetes,
95: 57
converting enzyme inhibitor,
trandolapril for left ventricular
dysfunction after myocardial
infarction, 97: 214
Ankle
arm blood pressure index decrease in
aged women, 95: 1
brachial index predicting survival in
peripheral vascular disease,
96: 198
pressure, falsely elevated, in leg
ischemia, pole test in, 96: 129
Annexin
V, in fibrin accretion after jugular vein
injury (in rabbit), 95: 29
Anomalies
renal artery, in horseshoe or ectopic
kidney, aortic reconstruction in,
97: 280
Antiaggregants
after carotid endarterectomy, 95: 338
Antibodies
anticardiolipin, myocardial infarction
risk and, in middle aged men,
96: 41
antiphospholipid (*see* Antiphospholipid
antibodies)

chimeric, to platelet glycoprotein IIb/IIIa
integrin in coronary intervention,
bleeding complications with,
97: 20
against endothelial cells and cardiolipin
in peripheral atherosclerotic
disease, 97: 11
against platelet IIb/IIIa integrin, for
coronary intervention for restenosis
reduction, 96: 26
Anticardiolipin antibody
myocardial infarction risk and, in
middle aged men, 96: 41
Anticoagulants
after carotid endarterectomy, 95: 338
oral
after chronic lower extremity
ischemia reconstruction, ischemic
and hemorrhagic stroke in, 95: 269
duration after proximal deep vein
thrombosis, 95: 390
Anticoagulation, 95: 20
effect of low dose of warfarin and
aspirin in stable coronary artery
disease, 96: 33
oral, six weeks vs. six months after first
episode of vein thromboembolism,
97: 416
in pseudoaneurysm, postcatheterization,
ultrasound guided compression
closure of, 97: 166
in pulmonary embolism, silent, with
deep vein thrombosis, 96: 408
in repetitive transient ischemic attacks
and high-grade carotid stenosis,
95: 337
vs. antiplatelet therapy, after coronary
artery stent placement, 97: 201
Antioxidants
consumption during exercise in
intermittent claudication, 97: 47
myocardial infarction and, 96: 3
Antiphospholipid antibodies
syndrome, thrombosis in, management,
97: 17
in vascular surgery, 96: 39
Antiplatelet, 95: 12
therapy
randomized trials, for vascular graft
and arterial patency maintenance,
95: 17
vs. anticoagulation after coronary
artery stent placement, 97: 201
Antisense
cdk 2 kinase oligonucleotides, inhibiting
intimal hyperplasia after vascular
injury, 96: 55

# B

Bacterial biofilm (*see* Biofilm, bacterial)

Balloon
coronary artery injury, endovascular
low dose radiation inhibiting
neointima formation after (in pig),
*96:* 57
dilatation, percutaneous, in central
venous obstruction, *95:* 412
expandable stent graft, for endoluminal
aortic aneurysm repair, *96:* 89
fenestration, for ischemic complications
of aortic dissection, *97:* 225
injured arteries, intimal hyperplasia
inhibition with photodynamic
therapy in, *97:* 52
occlusion, temporary, of carotid and
intracerebral arteries, brain blood
flow SPECT in, *95:* 320
pump, intraaortic, for repair of
cerebrovascular and coronary
artery disease, *95:* 295
test occlusion of internal carotid artery,
*95:* 318

Basilar
artery, effect of subclavian steal
syndrome on, *96:* 302

Basilic
cephalic upper arm loop for distal
bypass grafting, *97:* 386

Behcet's disease
arterial lesions in, *97:* 181
true and false aneurysms in,
ultrastructure, *95:* 137
vascular involvement in, *96:* 173

5,6-Benzo-[alpha]-pyrone
in lymphedema of arms and legs,
*95:* 430

Beta adrenergic blockade
in abdominal aortic aneurysm
expansion rate, *95:* 171
for aortic dilatation in Marfan
syndrome, *96:* 157
independent of altered lysyl oxidase
activity, in aortic aneurysm
development inhibition (in mice),
*97:* 77

Beta adrenoceptors
functional, on vascular sympathetic
nerve endings in forearm, *96:* 59

Beta carotene
long-term supplement, lack of effect on
cancer incidence, *97:* 221

Beta particle emitting stent
inhibiting neointima formation (in
rabbit), *97:* 98

Bifemoral
axillary bypass for blue toe syndrome,
*95:* 262

Biofilm, bacterial
arterial prosthesis infected by, in situ
replacement of, *95:* 346
infection in situ replacement in immune
deficient states, *95:* 345

Biology
molecular, *96:* 60
vessels, *97:* 68

Biomechanics
of vascular prosthesis, in myofibroblast
proliferation modulation, *95:* 37

Biotin, indium-111
with avidin
for scintigraphy for prosthetic
vascular graft infection detection,
*97:* 380
for vascular graft infection
localization, *97:* 379

Bleeding
aprotinin decreasing, in aspirin for heart
surgery, *96:* 38
complications
with chimeric antibody to platelet
glycoprotein IIb/IIIa integrin, for
coronary intervention, *97:* 20
late, in redo cardiac surgery, from
topical thrombin-induced factor V
deficiency, *95:* 33
suture line, during carotid
endarterectomy, fibrin sealant
reducing, *97:* 196
tendency, protein Z deficiency causing,
*97:* 26
(*See also* Hemmorhage)

Blockade
beta adrenergic (*see* Beta adrenergic
blockade)
ganglionic, vs. smooth muscle
relaxation in systemic hypertension
induced by aortic cross-clamping,
*96:* 199
thromboxane A$_2$, in outcome and
restenosis after successful coronary
angioplasty, *97:* 40
of vasospastic attacks by alpha$_2$
adrenergic antagonists, in
idiopathic Raynaud's disease,
*97:* 176

Blood
flow
augmentation in limbs with occlusive
arterial disease by intermittent calf
compression, *96:* 43

# Author Index

## A

Abebe W, 50
Abu-Own A, 328
AbuRahma AF, 413
Ackerstaff RGA, 146
Adams JG Jr, 45
Adelman MA, 347
Aguirre FV, 20
Ahlner J, 174
Ahmadi A, 102
Aisen AM, 125
Akkad A, 367
Akkersdijk WL, 162
Alexandrova NA, 341
Alfke H, 44
Allan PL, 432
Allen RC, 95
Allos SH, 271
Almgren B, 313
Amarenco P, 229
Anderson CA, 278
Andros G, 190
Anikin V, 439
Ankara, 243
Araki CT, 442
Arefi M, 258
Ascani A, 424
Ascer E, 414
Ascherio A, 41
Augustinsson L-E, 321
Ayanian JZ, 213

## B

Bacha EA, 226
Back TL, 442
Badimon JJ, 9
Baer RP, 176
Baert AL, 142
Bahra PS, 43
Baird RN, 161
Bandyk DF, 319
Banga JD, 405
Baptista J, 164
Barboriak DP, 395
Barlatier A, 61
Bastounis EA, 426
Battaloglu B, 243
Baum RA, 126
Baur WE, 86
Bayazit M, 243
Beard JD, 110
Beebe HG, 77
Belkin M, 273, 307, 308
Bell PRF, 367
Bendeck MP, 53

Bender MHM, 332
Bengtsson F, 449
Bengtsson H, 235, 255
Benjamin ME, 278
Berens ES, 111
Bergamini TM, 159, 293
Bergan JJ, 419
Bergelin RO, 423, 436
Bergmark C, 3, 11
Bergqvist D, 235, 255, 313, 317, 354, 409
Berk BC, 82
Berman PM, 141
Berman SS, 381
Berry S, 401
Besson I, 452
Bigatan E, 96
Birkmeyer JD, 208
Blebea J, 139
Bloemberg BPM, 2
Blom HJ, 57, 58
Blum U, 454
Blumenberg RM, 238
Bode-Böger SM, 44
Bodily KC, 397
Böger RH, 44
Boontje AH, 262
Bortman S, 10
Bosner MS, 191
Bove AA, 40
Bradbury AW, 432
Braithwaite BD, 23
Breen JC, 365
Bresticker MR, 269
Brevetti G, 315, 316
Brewster DC, 276
Brittenden J, 432
Brotzakis PZ, 129
Brown BG, 38
Brown PM, 237
Brown RD Jr, 356
Brown SL, 22
Bruyninckx CMA, 332
Buchanan SA, 359
Bucknell AL, 403
Buhl R, 428
Bui BT, 167
Büket S, 251
Bülach, 54
Bundens WP, 419
Buonaccorsi G, 52
Buring JE, 221
Burke AP, 33
Burmark US, 409
Buth J, 100

## C

Calligaro KD, 375
Cambria RA, 232, 437
Cambria RP, 115, 209, 276
Cao P, 348
Caplan LR, 365
Caps MT, 423, 436
Caracciolo EA, 211
Carlton L, 305
Castellano R, 379
Castrucci M, 117
Cavallari N, 50
Cave EM, 155
Chaikof EL, 95
Chalmers RTA, 185
Chang BB, 282, 302, 304
Chapman RL, 355
Chazel S, 124
Chen C, 382
Chernoff DM, 177
Cherry KJ, 280
Cherry KJ Jr, 373, 443
Chervu A, 256
Chiesa R, 379, 380
Chimowitz MI, 344
Chung SCS, 451
Cisek PL, 105
Clagett GP, 198, 256
Clair DG, 273
Cobbe SM, 28
Cohen J, 219
Cohen-Solal K, 71
Colditz GA, 67
Cone JB, 390
Conte MS, 307, 308
Cook NR, 219
Cook PS, 182
Cook TA, 127
Cooper GG, 339
Cornwell E III, 389
Cortelazzo S, 187
Coselli JS, 234, 251
Cosmi B, 415
Cowper D, 239
Coyle A, 401
Coyle KA, 355
Criado E, 337
Criado FJ, 336
Cronenwett JL, 34
Cross S, 217
Crowe D, 72
Cuadrado MJ, 17
Currie IC, 161, 287, 303
Curry R, 439
Curtin JJ, 144

529

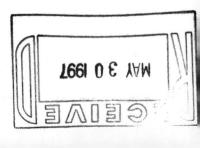